Mothers and Midwives
The Ethical Journey

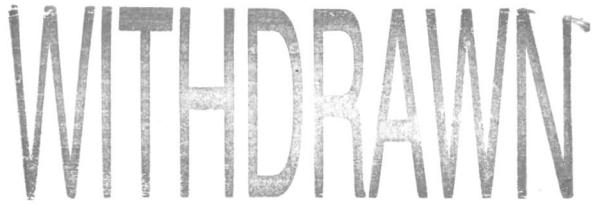

To my own parents, Lil and Les, who provided such a strong sense of virtuous character and ethical behaviour for me, and to all mothers and midwives who strive for these values in childbirth.

For Books for Midwives:

Commissioning Editor: Mary Seager
Development Editor: Catharine Steers
Project Controller: Joannah Duncan
Designer: George Ajayi

Mothers and Midwives

The Ethical Journey

Faye E Thompson PhD FRCNA MNSt DipAPSc (Nr Ed)

Foreword by

Mavis Kirkham PhD MA BA cert RU RN
Professor of Midwifery, University of Sheffield, UK

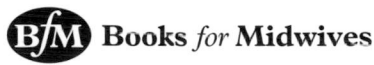 **Books _for_ Midwives**

EDINBURGH LONDON NEW YORK OXFORD PHILADELPHIA ST LOUIS SYDNEY TORONTO 2004

BOOKS FOR MIDWIVES
An imprint of Elsevier Science Limited

First published 2004

ISBN 0 7506 8776 2

British Library Cataloguing in Publication Data
A catalogue record for this book is available from the British Library

Library of Congress Cataloguing in Publication Data
A catalog record for this book is available from the Library of Congress

Notice
Medical knowledge is constantly changing. Standard safety precautions must be followed, but as new research and clinical experience broaden our knowledge, changes in treatment and drug therapy may become necessary or appropriate. Readers are advised to check the most current product information provided by the manufacturer of each drug to be administered to verify the recommended dose, the method and duration of administration, and contraindications. It is the responsibility of the practitioner, relying on experience and knowledge of the patient, to determine dosages and the best treatment for each individual patient. Neither the Publisher nor the author assumes any liability for any injury and/or damage to persons or property arising from this publication.

The Publisher

ELSEVIER SCIENCE your source for books, journals and multimedia in the health sciences
www.elsevierhealth.com

The publisher's policy is to use **paper manufactured from sustainable forests**

Printed in China

Contents

Foreword

Midwifery is ancient as a practice but very recent as an area of academic study. It has therefore suffered considerably from the application of concepts developed elsewhere. When we think of ethics we tend to think of concepts, developed by great men, which can be applied to any field of knowledge. Such ethics are decontextualised and described by Faye Thompson as 'the ethics of strangers'.

This study overturns the traditional approach to ethics and seeks 'an ethics of engagement', grounded in relationship. It is an account of a journey, with false trails but clearly charted, to explore the ethical nature of the mother/midwife relationship. The working metaphor of the journey demonstrates how ethics, like all enquiry, can be ongoing in our work not something completed by experts.

Faye Thompson makes a dialectical leap in her analysis by this turning over of the way we previously saw ethics. She reveals a distinctive midwifery ethic 'implicitly available in the lived realities and shared engagement of midwives and mothers'. The implications are challenging and require us to transform our understandings, relationships and working culture.

This book challenges our assumption in theory and in practice. It is also highly accessible being grounded in the experience of mothers and midwives. It has changed the way I see midwifery ethics.

Mavis Kirkham
Professor of Midwifery
University of Sheffield

Acknowledgements

I would like to personally thank the following mothers and midwives for so generously giving their time and sharing with me their experiences of childbirth and midwifery practice. Thanks, too, to their families for their consent and cooperation. Without their invaluable contribution this research would not have been possible.

Mothers (pseudonyms): Ellie, Caroline, Arline, Megan, Judy, Brenda, Maree and Kay.
Midwives (pseudonyms): Gemma, Bev, Ann, Ruth, Katie, Kerry-Anne, Diane and Madonna.

I also wish to thank Mrs Marina Noud for taking the time to read the final draft of this book from a midwifery practitioner's perspective.

Introduction

Is there such a thing as the ethics of midwifery? I believe there is, and the personal narratives of mothers and midwives convincingly tell us that there is. Different contexts require different ethical responses. Based on PhD research conducted in Australia, this book sheds light on the ethical nature of midwifery practice and identifies the distinctive features of a midwifery ethic.

Midwifery is currently promoting a partnership model of practice; a partnership built on the relationship between the childbearing woman and the midwife practitioner (Guilliland & Pairman 1995). The first problem associated with such an endeavour is that until now midwifery has officially adopted mainstream healthcare ethics which historically, are based on bioethics and Western moral philosophy. The moral philosophical approach adheres to normative theory and universal principlism which deliberately ignore context and relationships in their quest for generality and objective decision-making. Bioethics with such a framework, therefore, appears to be an inappropriate guide for a partnership model of midwifery practice.

Secondly, despite much discussion in the literature and amongst practitioners about the theory-practice gap in midwifery education, what is lacking in the discourse on ethics and midwifery are the voices of childbearing women and midwives, in the context of the mother-midwife relationship. Mavis Kirkham (2000) as editor of *The Midwife-Mother Relationship*, writes

If midwifery is conducted in and through the relationship between the woman and the midwife, it is strange that this is, to my knowledge, the first book on that relationship. However ... it becomes clear that the organisational context of midwifery care has served to divert midwives from this fundamental relationship (Kirkham 2000 p.xiii).

This lack of input and investigation represents a serious gap in knowledge required for identifying the ethical nature of the mother-midwife relationship and through that an appropriate ethical response to 'being with woman' in midwifery practice.

To address the problem, personal narratives from a small group of mothers and midwives told during in-depth interviews, are analysed and taken-for-granted assumptions and 'ways of seeing' are examined, in relation to (i) the established theory, (ii) official policies such as codes, and (iii) the profession's literature. A feminist-narrative and interpretive constructivist framework reflects my own values and beliefs, and listening to the voice of the 'other' (in this instance, childbearing women and midwifery practitioners), focuses the outcome on the collective interests of those women, situating emerging theory within the practice of midwifery.

This analysis brings out into the open for the first time the ethics that are *implicit* in practice (that is, the ethics personally experienced and practiced by individuals) and compares them with the ethics that are made *explicit* by the profession of midwifery (for example, in literature and codes).

What characterises ethical midwifery practice is the mother-midwife relationship. The ethical nature of that relationship is one of human engagement within a partnership of mutual trust and respect between an able mother who, in the vast majority of instances, is well-designed to birth her baby, and a midwifery practitioner who is a friend – a professional-friend. It is a relationship wherein the balance of power moves fluidly between mother and midwife depending on context, and it exists over time. In the ethical mother-midwife relationship the midwife is not an elite expert. S/he is a skilful practitioner who is also a friend for the specific duration of pregnancy, birth and several weeks after birth. This friendship endures and, as testimony to the importance and strength of that relationship, the mother seeks to reunite with 'her' midwife not only after the birth (for example in the postnatal ward or village shopping centre) but also for subsequent pregnancies.

The ethics of midwifery practice exist in the engagement between mother and midwife, and the exercise of power within their relationship. These ethics are not restricted to a set of principles brought out only at the time of a dilemma, and used for deciding which is the right or wrong 'action' to take. Childbirth and midwifery have their origins in the social contexts of community rather than the sterility of a laboratory or abstract academic debates. Understanding the mother-midwife relationship helps to relocate the ethical response of midwives from that of other practices and orientations such as scientific research and philosophy, to one that reflects the essence of midwifery practice – 'being with' woman during childbirth.

An ethic developed from within practice addresses the practical concerns of people who are directly involved in it. A distinctive midwifery ethic, therefore, offers a more adequate ethical response for mothers and midwives than traditional bioethics, because it is based on the values and beliefs of the women who experience childbirth as well as those who practice midwifery.

This journey I take alongside mothers and midwives looking for the everyday ethics of childbirth and midwifery, begins with the question 'What does ethical midwifery practice look like?' Chapter 1 attempts to explain why we need to identify a midwifery ethic of practice.

The next question is 'How have existing ethical frameworks directed the ethics for midwifery?' Chapters 2, 3 and 4 examine familiar territory; the historical development of contemporary midwifery ethics and the influence of medicalised healthcare on practice. Traversing bioethics turns out to be a false trail, given that the aim of my journey is to discover the ethical nature of the mother-midwife relationship and an adequate ethical response for midwifery practice. The trail leads through medicalisation and situations stripped of context. Instead of identifying relationships, experts direct the stranger past dilemmas towards principles that are abstract from lived reality and, therefore, not easily transformed into practice. Codification of practice has developed around those principles to ensure standards and provide consumer charters, but many of the codes only explain why action should be taken; they do not offer strategies for how one might approach a practice or behave when one comes across human engagement.

Subsequent chapters set out to explore uncharted terrain; the ethical nature of the mother-midwife relationship. Mothers and midwives tell their personal stories of what it is ethically like to birth a baby and to assist a woman with that experience. Listening to the voices of these mothers and midwives provides the necessary direction for re-orienting an ethic of midwifery: midwifery ways of seeing (and 'being') in the profession. The research methodology is based on feminist-constructivist values and assumptions, and feminist ethics guide the analysis – our 'course'. The 'course' or meaning is constructed by the mothers, midwives and me as co-researchers, and is checked against the values and philosophical foundations of midwifery practice, explicit in literature.

I journeyed from 'Practice Estate' and eventually found the pool of ethics. The final chapter endeavours to chart the return trip, from the pool (or billabong) back to 'Practice Estate', by travelling in tandem with those mothers and midwives who participated in the study (Thompson 2001). Findings indicate that there is a distinctive ethical response in midwifery practice, and this discussion proposes a mapping strategy for constructing a new ethic for midwives. The impact of human engagement on practice, and the centrality of concepts identified in the present narratives, are integral to such a strategy.

REFERENCES

Guilliland K, Pairman S 1995 The midwifery partnership: a model for practice. Victoria University of Wellington, Wellington NZ

Kirkham M (ed) 2000 The midwife-mother relationship. Macmillan Press Ltd, Basingstoke

Thompson F E 2001 The ethical nature of the mother-midwife relationship: a feminist perspective [unpublished PhD dissertation]. University of Southern Queensland, Toowoomba, Queensland, Australia

The need for a midwifery ethic of practice

If bioethics is not appropriate for midwifery practice, what, if any, are the alternatives? Are there ethics other than those we have been formally taught in schools of nursing and midwifery? Is there a pool (or 'billabong') of ethics, a body of knowledge about different ethical orientations and theories, from which one might choose the most appropriate ethical response for any given situation?

THE METAPHOR

Based on personal experience as a midwife and active involvement in the professional activities of midwifery, the metaphor I use is that of journey; in particular the journey of childbirth. Literature reviews and research data for the present project confirmed this as a metaphor common to many mothers and midwives. My metaphor is not so much about roads, landscape and a pool of water as it is about the fact that making a journey is something one must do for oneself – someone else cannot do it for you, although they can do it 'with' you. In this respect, childbirth is also a journey. The midwife does not birth the baby, s/he is 'with' the childbearing woman while *she* grows and births her baby.

The metaphor of journey used in this book concerns the process of discovery and uncertainty, and the impact of experiences associated with that journeying. Some of these are unique to the individual; others are shared in common with companion travellers.

Pregnancy, birth and the early weeks of a baby's life can be seen as a journey. The midwife provides a map for the woman if she needs one, warning her at the same time that the journey includes uncharted landscapes for which there can be no planning. She points out the signposts for various alternative routes and warns of hazards to avoid or obstacles that can be circumvented or surmounted. Most importantly, she puts the woman in touch with other women who have recently explored the same terrain, as well as those who will be making similar journeys and may wish to share resources and support each other along the way. The midwife may be there for a part of the journey if it is particularly rocky, for she usually knows the terrain well ... The midwife knows that, for most of the journey, the woman will manage with the support of her chosen travelling companions, so she gives these people various tools that may be useful along the way (Leap 2000 p.15-16).

Metaphors used by participants in this research are also identified. Moral metaphors are culturally determined, highlighting certain features of experience while suppressing others. Advocacy metaphors conceal potential moral conflicts because they suggest that the advocate acts on behalf of only one party instead of cooperatively between people of equal position, thus implying that other health-care practitioners somehow do not act in the patient's 'best interests'. Academic metaphors which recommend rational decision-making (problem-solving) as a resolution to ethical dilemmas obscure moral reality and only partly acknowledge the realities of competing values such as power, in the clinical setting. The consequences of these metaphors are only seen in retrospect, but because moral metaphors can be the basis of moral and social action

we need to look beyond them ... to understand [them] and how they relate to the time in which we live (Wurzbach 1999 p.98).

Metaphors are important because they convey new insights by using a comparison. They can convey a truth not yet recognised or acknowledged by a particular profession.

LOOKING FOR THE POOL OF ETHICS: A PERSONAL JOURNEY

As I walked along Bioethics Road, on the boundary of Practice Estate and Academia in the State of Professionalism, I found a small pebble in my shoe. I had been aware of it for some years but in the recent past it had become more uncomfortable. When I removed it and looked closely, it had a name. It was called Ethics-in-Midwifery-Practice – not A Theory of Ethics, or a set of principles, but a way of seeing and practising.

It seemed different to the other stones in the vicinity. It seemed to have a lot of flexibility, depending on the context and the individual holding it. Yet it remained a pebble – albeit more like the Ethics-in-Practice stones of applied ethics than the Western-Philosophical-Ethics stones used in academic debate. I was very interested in finding more pebbles similar to mine because I felt sure that if more of these Ethics in Practice sorts of pebbles were brought together they would help me learn more about my pebble – Ethics in Midwifery Practice.

With each step I took, the discomfort left by that pebble prompted me. What had shaped and developed the nature of *this* pebble so that it looked a little different from other Ethics pebbles? What, if any, was the importance and influence of the practice environment on the ethical decision-making of midwives?

By this time I was convinced such a thing existed; that there was a bank of pebbles similar to mine; that the ethics which midwives use in midwifery practice were not those of mainstream (medical) bioethics.

The question was, how could I find this bank of pebbles, and who would help me on my journey? I also felt sure that if I could find the Pool (or 'billabong') of Ethics in Practice I would find the stones of the various 'territories' and practices, and recognise 'my' pebble's representatives.

I chatted with several nursing, midwifery and philosophy colleagues in search of this pool of combined thought and practice. My question seemed so basic that at first I was hardly game to ask it. I was surprised and somewhat distressed to find that no one seemed to know of it. Indeed, I wondered whether it was simply a vivid dream I had had whilst attempting to teach the subject of ethics to tertiary nursing students. The advice from colleagues was gently firm – a deeper knowledge of bioethics would resolve my dilemma. So the issue and I were dismissed. I had followed the suggestions and advice of these colleagues in that I walked further along (mainstream modernist) Bioethics Road, hoping to find the signpost to the pool. Alas, I still could not find the right road. Sometimes I would imagine I had caught a glimpse of the pool through the trees, but then again it seemed safer and more sensible to stay within the 'cleared', built-up area and not to venture through the thick and unknown forest.

One day, when I thought the pool was in sight, I decided to throw my pebble towards it. Sadly, it landed on the road. Again, no pool. It was only a mirage. Although my pace slowed from time to time, I walked on ahead with my pebble.

I was afraid of looking silly with this proposal. Who did I think I was, persisting with one pebble? A small dirt track led off at a sharp angle to Bioethics Road. I stood there at the junction for some time considering my travel plans. I wrote words in my unsealed dirt track, cleared the words from the dirt with my sole, and wrote yet another set of words. Eventually, general questions and direction emerged. Some of the questions were: What is the contextual nature of ethics in midwifery practice? What do the stakeholders of maternity services consider to be the ethical issues in midwifery practice?

How do midwives respond when they are faced with an inner values conflict as the result of a decision made by another?

So I planned to ask mothers and midwives if they would tell me, in detail, about a clinical situation in which they personally were involved and which they considered involved ethics and midwifery.

I continued walking along this path, chatting to various people and reading various literature, for nearly 12 months until early morning, and just as the sunrise broke through so too did the pool come into view. There *is* a Pool of Ethics and there is a variety of ethics types and 'territories' within this pool of thought and practice. One type (modernist-principlism) I quickly recognised, noting both its public and private spheres; the feminist ethics, whilst less familiar, was easy for me to relate to with its relationship, caring and woman-centred characteristics, and its criticism of how the dominant paradigm effectively silences the vulnerable and disempowered. Another type, unfamiliar to me but similar to feminism in many aspects, also held great appeal and that was postmodernism. Feminists had also begun reviving Aristotle's virtue ethics, which brought moral character to the foreground.

I was encouraged. I looked around the water's edge for where it was lapping on the Midwifery Practice pebbles. Disappointed, I noticed what I had suspected at the beginning of my journey. All the *Ethics-in-Midwifery-Practice* pebbles were on the bank. No one, it seemed, had thrown any into the Pool of Ethics.

No wonder my colleagues on Bioethics Road knew nothing of 'my' side of the pool. My unsealed road was seldom used and easily overlooked when travelling at high speeds on their sealed road. Also, trees and reeds had grown up around the edges of the stones of modernism, obscuring the far banks where the stones of postmodernism, feminism, nursing and midwifery were situated – where they were embedded in context.

It was very quiet and a little scary being there all alone, but I so much wanted to throw my *Ethics-in-Midwifery-Practice* pebble into the water. This would require courage – not only for this early part of the journey (because I risked losing my pebble) but also for the future when findings would be viewed by others and the ripples felt.

By 'feeling the ripples' I mean that I am criticising that which traditionally forms the basis of healthcare (biomedical) ethics – (modernist) principlism. The principlist approach to ethics does not accommodate everyone, as its universal principles claim, but rather it legitimises the privileged (white) male dominance within institutionalised healthcare. Questioning the appropriateness for midwifery practice, therefore, of these long-held traditions of abstract universalism which guide deontology and utilitarianism, was certainly risky. Yet I took heart knowing that in the past 15-20 years postmodernists and feminists have criticised this traditional approach, and contemporary philosophers support critical examination of traditions, claiming that:

a way of seeing the world is given by tradition, but since traditions change it must be possible to see the world in different ways ... [tradition does not deny creativity or change, indeed] they are made possible by tradition ... what we see depends, quite literally, on the way we have been taught to see ... Seeing depends on a way of seeing which is acquired from others, and ways of seeing are the property not simply of individuals but of communities which have traditions and histories (Langford 1985 pp.8,13)

– communities, I suggest, such as midwives.

As a midwife myself, I embarked on an examination of ethics in midwifery practice from within the practice, by analysing the experiences of childbearing women and other midwives. For this reason, two philosophical issues arose for me in relation to this self-criticism (this criticism from within the practice) (Langford 1985): (i) if the tradition is a conservative tradition, then the tradition is accepted by the practitioners as the best way to do things (so no change is possible or likely – I'm hoping this is not true for midwifery) and (ii) how is it possible to have critical traditions (i.e. traditions which allow criticism from within) if tradition itself provides the only guide to practice?

My reply to the latter issue is that practice

and tradition can be criticised and developed from within by practitioners on the basis of personal vision. Our personal vision develops as we acquire a way of seeing from the tradition, and generally accept what the purpose of the tradition is and ought to be. So that while we have been inducted into the practice of midwifery by others, the innovation of the individual midwife can and does move the practice forward. Secondly, the ethics of midwifery ought to be determined not alone by 'outside experts' such as philosophers (who also are mostly male) but by the many individuals and practitioners within the practice, according to the traditions and shared social values of the practice (i.e. it should be embedded and embodied). This raises questions such as: What is the ethical nature of the mother-midwife relationship? Within our healthcare contexts? Shouldn't it be woman-centred? Is it a partnership? Do we need a different ethic for midwifery practice?

For the latter part of my journey I was camped alongside Bioethics Road, on the margin of Practice Estate and the forest, gathering more pebbles (the personal experiences of mothers and midwives, and discussions published in literature) from the Midwifery Practice bank. After examining the individual stories for context and character I analysed the relationship between them (including my own pebble). Hopefully, the ethics which these mothers, midwives and I jointly developed will contribute at least one valid version of *Ethics in Midwifery Practice* to the Pool of Ethics and who knows, in years to come Practice Estate may expand through the forest, up to 'our' side of the pool, clearing some of the uncertainty that lies between practice and ethics.

WAYS OF SEEING: WAYS OF ACTING

The social construction of our world

The way we see or interpret our social world determines how we are and how we act (our 'being with') in that world. The being of persons as persons is only possible through how they see themselves and how others see them (Langford 1985). As humans we make sense of our world through our knowledge and understanding of concepts, and through our beliefs. These are the terms of reference for our learning, including our ethical learning. I will define orientation or 'way of seeing' as our knowledge and interpretation of a particular field. Because our world as we see and understand it is a social construct, prior knowledge and socialisation into particular fields such as a professional practice are integral to any decision and response that we make about the appropriate way in which to behave in certain situations.

Training in ethics is as much about learning to think in a particular analytical way as about identifying what may or may not be moral in any given circumstance (Pritchard 1996 p.194).

If one accepts the definition of midwife as that of 'being with woman' during childbearing, then the concept of our orientation becomes crucial not only for how midwives are socialised into their practice, but also for how midwives see the childbearing woman and how they see themselves as the midwife – their 'being with' and 'being for' in that practice. Tension and conflict may arise, for instance in clinical decision making, when practitioners view childbirth and their role in that process from differing philosophies of care (Way 1998), from different 'gazes'. For example, from a feminist and a woman-centred midwifery view, childbirth is seen as a normal life-and-physiological 'experience' rather than a high-risk, physical 'problem' or 'event' as the medicalised approach suggests.

The nature of 'practice'

The practice is the place from where the power flows. The dynamics of power gives rise to and expresses the ethics. Practices are settings defined by power and relationships, and the role is defined around certain notions of power; for example, one is entitled to do 'x' and has certain obligations to others. Role can only be understood in the context of power (Thompson, Melia & Boyd 1994). Given that the nature of a practice is the basis for its ethics (Walker 1993), the midwife's interpretation of her role in childbirth will determine her ethical approach to, and relationship with, the mother – and of course other stakeholders such as the woman's family, other midwives, the medical and allied health professionals, and the employer. Inherent in the role of midwife is the ethical orientation of both the individual practitioner and the profession within which she practices.

When we enter a practice, we adopt the ethics of that practice as part of the commitment (Isaacs 1998; Toulmin 1986; Pritchard 1996). It is important, therefore, that the ethics espoused by the profession resonate with the ethics of the lived reality within the practice.

Western thought tends to view the world in terms of continuity, generality, and logical features, such as 'all women'. This approach links ethics to philosophy. Perhaps a parallel way of approaching ethics for the practice of midwifery is to consider the 'particularity' of the practice. This latter approach focuses on lived reality, not matters of logic.

In conclusion, because our 'ways of seeing' determine to a large extent the way we practice, and because when we are inducted into a practice we are taught our ways of seeing within that practice, a major requirement of ethical midwifery practice is to examine the underlying assumptions and values – the concepts – of midwifery.

REFERENCES

Isaacs P 1998 Advanced seminar in applied ethics research methods. School of Humanities, Queensland University of Technology

Langford G 1985 Education, persons and society: a philosophical inquiry. Macmillan, London

Leap N 2000 The less we do, the more we give. In: Kirkham M (ed) The midwife-mother relationship. Macmillan, Basingstoke

Pritchard J 1996 Ethical decision-making and the positive use of codes. In: Frith L (ed) Ethics and midwifery: issues in contemporary practice. Butterworth-Heinemann, Oxford, pp. 189-204

Thompson I K, Melia K M, Boyd K M 1994 Nursing ethics, 3rd edn. Churchill Livingstone, Melbourne

Toulmin S 1986 How medicine saved the life of ethics. In: DeMarco J P, Fox R M (eds) New directions in ethics. Routlege and Kegan Paul, New York

Walker M U 1993 Keeping moral space open: new images of ethics consulting. Hastings Centre Report 23 (2): 33-40

Way S 1998 Social construction of episiotomy. Journal of Clinical Nursing 7 (2): 113-117

Wurzbach M E 1999 The moral metaphors of nursing. Journal of Advanced Nursing 30 (1): 94-99

2

On the sealed highway – mainstream ethics, medicalisation and midwifery

Given that the nature of a practice is the basis for its ethics (Walker 1993), this chapter begins by outlining what I believe to be the nature of midwifery practice, thereby situating myself as both researcher and midwife within this discussion – establishing my point of departure for this journey.

The present lie of the land for midwifery ethics is noted. Because the ethics for midwifery practice are currently based on the ethics of other practice areas such as moral philosophy, medicine and nursing, the first assumption drawn is that a distinctive midwifery ethic is not explicitly available. The next step in my journey, therefore, is to explore how the ethics of those other practices have directed ethics for midwifery. To this end, the second part of the chapter investigates the questions, 'What are the mainstream ethical frameworks available to midwives?' and 'Why would midwives be turning to these ethical frameworks?'

Chapter 9 discusses whether or not the ethics discourse in midwifery – that tract of land with other pebbles similar to mine – parallels these mainstream frameworks or whether we might need to check our course and travel in another direction to reach the Pool of Ethics.

THE NATURE OF MIDWIFERY PRACTICE

If the aim of a practice is a shared tradition and the nature of a practice is the basis for its ethics, then concepts, values and beliefs that demonstrate what ethically matters to both mothers and midwives during childbirth will reflect the ethical nature of the mother-midwife relationship, and thus the nature of a distinctive ethical response for midwifery practice.

Moral philosophy, medicine and the curative-based areas of nursing are different in nature from midwifery, and therefore ethics derived from those practices are not appropriate for midwifery practice. Science, technology and objective decision-making form the basis of medicalised healthcare which is largely interventionist and problem-oriented with a utility focus. Ethical decision-making within such practice surrounds dilemmas and a 'dilemma' is defined as being a choice between two equally undesirable alternatives – often unresolvable (Thompson, Melia & Boyd 1994), often in life-threatening situations.

Everyday ethical midwifery practice is not based on dilemmas and life-threatening situations. There is more to it than that. There is ethical practice prior to the point of any dilemma and in addition to any dilemma.

The nature of midwifery practice is similar to that of mainstream Western medicine and the curative areas of nursing in that it is a profession of skill and expertise. It differs from them in that childbirth is primarily 'creative' not 'curative'; not a health 'problem' affecting the 'patient' or a condition that needs prophylaxis, treatment and/or counselling. I acknowledge that family planning techniques can often prevent unwanted pregnancies, pharmacology controls coexisting medical conditions, surgical intervention rescues mother and baby from complications of birth, and counselling enables mothers to restore their mental health postnatally. However, generally childbearing is a creative, 'normal' life experience for both the childbearing woman and the baby who is being born. So too, I propose, are its ethics concerned primarily with ordinary everyday practices and only less frequently with dilemmas.

Unlike health 'problems', in most cases childbirth when left to progress without medical science and technology does not deteriorate to a state of ill-health and possibly death of the patient. Usually, childbirth progresses towards the creation of a new life, a 'beginning' process, and the purpose of midwifery practice is to assist a healthy, able woman with 'her' birthing process.

The achievement of childbirth ought to be accompanied by a positive mental state with the mother ultimately retaining her self-determination, and the midwife sharing power and codependence from time to time during the process. Childbirth ought not be seen as an 'end', or the fixing of a 'problem' and 'doing for' the unable patient; that is more akin to the traditional 'empathetic-expert' approach towards the ill and dying. The way we see our practice and its purpose determines how we practise it – our 'being with woman'.

Another feature of childbearing which is integral to the ethics of midwifery practice is that of relationship. Childbirth is not concerned with 'the' patient. For the midwife there is a triad between mother, baby and herself but there is an inseparable dyad between the mother and her baby – some argue that the mother's prime relationship is with the baby whilst the midwife's prime relationship is with the mother (Guilliland & Pairman 1995).

There are two (or more with multiple pregnancy) individuals directly involved in the birthing process; that is, the mother and the baby. Then there is the mother-midwife relationship. The problem with a medicalised approach to childbirth is that it either implies that the fetus is a parasite, which is disease-relat-

ed terminology, or it sets up the mother and the baby as adversaries of each other, as a 'problem' to be fixed. With illness, disease, and other actual or potential health problems it is only the one person's body that is directly involved. The relationship for the health professional in the latter situation is first and foremost a dyad between two people, the practitioner and the patient or client, unlike the triad of mother, midwife and fetus/baby. Significant 'others' are involved in a supportive way and colleagues with each other, but the focus for the health professional in the curative or 'problem' situation involves the health-related-problem and the patient's body.

Both the patient/client and the nurse/doctor of the dyad have their prime focus on the aspect of 'combating' the 'enemy' which is one's actual or potential health problem. The patient-problem connection is adversarial. This patient does not develop a bond or sense of 'being part of', and 'being responsible for, for a life time' their actual or potential health problem in the same way that a childbearing woman does with her baby. The baby is not her enemy and the mother is not aiming to combat it – quite the reverse – she wants to protect and help her baby to grow and develop.

As Ellie, one of the mothers interviewed, says:

They brought me the baby and said feed the baby which I was only too willing to do. All mothers in that state would get out on a flag pole if they told them that the milk was actually located at the end of the flag pole six flights up and they had to crawl out there and get the milk and retrieve it. So, you feed the baby, you are utterly desirous of feeding the baby, you'd do anything for the baby, you'd die for the baby at this stage.

It is this special relationship between mother and baby, and the relationship between mother and midwife, that I believe forms the distinctive nature of midwifery practice.

To apply the dualism of positivist ethical decision-making to mother and baby, categorising them as adversaries, as two separate individuals who compete against each other for survival, is to offer an inaccurate and inadequate ethical response not only to the mother-midwife relationship but also to the mother-baby relationship.

Firstly, it creates a tension that is potentially a dilemma for the midwife by posing the inappropriate question of 'With whom does my first duty lie, who is my client/patient?' The midwife does have a close relationship with the baby but rather than being in opposition with the mother-midwife relationship, the baby-midwife relationship exists 'through' the mother-midwife relationship.

Secondly, separation of mother and baby as two 'patients' and having expert health professionals claim prime responsibility for each fails to acknowledge, at that pregnancy-birthing stage, the existence and primacy of the mother-baby relationship, and denies the childbearing woman an active role in 'her' birthing of her baby. It disrupts, at that very early stage, the effective establishment of the mother-baby relationship.

Furthermore, although childbirth is a critical life experience for the woman, the baby and her family, it is essentially a 'normal' life process. To label the healthy members of this duo as patients is to linguistically and conceptually, falsely categorise childbirth as a medical illness or disease condition.

The way we see our social world depends upon what we are taught to see. If we are taught to see a physically tired, less agile pregnant woman as needing to be hospitalised, 'cared for' in bed, and treated by experts with surgery and medication to 'get over' and 'be saved' from this high-risk, life-threatening episode, then our 'gaze' of childbirth will be that of illness and injury, death and disease, fear and feebleness. It is medicalised.

This way of seeing becomes the childbearing woman's gaze, too, when it is the only practice available to her. As Erving Goffman (1961 cited in Symonds & Hunt 1996 p.13) said in relation to the institutionalisation of human behaviour in mental hospitals, once a label has been given, a person's subsequent life and actions are interpreted by others within the light of that definition.

THE INFLUENCE OF MORAL PHILOSOPHY AND NURSING ETHICS

Moral philosophy and mainstream ethical frameworks available to midwives

Which ethics are accessible to midwives? On the sealed highway, Bioethics Road, only two signposts are encountered. The first directs the traveller to continue forward, towards the mainstream ethical discourse comprised mainly of normative theories. This main road, Bioethics Road, takes the problem-solving approach of moral philosophy, principlism and reflection from moral philosophy as adopted by bioethics. The second signpost stands a little distance further along where a side road branches off the main road. The side or 'service' road follows the traditions of professional practice with their accumulated wisdom and knowledge of practice, and the application of codes of practice, as in nursing ethics. This side road arcs around to rejoin the main Bioethics Road, in as much as codes themselves draw on ethical principles and act as a set of 'rules' to guide practitioners in their decision-making.

Western moral philosophy, the Church, and midwifery

What has shaped and developed mainstream ethical frameworks? Firstly, the problem-solving approach of Western moral philosophy has its origins in ancient Greece with philosophers such as Socrates, Plato and Aristotle, all of whom lived circa 5th century BC. Its nature has remained essentially unchanged in that as a branch of philosophical inquiry, these ethics seek rational clarification and justification of what is deemed morally acceptable behaviour, and ask why a particular act is considered right or wrong (Johnstone 1994, p.39). Another orientation described in the ethics discourse is 'common-sense ethics' which is derived from habit, custom, convention, and tradition, and which justifies action or behaviour on the basis that it has always been so. Because this latter approach lacks the critically reflective moral schema of philosophical inquiry, it is regarded as suitable only for social schema and is given no ultimate moral authority in deciding complex matters (Weber 1964 p.60 cited in Johnstone 1994 p.40).

After the fall of the Roman Empire, circa 4th century AD, the main source of knowledge about the human body was the Church, and the religious demands were that science and medicine should not challenge Christian biblical teachings (Davis 1995).

In the middle ages (14th-17th century), women who were identified as witches were considered evil and burnt alive at the stake. The Church believed that the power of all witches was derived from their sexuality, and that witches had had sexual intercourse with the devil. The devil always acted through the female. The European 'witch craze' began in feudalism and lasted into the 'age of reason'. It was a campaign of terror directed by the ruling class against the female peasant population because witches represented a political, religious and sexual threat to the Protestant and Catholic churches and the state. Superstition, therefore, linked midwives to power and evil because of their 'magic' herbs and intimate involvement with reproduction (Ehrenreich & English 1973 p.7). The Church controlled the licensing and behaviour of midwives, and supported witch hunts for them, whilst at the same time scientific and rational thought was providing prestige to male medicine (Donnison 1988). Much later, in America, it was a similar story.

In 1910, about 50 percent of all babies were delivered by midwives – most were blacks or working class immigrants. It was an intolerable situation to the newly emerging obstetrical specialty: For one thing, every poor woman who went to a midwife was one more case lost to academic teaching and research. America's vast lower class resources of obstetrical 'teaching material' were being wasted on ignorant midwives (Ehrenreich & English 1973, pp.33-34).

The proclaimed modern approaches of Western moral philosophy (modernity) continue to promote the superiority of (male) intellect and the inferiority of ('feminine') experience and feeling, of 'so called' objective science versus skilled practice and wisdom gained from experience. Deontology with its teachings of reason from Immanuel Kant (1734-1804) is an ethic of moral duty also espoused by theologians. Utilitarianism, the main teleological theory with its teachings from Jeremy Bentham (1748-1832) and John Stuart Mill (1806-73) (Johnstone 1994 pp.68,86) is compatible with the outcome emphasis of science. The theories differ in that 'duty', 'obligation' and 'rights' form the basis of the deontological argument and the consequences of one's action in balancing the greatest amount of pleasure (good) against the greatest amount of pain (evil) is the basis of the utility argument for the latter (Veatch 1989; Johnstone 1994; Singer 1994; Beauchamp & Childress 1994). Whilst these main theories reject each other's arguments of why one ethically ought to do 'x', the superiority of intellect over feelings and of mind over body are integral to both. Another commonality is the absence of female values and thought.

With capitalism and Protestant reformation, the power shifted from the Church to the state and economic organisation. Faith was superseded by rational, logical 'truth', demonstrated with objective scientific experiments (positivism/logico-empirical science). Nature could be controlled and mastered (Davis & George 1988 cited in Davis 1995).

Today, the Church, Western moral philosophy and medical science are closely linked.

[for deontologists] a 'rights' claim involves the protection of one's own interests whereas a 'duty' claim is based more on the consideration of another's interests ... [for teleological theorists though] duties are primarily concerned with avoiding intolerable results ... [and are] more morally compelling than are obligations (Johnstone 1994 p.85).

Deontologists say that one ought to take a particular action because of the inherent 'goodness' in the action, because it is one's moral duty, a stance frequently followed by theologians. These rule-based ethics are concerned with antecedent grounds for moral action, with the means used to promote others' wellbeing, whereas utilitarianism focuses on goals, outcomes and the effects of actions (Thompson, Melia & Boyd 1994) – also a basic tenet of science. People's collective and overall interests take precedence for utilitarians, rather than the particular welfare of individuals, but

because rational persons are the best judges of their own best interests individual independence and freedom of choice are essential elements of the theory (Johnstone 1994 pp.86-7).

The sacrifice of the individual is justified by the greater good it produces. 'Public' debates over sanctity of life versus quality of life, and the woman's right to decide what happens to her own body versus the right of the fetus to life, continue unresolved in most Western countries. Such debates, however, occur at the wider societal level and do little to guide the everyday practice of midwifery. The ethics of the particular and the personal tend to be relegated to the so-called 'private' sphere, and thus are excluded.

More recently, Beauchamp and Childress proposed that healthcare practice should reflect the four primary ethical principles of respect for persons (autonomy), do no harm (non-maleficence), do good (beneficence) and be fair (justice), plus secondary principles such as veracity, fidelity, privacy and confidentiality – principlism (Beauchamp & Childress 1983 cited by Childress in Veatch 1989). Using these universal principles, one can decide objectively on the right or wrong ethical 'action' to take on this occasion and for other same or similar 'issues'. This approach does not conflict with the Church, deontologists or utilitarians because whilst it allows for the Golden Rule of 'do unto others as you would have them do unto you', that rule is viewed only as a necessary principle, not a sufficient principle (Childress 1989 in Veatch 1989). The normative principles approach uses a set of what are claimed to be universally applicable principles as 'rules' to guide or 'prescribe' behaviour, and these form the basis of professional codes of practice. This leads into the matter of professional codes of practice and the codification of practices.

The emergence of professional codes

As late as the 1980s, a popular worldwide view of ethics was that moral obligation and ethical decision-making were relevant only for doctors (Johnstone 1994).

When ethical issues were presented to nurses, they were taught from a medical perspective. When ethical issues were reported by the media, the nursing perspective was often omitted or represented as the 'emotional' aspect of moral dilemmas. It is misleading to think that nursing practice is devoid of moral complication, that nurses should not have any independent moral responsibilities when caring for patients and that nurses are not required to make independent moral judgments in the nurse-patient relationship (Johnstone 1994). Similarly, midwifery ethics ought not be subsumed under the umbrella of either 'medical' or 'nursing' ethics.

As a result of atrocities during World War II, the Nuremberg Code of 1947 and the Universal Declaration of Human Rights (published in 1949) were established. Intense focus was directed at the ethical and unethical practices associated with medical practice and research into humans. Essential considerations were the requirement for informed consent, confidentiality, justice, and a cost-benefit analysis regarding an acceptable upper limit of harm. Controversial areas were, and still are, highly risky research, vulnerable participants, and the use of deception – for example, in clinical trials. Such focus highlighted the ethical agenda in nursing too and in 1953 the International Council of Nurses (ICN) first adopted a code of conduct.

Despite such documents, practices in some hospitals and clinics caused great concern, not only at national level but also among individual nurses (and midwives) who were not able to defend patients' rights and who wanted to know to whom to report these matters. Events in a New Zealand hospital in the 1980s are well documented examples. Women were unconsenting subjects in medical experiments when cervical cancer was randomly treated and not. Fetal cervices were collected from stillborn baby girls for histological studies without parental consent, and female babies were subjected to vaginal swabbing not only without parental consent but also unnecessarily because the nurses were not informed that the research had been discontinued. Another disturbing practice revealed through the same inquiry was that of encouraging medical students to practice invasive techniques such as vaginal examinations on anaesthetised women (Johnstone 1994). There emerged a growing need politically, practically and legally, for the professional bodies to provide guidelines for nurse practitioners on ethical conduct. This was also taken up by individual countries; for example, in 1993 the Australian Nursing Council Incorporated, the Royal College of Nursing Australia and the Australian Nursing Federation published the ANCI Code of Ethics for Nurses in Australia. The Code is complementary to the ICN Code for Nurses, 1973. Similarly, the UKCC Code of Professional Conduct was produced in 1992, the UKCC Midwives Rules in 1993, and in 1995 the Australian College of Midwives Incorporated (ACMI) published a Code of Ethics for midwives which was adapted from the International Confederation of Midwives (ICM) Code of Ethics, 1993.

Why midwives would be turning to mainstream ethical frameworks

Midwives have turned to mainstream ethics for four reasons:

- political dominance by men and medicine
- the route by which midwives enter their practice
- the widespread influence of logico-empirical science and medicalisation of healthcare, and
- the influence of the workplace in reinforcing the status quo.

Political dominance by men and medicine

This brief review uses highlights from early Australian history to demonstrate the political dominance by men and medicine in that region.

It is not intended to be a comprehensive account of world events. Examples from Britain and Australia act as a prompt for recalling similar impacts elsewhere, and shed some light on why midwives in the Western world would be turning to mainstream ethical frameworks. Historically and politically, the practice of midwifery has been subject to the same sort of oppression as have women generally, and their voices have not been heard. From early times male moral philosophy dominated Western ethics and socially controlled moral behaviour, and in the 19th century male dominant medicine began to influence philosophy (Toulmin 1986), and control nursing. For example, British and Australian nursing and midwifery were eventually developed on the basis of English Florence Nightingale traditions. Nightingale was dubbed 'the lady with the lamp' reflecting the repressive notions of 19th century ladylike behaviour and 'feminine mystique' (Kingston 1975). However, prior to the migration of those nurses, nursing in colonial Australia was considered as immoral as prostitution.

In the early days of the new penal colony of Australia, nurses were domestic servants in hospitals and infirmaries which were similar to gaols and insane asylums. Most hospitals were charitable institutions for contagious diseases and epidemics (Kingston 1975). The majority of women giving birth were either convicts or prostitutes, with the convicts' pregnancies often resulting from sexual abuse during transportation and after arrival (Summers 1981 cited in Barclay 1989). These women could not afford midwifery or medical services, and in any case they were regarded as not respectable. So it was the 'accidental midwife' who served women during this convict era. After this came the 'Aunt Rubina' period – an experienced married relative arrived before the baby was born and stayed some weeks. Only the destitute convict or single government employee went to hospital because most preferred to be ill or confined at home (Thornton 1972 cited in Barclay 1989). By the 1880s the midwife was an institution in the colony. Bush midwives and Aunt Rubinas were considered women of high integrity, valuable friends, rich in common sense, experience, kindness and with skilful hands: having families of their own allowed them to share the problems, concerns and joys of the families they serviced (Gillison 1974 cited in Barclay 1989).

Whilst the majority of women were birthing at home with their Aunt Rubinas, nursing and medical training was being developed around therapeutic care, in hospitals. Nurses were taught according to the Nightingale philosophy of dedication, rules, regulations, restrictions and inhibitions – similar to that of a religious order (Kingston 1975).

The Nightingale philosophy of subservience ensured that nurses would not compete but rather improve the service a doctor could offer (Barclay 1989 p.136).

History reveals similar power relationships to those that continue today. In earlier times in Australia and England most community midwives were middle-aged to elderly married women or widows, and mothers, who relied on their work to support their families (Summers 1997; Mcintosh 1998). This was an unsuitable image for the new profession of nursing and the obstetric nurse.

Under the guise of professionalism and safety, medicine and nursing combined to marginalize the community midwife... childbirthing with the medical profession was safe, while childbirthing with community midwives was unsafe (Summers 1997 p.15).

Secondly, the campaign created an unfavourable physical image of the community midwife. She was depicted as obese, dirty, drunk, incompetent, garrulous and stupid, and nicknamed 'Sairey Gamp' after the 1843 Charles Dickens character. Sairey Gamp was everything the Victorian wife should not be and there was dichotomy to her character. On the one hand she was optimistic, hardworking and able to endure, a good business woman and totally reliable for her patients. On the other hand, she was an expert in the sordid ways of the world.

She refused to be subservient to her husband 'alive or dead' and she was economically independent as a midwife who assisted women in the face of men's helplessness in this basic life situation. She would not be dominated, coerced or ignored or, to put it into her words, 'impoged upon' (Summers 1997 p.16).

Eventually the label of the fictitious 'Gamp' stuck. Indeed, the medical profession still revert to the reference when tightening their control over midwifery practice (Summers 1997).

When the £5 Baby Bonus was introduced into Australia by the Commonwealth Government in 1912, authorities asserted that it would increase the declining birthrate, diminish maternal and infantile mortality, and make childbearing safer for women. In the nine years following its introduction, the birth rate steadily decreased. There was no substantial reduction in the maternal or infantile death rates, and the number of women attended in childbirth by a doctor greatly increased – medical attendance was greater in the State of Victoria despite the Midwives' Act in Victoria (Kingston 1977 pp.142-45).

Midwives were seen as a threat to medical practice because, like the optometrist who was skilful enough to prescribe glasses, midwives were often trained by extensive practical experience and could provide, in many cases, a superior service than doctors (Pensabene 1980 cited in Barclay 1989).

[A]n effective manner of dealing with the threat posed by midwives was to increase their links with nursing until 'incorporation' occurred (Barclay 1989 p.136).

The first hospital-trained midwives occurred in Australia in 1862 at The Women's Hospital in Melbourne (Thornton 1972 cited in Barclay 1989).

The route by which midwives enter their practice

Using Australia as a case study for instance, prior to the 1990s, all of the State and Territory governments legislated that only registered nurses would be admitted to a midwifery course (for example, Queensland Nursing Act By-Law 1993). Even now, individuals who have completed a 'direct entry' midwifery course may have their practice license restricted to areas where there is nursing/medical supervision.

When we enter a practice, we adopt the ethics and traditions of that practice as part of the commitment. The influence of nursing ethics on midwifery occurs when midwives are inducted into their practice via nursing, and nursing derives its ethics from bioethics which itself is based on Western moral philosophy. Midwives, therefore, adopt (initially at least) nursing ethics and traditions – 'ways of seeing'.

The widespread influence of logico-empirical science and medicalisation of healthcare

The third reason is the widespread influence of logico-empirical science and medicalisation. The influence of medicine and moral philosophy on society has occurred with the 'medicalisation of life' (Illich 1977 cited in Thompson, Melia & Boyd 1994). With the medicalisation of life came the medicalisation of childbirth and thus of midwifery practice.

This was done with the best of intention. The welfare of the mother and baby was paramount. Infantile epidemics such as diphtheria, whooping cough and bacterial gastroenteritis had high mortality rates, so to segregate newborns from everyone except doctors and gowned nursing staff (midwives were not identified as such outside the labour wards), who were trained in the art of hand-washing, was for the good of everyone. The detrimental effect on mother, baby and family from minimal contact was considered unimportant, if considered at all, compared with the disastrous effect of the diseases. The success of restrictive practices was reflected in popular obstetric texts. Beischer and Mackay (1986 p.119) note that according to 'a recent regional survey' only 7.1% of post-neonatal deaths were caused by infections. However, cause-related infant mortality rates are more difficult than total deaths to compare across years because of changes in national and international classification systems. Causes of death shown for the years 1972 to 1978 are classified according to the Eighth Revision of the International Classification of Diseases, 1965 (Australian Bureau of Statistics 1982). Infectious and parasitic diseases were responsible for 10/1,000 male and 4/1,000 female infant deaths in New South Wales in 1972, and 14/1,000 male and

8/1,000 female infant deaths in 1978. Yet in 1982, using a different classification system, only 3/1,000 male and 0/1,000 female infant deaths occurred from infectious and parasitic diseases.

The absolute belief in and dominance of 'the' scientific truth determined the status quo for childbirthing practices in Australia and the rest of the Western world. It silenced the voices of the women who were being practised upon. Families, too, were persuaded of the benefits of medical science, especially as it meant having a safe childbirth and 'getting' a healthy baby. Medical research supposedly showed that pushing on an intact perineum attributed to urinary incontinence and/or uterine prolapse for the woman in later life, and it was widely believed that suturing the neat straight edges of a surgical incision resulted in better healing than a torn perineum. Beischer and Mackay give the advantages of an episiotomy as

The risks of trauma to the fetal head and fetal hypoxia are reduced by hastening the birth of the baby, overdistension of maternal tissues is avoided thus minimising the risks of genital prolapse, and perineal and vaginal lacerations are prevented; these are often more painful than an episiotomy, and are more difficult to suture (Beischer & Mackay 1986 p.690).

Subsequent research however, negates these views:

Six studies were included. In the routine episiotomy group, 73.4% of women had episiotomies, while the rate in the restrictive episiotomy group was 26.6%. Compared with routine use, restrictive episiotomy involved less posterior perineal trauma, less suturing, and fewer healing complications. There was no difference in severe vaginal or perineal trauma, dyspareunia, urinary incontinence or severe pain measures ... Reviewers' conclusions: Restrictive episiotomy policies appear to have a number of benefits compared to routine episiotomy policies (Carroli, Belizan & Stamp 1999).

The increasing influence of medical science and technology is seen also in restricting the woman's movements and oral intake. The advice in midwifery texts of the 1960s was concerned with the woman's suffering and comfort, with care being guided by the woman's changing responses to the process of childbirth, and with assisting the woman to 'deliver herself' of her baby. For example, for the woman to be in bed, lying on one side, meant that the woman was resting and conserving energy:

When the intensity of the contractions gives rise to suffering, the woman should of course be in bed so that she can relax and conserve her strength and in order that sedatives may be given to relieve the pain ... If the woman is well nourished during the early part of labour she will stand up to it better ... [but] food should not be given when the woman is in strong labour (Myles 1964 p.290-1).

On the other hand, twenty years later the medical texts of the 1980s were directed towards intervention and outcome. The woman had been replaced with 'the patient': she was not allowed to eat during labour in case she vomited and suffered all the complications associated with that.

It is now accepted that, once painful contractions are established, little food is absorbed by the patient. If meals are given, they will either be vomited or will provide a hazard should anaesthesia be required. In early labour, fluids, barley sugar and puree-type foods may be tolerated, but thereafter oral intake should be restricted to sips of fluid to keep the mouth moist. An intravenous infusion should be set up if the end of labour is not in sight by 12 hours. Two litres of 5% dextrose and one litre of normal saline should be administered over a period of 18-24 hours (Beischer & Mackay 1978 p.236).

More recently, this approach has been challenged.

There is no guarantee that withholding food and drink during labour will result in an empty stomach when general anaesthesia should become necessary. No time interval between the last meal and the onset of labour guarantees a stomach volume of less than 100 ml (Enkin, Keirse & Chalmers 1995 p.202).

Current policy on food and fluid intake during labour in The Netherlands is that 75% of midwives and obstetricians leave the decision to the women themselves:

Despite the non-restrictive policy in The Netherlands, the mortality due to the Mendelson-syndrome is not higher than in countries where a restrictive policy is followed. During normal labour there are no conclusive reasons for food or fluid-restriction. From a metabolic point of view it is

hypothesized that the intake of energy-rich substrates may have a positive influence on labour progression (Scheepers, Essed & Brouns 1998 p.37).

To have mother lying on her side in the left lateral position meant that the heavy uterus would not press on major maternal blood vessels, and maternal hypotension would be prevented. It also meant that circulation to the placenta would not be impeded and the optimum amount of oxygen would cross the placenta to the unborn fetus. This makes objective scientific sense and may remain true, but as post-structuralism and feminism argue, there is more than 'one' truth. Available data now cast doubt on the wisdom of the policy to restrict birthing women to bed. The supine position causes a significant reduction in cardiac output, contraction intensity is consistently reduced, contraction frequency is often reduced, and the ability of contractions to dilate the uterine cervix is reduced (Enkin, Keirse & Chalmers 1995). A Cochrane Systematic Review of 18 trials on positions for women during second stage of labour indicates that the use of any upright or lateral position, compared with supine or lithotomy positions, is associated with:

1. Reduced duration of second stage of labour (12 trials)
2. A small reduction in assisted deliveries (17 trials
3. A reduction in episiotomies (11 trials)
4. A smaller increase in second degree perineal tears (10 trials)
5. Increased estimated risk of blood loss >500ml (10 trials)
6. Reduced reporting of severe pain during second stage of labour (1 trial)
7. Fewer abnormal fetal heart rate patterns (1 trial).

Reviewers' conclusions are that women should be encouraged to give birth in the position they find most comfortable. Until such time as the benefits and risks of various delivery positions are estimated with greater certainty, when methodologically stringent trials data are available, then women should be allowed to make informed choices about the birth positions they might wish to assume for delivery of their babies (Gupta & Nikodem 2002).

Pre-medicalisation texts, written by midwives, advised that supine and lateral positioning of the birthing woman in bed impedes labour because of the mother's inactivity and the lack of gravitational force on the cervix:

There is a distinct advantage in the assumption of the upright position [for the woman to 'deliver herself' of her baby]; the foetus sinks into the lower pole of the uterus and by pressing on the cervical nerve endings stimulates good uterine action. It also facilitates dilatation of the os. In the erect position the antero-posterior diameter of the pelvic brim is enlarged because a certain degree of movement takes place at the sacro-iliac joints (Myles 1964 p.290).

Again, this 1960s woman-centred midwifery advice was superseded during the 1970s and '80s by the scientific, medicalised approach to birth which had the 'patient' in bed, depersonalised in a hospital gown, and compartmentalised in labour ward until she and the baby were transferred to the postnatal ward area. The woman had little say in what happened to her but she willingly relied on medical experts, who knew best, to 'give her a healthy baby.' Given that the caesarean section birth rate has increased to more than 20% in Australia (Australian Federal Government 1999), 21% in England, 24% in Wales and Northern Ireland, 22% in Italy, and 19% in Scotland (Thomas & Paranjothy 2001) this is what often happened – the woman did not experience birth, rather she was handed her baby when she awoke from general anaesthesia and abdominal surgery. It was not until the mid- to late 1980s that 'alternative birthing positions' were widely promoted, often by what had become known as Birthing Centres, and the woman was once more the focus of the birthing process. Birthing women were encouraged to adopt the positions and mobility that were most effective for them. Unfortunately, many maternity units and many attending professionals continue to enforce the policy that the woman is lying down in labour (Enkin, Keirse & Chalmers 1995).

Artificial rupture of membranes (ARM) shortened the labour for most women and was thought to be better for both mother and baby (Beischer & Mackay 1986) but present day criticism is that each technological intervention tends to result in needing another – 'the cascade of intervention' (Wagner 1994). For example, surgical induction of labour (ARM) frequently leads to medical induction with oxytocin via insertion of intravenous therapy. Women complain that the artificially induced contractions are more painful than those that occur naturally, and thus the incidence of epidural anaesthesia tends to increase with induction of labour. Effective epidural anaesthesia eliminates all sensation in the pelvic region, not only pain, and this often necessitates forceps or vacuum extraction of the baby when the mother lacks the urge to push in coordination with contractions. And so on.

[A]rtificial rupture of the membranes has been used to augment labour for decades, but whether the procedure confers more benefit than harm is still undetermined (Enkin, Keirse & Chalmers 1989 p.207).

Generally, obstetricians in the 1960s and late 1970s considered infant feeding and breast care to be less important than the more glamorous areas of pregnancy, birth, technology and science. It was left to midwives to deal with babies and breastfeeding, and even they tended to think of postnatal care as 'unscientific' and thus one of the less important aspects of childbearing. Despite this ascribed lower status, the medicalisation of and institutional influence on breastfeeding were evident in policies and rules. Feeding baby more often than every three or four hours, or for longer than 10-15 minutes on each breast was forbidden because the excessive trauma on the nipples would crack them and because baby should not be encouraged to 'play' at the breast (Beischer & Mackay 1978). Feeding was work. Medicalisation marginalised breastfeeding. It was positioned in the 'private' arena and subordinated, but it was controlled in the public arena using the cloak of scientific 'fact' to render relationship invisible. 'Test-weighing' the baby involved weighing a clean, dry, wrapped baby prior to breastfeeding and, with no alteration to clothing or cleanliness, weighing the baby again after the feed. This gave a mathematical and tangible calculation of the quantity of milk the baby had consumed (for example, Beischer and Mackay 1986 p.565). Mothers and healthcare practitioners alike became obsessed with this protocol. 'Discharges home' were delayed or cancelled and mothers were found sobbing because of baby's insufficient weight gain.

[When] normal birth moved into hospital the reality behind definitions changed. Previously all pregnancies were seen as normal until judged otherwise, a judgement usually made initially by the midwife. The reverse is now true, as all pregnancies are under medical management and are 'normal' only in retrospect (Kirkham 1986 p.37).

Conducting healthcare and childbirth according to strictly objective and standardised criteria was a worldwide trend based on the belief that science provided the absolute truth and that mothers' knowledge was subjective and not legitimate. As a result, mortality and medically diagnosed morbidity statistics directed both medicine and politics. Statistical data showed improvements in maternal and neonatal mortality. For example, in 1898 the Australian infant mortality rate was 1 in 9 births (Australian Bureau of Statistics, 1998, catalogue 3302.0, Section 3, p. 50). In 1875 the infant mortality rates for France, Germany and UK were 170, 242 and 158 infant deaths per 1000 live births, respectively, and by 1910 the rates had reduced to 111, 162 and 105 per 1000 live births, respectively (www.aug.edu/~hishpv/World/E/E1b4.html). The Australian rate dropped markedly between 1898 and 1948 when it began to level out. Infant mortality continued to improve until by 1998 it had declined by 96% in Australia over the hundred years. The 1979 maternal mortality rate from complications of pregnancy, childbirth and puerperium was less than 0.5 (Australian Bureau of Statistics, Causes of Deaths, Australia 1979). The generally accepted explanation for the declining mortality rate was the use of modern medical practices and scientific technologies. As technology dominated decision-making more and more, discussions ensued around the life-saving benefits and economic efficiency of such advances, and the duty to provide healthcare to all people in need. The only real ethical debate was the greatest good for the greatest number versus equity of access and the obligation of duty.

Childbirth practices and technologies have altered since the 1980s. The postnatal stay in hospital has been reduced in the past decade from 1-2 weeks to usually 1-2 days depending on obstetric complications and category of care, whether it be private or public patient status, with or without healthcare insurance. Earlier discharge from hospital allows mother and baby to be reunited earlier with their family. Nevertheless, childbirth today remains medicalised and renders invisible the ethical nature of everyday practice – that is, the nature of relationships and the imbalance of power.

Because the bioethical approach provides a forum for dealing with ethical dilemmas surrounding 'issues', there is a taken-for-granted assumption that the bioethics of medicine are appropriate for all healthcare practices which encounter these 'issues', including midwifery. Moreover, the question that these ethics may not be adequate, and that midwifery may require its own distinctive ethic for practice, does not even appear in the mainstream ethical discourse.

This taken-for-granted assumption is reinforced through formal and informal education. The theoretical instruction on ethics for midwives in midwifery courses is taken almost entirely from nursing and medical bioethics (Beauchamp & Childress 1994; Johnstone 1994; Thompson, Melia & Boyd 1994; Bandman & Bandman 1995). The student/ practitioner is presented with the two main theories of utilitarianism and deontology, and then left to decide which theory s/he mostly agrees with, because both are recognised as legitimate and defendable stances. When other kinds of ethics are mentioned in texts, they are frequently given little credence.

In conjunction with these theories, practitioners are advised that ethical practice should be guided by ethical principles that act as a set of rules-of-thumb. Scenarios depicting extracts from clinical practice are constructed around dilemmas involving one or more of the ethical principles (autonomy, beneficence and non-maleficence, or justice), usually in life-threatening situations. Allocation of scarce resources, balancing the quality of life against the duty to treat, and the greatest good for the greatest number are common problem-solving exercises intended to develop the student's skill of objective decision-making. However, because of the centrality of objectivity within Western moral philosophy, normative principles alone do not allow for the inclusion of context, relationship and subjective feelings in ethical decision-making. Something more is required if the student/practitioner is to consider 'relationship' as well as principles. A framework of principles needs to be used as a means of actualising relationships in an ethical way. By capturing the practitioner's core ethical obligations towards the patient, the profession and society, the relationship would be utilising the expert's power 'for' the benefit of others.

The influence of the workplace in reinforcing the status quo

Finally, the fourth reason why midwives might be turning to mainstream ethics is that the workplace reinforces the status quo. On successful completion of the course, the graduate is registered or endorsed to practise midwifery and with the majority of childbearing in the Western world occurring under tertiary level medical supervision, most midwives are employed as nursing staff, in hospital settings, by healthcare organisations. These organisations usually have as Board members and senior staff, medical officers who embrace the Hippocratic Oath (c.420 BC) (Thompson, Melia & Boyd 1994) and either deontological or teleological ethics (Veatch 1989). The workplace ethics for most midwives in such societies, therefore, are the frameworks of normative Western moral philosophy, abstract principlism and dilemmic problem-solving. These frameworks focus on 'issues' not relationships. Because they strive for objectivity and universalism in decision-

making, they necessarily exclude casuistry's notions of cases and precedents, and context, character and power relationships which are the focus of feminist ethics – and everyday midwifery practice.

SUMMARY

The conclusion drawn so far is that a distinctive midwifery ethic is not explicitly available. The ethics for midwifery practice are currently based on the ethics of other practices such as moral philosophy, medicine and nursing. It has been argued that if the nature of a practice is the basis of its ethics, midwifery needs a different type of ethic to that of bioethics. The ethical nature of everyday midwifery practice differs from other health-related practices in its goals as well as its means and context. Midwifery is not based on dilemmas and life-threatening situations, but rather on the human, 'normal' and creative life experience of childbirth, and thus bioethics is not adequate. Ethical midwifery practice exists prior to the point of any dilemma and in addition to any novel health problem. A further feature of childbearing which is integral to the ethics of the practice has to do with the nature of its relationships. The midwife's prime relationship ought to be with the childbirthing woman, while the mother's prime relationship is with her baby. It is through the mother-midwife relationship that the midwife-baby relationship exists. The midwife has a working relationship with her colleagues and the mother's significant others, but these are not her prime relationships. The special relationship between mother and baby, and the relationship between mother and midwife, form the distinctive nature of midwifery practice.

In response to the question, 'What are the mainstream ethical frameworks available to midwives?' the conclusion is Western moral philosophy and contemporary applied ethics, doctrines of the Christian church, and the logico-positivist approach of principles-based, problem-solving bioethics. The superiority of intellect over feelings and of mind over body is the basic belief of both deontology and utilitarianism. Capitalism and Protestant reformation shifted the power from the Church to the state and economic organisation. Rational, logical 'truth' replaced faith. In response to Second World War atrocities and intensified scientific experimentation, professional bodies developed codes of practice and the codification of practices began.

Why would midwives be turning to these mainstream ethical frameworks? Four reasons emerged: political dominance by men and medicine, the route by which midwives in Western societies enter their practice, the widespread influence of logico-empirical science and medicalisation of healthcare, and the influence of the workplace in reinforcing the status quo.

REFERENCES

Australian Federal Government 1999 Who's rocking the cradle: Senate inquiry into childbirth practices. Australian Federal Government, Canberra, Australia

Bandman E L, Bandman B 1995 Nursing ethics: through the life span. Appleton & Lange, Norwalk, CT

Barclay L 1989 What are the origins of the regulation, training and practice of midwifery in Australia. Midwifery, back to the future. 6th Biennial Conference, Australian College of Midwives Incorporated, Darwin, Northern Territory, Australia

Beauchamp T L, Childress J F 1994 Principles of biomedical ethics. Oxford University Press, New York

Beischer N A, Mackay E V 1978 Obstetrics and the newborn. W B Saunders, Sydney

Beischer N A, Mackay E V 1986 Obstetrics and the newborn. W B Saunders, Sydney

Carroli G, Belizan J, Stamp G 1999 Episiotomy for vaginal birth (Cochrane review). The Cochrane Library, 2000

Davis D 1995 Ways of knowing in midwifery. Knowledge and wisdom: the keys to safe motherhood. Australian College of Midwives Inc. 9th Biennial Conference, Sydney, Australia

Donnison J 1988 Midwives and medical men: a history of the struggle for the control of childbirth. Historical Publications, London

Ehrenreich B, English D 1973 Witches, midwives and nurses: a history of women healers. Feminist Press, New York

Enkin M, Keirse M J N, Renfrew M, Neilson J 1995 A guide to effective care in pregnancy and childbirth, 2nd edn. Oxford University Press, Oxford

Enkin M, Keirse M J N C, Chalmers I 1989 A guide to effective care in pregnancy and childbirth, 1st edn. Oxford University Press, Oxford

Guilliland K, Pairman S 1995 The midwifery partnership: a model for practice. Victoria University of Wellington, Wellington, NZ

Gupta J K, Nikodem V C 2002 Position for women during second stage of labour (Cochrane Review). In: The Cochrane Library, 2000, Issue 2. Update Software, Oxford. http://80-cochrane.hcn.net.au.ezproxy.library.up.edu.au accessed 07/05/02).

Johnstone M J 1994 Bioethics: a nursing perspective. W B Saunders, Sydney

Kingston B 1975 My wife, my daughter, and poor Mary Ann: women and work in Australia. Thomas Nelson (Australia) Ltd, Melbourne

Kingston B (ed) 1977 The world moves slowly: a documentary history of Australian women. Cassell Australia Ltd, Stanwell, NSW

Kirkham M 1986 A feminist perspective in midwifery. In: Webb C (ed) Feminist practice in women's healthcare. John Wiley & Sons, Chichester

Mcintosh T 1998 Professsion, skill, or domestic duty? Midwifery in Sheffield, 1881-1936. Social History of Medicine 11 (3): 403-420

Myles M F 1964 A textbook for midwives. Livingstone Ltd, Edinburgh

Scheepers H, Essed G, Brouns F 1998 Aspects of feed and fluid intake during labour – policies of midwives and obstetricians in The Netherlands. European Journal of Obstetrics Gynecology and Reproductive Biology 78 (1): 37-40

Singer P 1994 Utilitarian theories of ethics. Centre for Human Bioethics Intensive Bioethics Course, Mt Buffalo, Victoria and Centre for Human Bioethics, Monash University, Melbourne

Summers A 1997 Sairey Gamp: generating fact from fiction. Nursing Inquiry 4: 14-18

Symonds A, Hunt S C 1996 The midwife and society: perspective, policies and practice. Macmillan, London

Thomas J, Paranjothy S 2001 National sentinel caesarean section audit report. Royal College of Obstetricians and Gynaecologists Clinical Effectiveness Support Unit/RCOG Press, London

Thompson I K, Melia K M, Boyd K M 1994 Nursing ethics. Churchill Livingstone, Melbourne

Toulmin S 1986 How medicine saved the life of ethics. In: DeMarco J P, Fox R M (eds) New directions in ethics. Routledge and Kegan Paul, New York

Veatch R M 1989 Medical ethics. Jones and Bartlett Publishers, Boston

Wagner M 1994 Pursuing the birth machine: the search for appropriate birth technology. ACE Graphics, Sydney

Walker M U 1993 Keeping moral space open: new images of ethics consulting. Hastings Centre Report 23 (2): 33-40

3

The false trail – a critique of bioethics and the problem-solving approach for midwifery ethics

This chapter discusses the inadequacy of traditional biomedical ethics for midwifery practice. Firstly, the development and criticisms of bioethics are reviewed, then a critique of the problem-solving approach of contemporary Western applied ethics and bioethics is presented. The critique identifies those underlying assumptions which are particularly relevant to midwifery practice, and makes them 'visible' as feminist theory encourages. This reflects my personal values, beliefs and choice of feminist theory for the research, and links my journey of dissatisfaction with the use of principles-based decision-making for ethics in midwifery.

As discussed in Chapter 2, medicalisation of healthcare has directed the preparation and practice of nursing and midwifery in recent years, and bioethics has guided their ethics. Bioethics is based on moral philosophy, and gained prominence in relation to medical and scientific experimentation. Because medicalisation and bioethics arose out of modernity, they consider human intellect and reason as being superior to feelings and personal knowledge. On the other hand, midwifery is a practice conducted within the context of feelings, experiential knowledge and relationship.

Bioethics as we have known it through logical positivism (and the scientific method), aims to objectively identify and resolve dilemmas or problems, and, through rational decision-making, take action. Its problem-solving is based on knowing which is the 'good' and 'right' action to take in certain circumstances, according to a theory of values and ethical principles that are said to suit any similar circumstance, and represent society's norms ('universal'). The theories are usually deontology and utilitarianism, and the principles are universalism, utility, autonomy, justice and beneficence/non-maleficence. Having the origins of bioethics in rational, objective logic and scientific experimentation has meant that the dominant mode of 'doing' ethics in nursing and midwifery has focused on deciding which is the ethically right and correct action to take in the presence of a novel problem or dilemma. Educational texts and literature on ethics in midwifery usually discuss maternal versus fetal rights to life, and the ethics of using technology in childbirth. Nurses and midwives are advised as to their hierarchical position in the decision-making process and their duty of care surrounding the 'right' action to take. The kind of person or interaction required of ethical midwifery practice is not debated.

Ethics that address only dilemmas and problem-solving do not inform midwives or childbearing women about their roles and characters as moral agents, as the 'doers' of ethics. Yet ethical midwifery practice mostly involves everyday and 'ordinary' human interaction and only less frequently dilemmas and novel problems. It is this human engagement – the 'doing' of ethics – which is the site of ethics for mothers and midwives. A problem-solving approach that uses normative principles and concentrates on dilemmas tends to objectify situations to 'issues' and 'rights', excluding the nature of engagement between moral agents. Traditional bioethics does not provide the practitioner or the childbearing woman with strategies for engagement or inform them about the nature of the mother-midwife relationship.

Whilst moral philosophy is helpful for understanding concepts such as justice or non-maleficence, when normative moral theory is adopted as the paradigm of practice it struggles to take account of the contextual features of situations. The essence of ethical practice is not determined by identifying which features enter into an equation – for example, cost and benefit – or by being able to adapt the principles to 'fit' differing situations. Ethical practice occurs through human engagement, relationships, and the flow of power within those relationships. For example, Judy, a mother, says in her narrative:

They were really encouraging him to do whatever he could to help me, and when I didn't like him rubbing my back they just said 'Oh, that's fine' and they took over. They involved him in things, they asked him if he wanted to, or myself, if we wanted to cut the cord.

Midwife Kerry-Anne describes a very different 'relationship' between birth attendants and parents. The birthing woman was screaming during the birth: the obstetrician reprimanded the woman and sent the husband out of the room.

[after the baby was born] I had said something about 'Will I get her husband?' So he stitched her up, then he left the room, and then I went to get the husband. As the husband walked up the corridor he walked over to the doctor who was now sitting at the desk writing up the notes, put out his hand and shook hands with the doctor and said 'Thanks very much doctor' and the doctor said to him 'She just had to behave herself and once we got her under control she was OK'. And he said 'Thank you very much doctor', and came into the room.

BIOETHICS – ITS DEVELOPMENT AND CRITICS (THE POOL OF ETHICS)

Moral philosophers of the early 20th century largely isolated themselves from practical or applied ethics, concentrating on discerning meanings of terms such as 'good' and 'right', and remaining at the philosophical and theoretical debate level (Singer 1993; Callahan 1988; Winkler 1993). Theoretical analysis was divorced from factual judgment and factual judgment from value. Moral value was seen as being generalisable and universal. The individual, isolated moral judgment was seen as subjective and invalid (Almond 1987). During the 1960s, medical technology was developed that affected the beginning and end of life, there was increased civil disobedience with controversies over the Vietnam War, and business and corporate ethics grew (Almond 1995; Singer 1993; Beauchamp & Childress 1994).

The perceived problem with the philosophical approach to bioethics was that it narrowed the debate to the problem, issue and dilemma. Normative theory did not provide justification for deciding upon a certain action. It ignored the significance of context, a criticism which gave rise to casuistry. Virtues of character and the significance of the role of the moral agent were excluded for the sake of generalisably 'good' actions, and finally, questions of expertise and the use of power in an increasingly specialised society were not addressed. Contemporary Western applied ethics set out to redress these deficiencies by applying normative theories to practical moral problems (Singer 1993).

The purported moral decline of Western culture and demise of religious convictions, change and uncertainty from increased education, ethical relativism, medicalisation and advances in medical technology, the allocation of scarce resources, and more recently the phenomenon of AIDS have all contributed to the development of bioethics (Lewins 1996) as an emerging discipline.

Biomedical ethics evolved through formal codes of medical and nursing ethics, research ethics, and reports by government-sponsored commissions.

Healthcare professions typically specify and enforce obligation, thereby seeking to ensure that persons who enter into relationships with their members will find them competent and trustworthy ... Problems of professional ethics usually arise from conflict of values (Beauchamp & Childress 1994 p.7).

Furthermore, Beauchamp and Childress found that medical codes focused on non-maleficence and confidentiality, but few recognised the implication of other principles and rules. They introduced secondary principles such as veracity, respect for autonomy and justice.

Clouser and Gert (1990) argue that because the principles as proposed by Beauchamp and Childress (1994) lack any systematic relationship to each other, they often conflict with each other, and since they do not originate from a unified moral theory those conflicts are unresolvable. This is borne out in research which shows that although beneficence usually takes precedence over the other moral principles in bioethical discussions, for healthcare practitioners there is often a tension between beneficence (doing good) and autonomy, and between justice and beneficence (Robertson 1996; Woodward 1998). Clouser and Gert (1990) contend that the principles are primarily checklists for concepts that are worth considering. In addition, there are often two or more competing principles involved in a given case, and real duties that are created by special relationships and roles are not distinguished from what is morally required. Custom and practice often determine how a healthcare professional is morally required to act, and an adequate moral theory should set limits on what s/he is allowed to do.

Another argument is that in bioethics we ought to seek reflective equilibrium between our deepest moral convictions and our moral principles so we can compare that reflective equilibrium to the medical diagnosis. Where there is 'inconsistency' a complex principle or several different principles are required (Callahan, 1988). The inference here is that establishing such a balance through comparison can solve these ethical problems, but who is the authority who defines the ethical problem for the practice? Is it the philosopher or the practitioner? Dare one include the client-patient as one of the authorities?

Casuistry and context

In the 1960s, applied ethics started paying attention to the ethics of medicine (Toulmin 1986), scrupulously analysing particular kinds of cases. Debate redirected analysis to professions involved in human tasks and duties, and to equity, reasonableness and relationships – the ethics of Aristotle. A basic presupposition of modern Western medicine is that, mostly, human beings in all cultures share common bodily frames and physiological functions.

The central subject matter of medicine thus comprises those objective, universal conditions, afflictions, and needs that can affect human beings in every culture, as contrasted with those relative, subjective conditions, complaints, and wishes that are topics for anthropological study in any given culture (Toulmin 1986, p. 268).

Thus 'objective' standards of good and harm, and practical reasoning about moral issues, were reintroduced. Casuistry claimed, however, that to know the situation it was necessary to understand cases of conscience, cases that address the concrete detail of actual moral quandaries of real people, and to analyse the circumstances of both the agent and the act. Casuistry, therefore, discusses how the circumstances of particular cases or precedents of moral perplexity fit general norms, rules, standards and principles of morality. Moral discourse talks cases, and cases are the substance of medicine (Jonsen 1995).

Problems arise not at the level of the principles themselves, but at the point of applying them (Toulmin 1986). Duties are central. Firstly, moral obligations are not purely universal. Our position in relation to others means that different people are subject to different moral claims. Professional affiliations and concerns shape one's obligations and commitments. Radical individualism overlooks the interaction of mediating structures and intermediate institutions such as family and profession, in the larger scale context of the agent's action. Secondly, those who undertake a certain profession are obliged to perform the special duties of their profession as part of that undertaking. These professional roles and commitments have replaced our communal roles and commitments (Toulmin 1986; MacIntyre 1984). The concepts of 'friendship' or 'relationship', and 'equity' are closely connected in that we expect markedly different conduct depending on who is affected and what the relationship is between the parties. Mothers and midwives in the present narratives also highlight the distinctiveness and ethical importance of a 'professional friendship' within the mother-midwife relationship, compared with an 'objective' and what they see as impersonal approach of 'system workers'. Arline, a mother, discusses the character of the midwife who cared for her during pregnancy and birth, and the importance for her of a professional friendship.

The fact that I had birthed our first child and she was our midwife and just through all the antenatal care I respected her professionalism. I respected her as a midwife and I'm sure she respected me as a person and as a mother that was able to birth, so yeah I think that's how I come to know that I respect her judgement because I trust her and that's because I had formed a relationship with her which is the key, for me anyway. She's very professional but very casual at the same time. You know like yeah we ended up forming a friendship. We were renovating our house at the time when we were expecting [first child's name] and when we were building this house we were expecting [second child's name] so she used to come over for a cup of tea and during the time before [second child's name] was born she met this fellow and was getting married and so it was kind of like where you catch up and have a cup of tea and a chat and she'd tell me all the 'goss' about this fellow and so yeah. So that was nice to form a friendship together.

Pairman (2000) found similar expressions in her research and concluded that although the professional and friend initially seemed to have different meanings they in fact meant similar things – it was the setting that influenced the women's descriptions of the midwife.

Gemma, a midwife, speaks despairingly of what she sees as a trend within the hospital where she worked.

They can help by not being complicit in it all, and in fact they are complicit in it all. I mean I just have to walk this place and go down to any woman that's having an induction and ask her what she knows about her induction and it would be very little. And that may be that she doesn't want to know but mostly it's because as 'system workers' we've failed these women ... Well people employed within large institutions like this one, we tend to get into routines and just do what we have to do in order to get through the day rather than actually thinking about the needs of the individual women, and if she's having a procedure done what does she understand by that?

Rather than considering it fair to treat everyone equally, in the case of close friends and relatives it is considered perfectly reasonable and equitable to show a degree of partiality. So for Toulmin (1986) and writers on applied ethics, the ethical problems of medical practice and research, and the interaction with law and other professions, have revived ethics. Academic theory is no longer adequate and ethics has to debate practical, concrete and political issues.

Quandary or dilemma-based ethics

May (1994) refers to case-oriented ethics as quandary ethics; the search for rules and principles as guidelines for decision-making. This dilemma-based approach has dominated professional ethics because of its intrinsic philosophical and theological prestige, and cultural convenience. Mass media focus on headliner (or 'neon') quandaries and professional education organises itself around the case study. The approach emphasises the perplexities that the individual practitioner faces, but does not critically examine systems, institutions and structures. Practitioners are reluctant to accept responsibility for a colleague's behaviour because they are not their colleague's keeper, and quandary is intellectually more interesting for ethicists than self-discipline. May (1994) criticises the reluctance to discipline the bad performer, given the amount of power that professionals wield, and the relations between institutions, ethos and virtue. Bureaucracies have made society hostage to the virtue of professionals who work for them, and increased specialisation has meant that fewer other people know what the expert is up to, and thus cannot discredit her/him. When knowledge is power, ignorance is powerlessness. Despite the use of institutional mechanisms to limit the abuse of specialised knowledge, it is the virtues in those who wield the power that results in 'being good', not simply 'producing good' in a utilitarian way. We habitually learn what we ought to do through experts and powerful role models. For instance, we can learn that the virtue of behaving benevolently is morally subordinate to the principle of beneficence according to the professional expert's definition of 'doing good'. Or we can learn the opposite. Rather than ask what one can do about a problem, it is sometimes more appropriate to ask how one should behave toward it. This distinction is seen

between the more glamorous systems of cure and the humbler action of care ... [when challenged with what we ought to 'be', self-definition] we are not simply agents producing deeds but, in part, authors and co-authors of our very being (May 1994 p.78).

A virtue is not an inherited temperament. It is an acquired human quality which enables us to achieve the internal 'goods' of a practice. The lack of it prevents us from achieving those goods. The 'goods' that are external to a practice, such as rewards or results are secondary to the practice (MacIntyre 1984). May (1994) does not reject principles or ideals. Rather, the imperative is to approximate the ideal and to respect the difficulties of its realisation in an imperfect world. In that way, virtues reflect commitments to principles and ideals but also to narratives which are the exemplary lives of others.

Writers such as Bandman and Bandman (1995) also think that rights and virtues fit together. Given that their structure and functions have been carefully thought through, they are not necessarily oppositional. Indeed, in their latest edition Beauchamp and Childress (2001) address virtues and character in the early part of their discussion and then conclude with theory. This reflects a change from the deductive approach of firstly developing a theory and then providing examples to support it, to an inductive approach that draws on practice and reality to inform theory – the latter approach is also adopted by the present analysis.

Contextualism

Winkler (1993) challenges the adequacy of saying that bioethics consists of three main principles – autonomy, beneficence and justice. Applied ethics treats biomedical ethics as if it is not a special kind of ethics, as if it is governed by the same general normative principles and rules as are effective in other spheres of human life. Trying to bridge the gap between the abstractions of philosophical theory and the complexities of actual situations merely leaves the ethicist to 'broker' moral options as defined by this or that theory.

Furthermore, due to the dominance of paradigm theory, the practitioner works and thinks contextually but is surrounded by conferences, classes and programmes that preach autonomy, beneficence and justice. Winkler (1993 p.353) asks to whom do these principles apply, and on what basis: 'What must something be like in order to qualify as a subject of serious moral concern in its own right?' The standard theory is dependent on some supplementary account of moral status.

The following is from Kay's narrative. The obstetrician who supervised her pregnancy undoubtedly believed herself to be practising according to the principles of beneficence and non-maleficence, affording Kay her autonomy. There were no serious moral concerns. Lives were not endangered. However, Kay considers that her wishes were not heard or respected and she was not able to establish realistic expectations for her birthing experience. Does this kind of relationship and lack of engagement qualify as a subject for serious moral concern in its own right? Kay says:

As we [doctor and mother] met throughout my pregnancy I would raise the subject of wishing to have as natural a childbirth as I could manage and the conversation didn't develop on that. It was quickly switched to other issues not related necessarily even to the birth. Very little time was spent discussing the birth.

Ann, a midwife in a traditional hospital ward, tells of a young couple who came to the hospital worried, wanting something done. They felt that something was wrong with the baby but were told there was nothing wrong and sent home. Ethical theory and principles may retrospectively explain or justify actions taken, but interpretation of the contextual features of their engagement with health professionals is integral to our moral deliberation on the situation.

I can remember one of the young registrars who was involved came to see me a bit later and he was a little bit upset by the fact that he couldn't help these people because he was told by his consultant that no they weren't to be delivered at this stage, that [the policy was] they would reassess them in 10-12 days and then she would come in for an induction at that time. Well that didn't happen. The meconium happened before that time so he felt very helpless because he was governed by another person further up.

Applied ethics is deductivist: it is 'top-down' in its conception, and mistakenly sees bioethics as constructing and applying principles to resolve difficult cases. Winkler (1993) says that rather than adapting the principles to the situation, in practice it occurs the other way around. We use wide reflective equilibrium and the complex processes of interpretation to inform our understanding of principles. Instead of a paradigm theory Winkler proposes 'contextualism', a dominantly case-driven model of actual moral reasoning:

Moral problems must be resolved within concrete circumstances, in all their interpretive complexity, by appeal to relevant historical and cultural traditions, with reference to critical institutional and professional norms and virtues, and by utilizing the primary method of comparative case analysis. Applicable moral principles will derive mainly from these sources, rather than from ethical theory on the grand scale (Winkler 1993 p.344).

Principles do not play a major part in decision making. Interpretation is more important in moral reasoning. A universally valid ethical theory is inconsistent with the concept of a social morality; a morality that

serves certain very general ends, within the context of real time, pervasive uncertainty, and continually evolving historical circumstance (Winkler 1993 p.360).

Principles are nothing more than generalisations of decisions made within certain kinds of moral contexts. Finally, contextualism does not totally deny the normative relevance or impor-

tance of moral principle, but rather than being instrumental in resolving difficult cases, conformity with the stated principle 'explains' the morality of the case. It justifies the moral conclusion, and gives the reason why the particular case and all relevantly similar cases have the moral quality they have; that is, why they are right or wrong.

Lutzen (1997) supports the notion of contextualism and argues that a context-sensitive approach to the understanding of ethical issues in nursing practice is also needed for the next millennium. By that she means that the idea of universalism must be questioned because ethics is an interpersonal activity, set in a specific context.

Similarly, Lewins (1996) criticises the existing approaches to bioethics, saying that a social and contextual model of bioethical behaviour is required. He suggests that bioethics needs to incorporate links with other disciplines because, to date, bioethics has focused on codifying and controlling healthcare practice rather than posing important questions and generating public discussion of issues. Bioethics and its current lack of homogeneity can only be explained by examining its social context. The lack of cohesion is evident because the academic approach raises questions such as 'When does life begin and end?' – questions that require answers but lack certainty. Conversely, the imperative approach occurs in actual healthcare settings and political circles, and sets out to provide certainty through codification and control of professional behaviour (Lewins 1996).

In summary, the emerging tensions within the practice of applied ethics are two-fold: the significance of the embedded nature of relationships, and the implications for methodology. The embedded nature of relationships highlights the need to recognise context, the significance of practice, institutional structure, role relations, and the link between the virtues and role of the moral agent. The implications for methodology are the significance of philosophy beyond the moral, the significance of both empirical and historical social inquiry, and the problem that the traditional applied ethics model does not address evil (it concentrates on 'good') whereas, significantly, social critique does. Traditional models are also inadequate, in not proposing a transformative response. The altered way of seeing and being is not available or explained. Lastly, contemporary Western applied ethics does not recognise justification of the ethical response in practice as distinct from justification in theory.

The relational ethic of care associated with feminist writers such as Carol Gilligan (1982) and Nel Noddings (1984) emphasises context, detail and responsibility to particular others, rather than abstract principle and justice. Similarly, virtue ethics seeks the good in particular situations and the development of virtues such as personal character. Feminist approaches to ethics also analyse the power structures in society which they claim are incompatible with individual freedom of action, itself a necessary condition of morality (Tong 1993).

Normative principles-based problem-solving deliberately ignores context and temporality for the sake of being 'objective'. Context and temporality influence relationship. Character and values, which are dependent upon a relationship, are the focal points of feminist and virtue ethics. What ethically matters to mothers and midwives involves character and values, context and relationships. Therefore, it seems that feminist-virtue ethics would be a more appropriate theoretical basis than normative bioethics and principlism for teaching and practicing ethics in midwifery.

A CRITIQUE OF THE NORMATIVE, DILEMMIC/PROBLEM-SOLVING APPROACH OF BIOETHICS FOR MIDWIFERY

Echoing the discussion above, contemporary writers also criticise the traditional biomedical approach to nursing ethics for its

abstraction, focus on universality, and paucity of terms for describing moral character and the morality of relationships (Robertson 1996 p.292).

It lacks context and utilises a top-down perspective. Thus normative theory and dilemmic problem-solving are seen as particularly inadequate for ethics in midwifery practice.

In addition to criticisms already raised, bioethics and ethical theory derive from Western moral philosophy that strives for objectivity, excluding other ways of 'knowing' as not legitimate; for example, women's ways of knowing and seeing, and the non-expert's experience. These problems and assumptions are particularly relevant to feminist ethics and midwifery.

A principles-based approach to ethical decision-making judges the rightness and wrongness of acts independently of the particularity of the situation and the moral agency of the people involved. In doing this, the situation is disembedded (stripped of context), and the subject is disembodied (depersonalised). Decision-making is based on abstract, universal principles which do not take account of motivation, changes over time, events and influences in the past or cultural differences; they subordinate the means for the ends, and are atemporal and acultural. Experts define ethical meaning and make the decisions. Moral character such as virtue and the morality of relationships are not addressed.

When the situation is stripped of context

When the situation is disembedded, it is stripped of context. Narratives gathered from mothers and midwives demonstrate that midwifery uses knowledge gained from personal experience, that context including language is important in ethical deliberation, and that childbirth is a social construction not merely a physiological event. They reflect that midwifery has its own way of seeing, and practitioners are embedded in practice traditions.

Positivism (for example, the scientific method and a striving for 'rational' decision making) argues that to strip away the context and subjective experience of a situation increases the objectivity, validity and reliability of information and, therefore, of decision-making itself. However, ethical deliberations draw on social construction for meaning. To decontextualise a situation disembeds it from features that have helped to create its social construction. Features such as the roles and interaction of moral agents and the importance of relationships between them indicate the flow of power between individuals, groups and institutions (Thompson, Melia & Boyd 1994). The knowledge base or epistemology of a practice is defined according to how members conceptualise their reality and images of the world (Denzin & Lincoln 1994). Midwifery practice incorporates information from multiple sources, including personal experience. To consider only a part of the information available is to offer an inadequate explanation and ethical response.

Locke proposed that a person is made up of a mind and a body separately, with the mind being the more important. The mind is like a mirror. External reality imposes itself directly on the passive mind of the individual, and the mind then rearranges the 'information' according to mechanical principles; our ways of seeing, therefore, need not be influenced by social tradition. Langford disagrees, claiming that

what we see depends, quite literally, on the way we have been taught to see (Langford 1985 p.13).

Examples of socially constructed meanings and taught ways of seeing include ambiguous images depicted within the same picture on the page, such as the 'duck/rabbit', the 'goblet/two faces', and the 'young woman/old woman' combinations. Members from cultures and societies that do not have these items and concepts would interpret the images differently. How we interpret our reality and the world around us is socially and culturally related. Context is important. Similarly, a practice such as midwifery is not merely an expression of personal vision. Features of the practice such as being emotionally supportive of the birthing woman, valuing her ability to birth her baby and respecting the centrality of the parent-child relationship rather than the dominance of science, technology and institutional might, may be seen as subjective features by advocates of logical positivism. Nevertheless, childbirth and the roles and relationships connected with it are

social constructions embedded in social context, carried out in accordance with social practice. The practice of midwifery is not only about skills and techniques; it is also a way of seeing. The practice provides the skills and techniques, and a certain way of seeing: the way of seeing guides and structures the use of those skills and techniques. The individual decides what to do and how to act, but the tradition provides the opportunity, and guides and constrains the action according to its way of seeing and doing (Langford 1985). The practitioner is embedded in the practice, and the practice is embedded in its lived reality and social construction.

Whilst the objective, valid and reliable data may guide some physiological management or practice decisions for childbirth, it is not adequate in guiding ethical deliberation and practice. The contextualised situation reads differently, and it is the context which guides ethical practice. An integral part of the context is the language used. Franco Carnevale argues that

bioethics discourse typically disregards the context from which controversies emerge and the processes that inform and constrain such discourse ... [and] medical futility was constructed, in part, as a means of enhancing physician domination of a context wherein medical authority was threatened (Carnevale 1998 p.509).

Support of constructivism as an alternative approach therefore, stems from a belief that the public space between us is founded on and shaped by our language.

Bioethics discourse, Carnevale says,

typically examines a biomedical problem from rival moral frameworks, struggling with how to construe and pursue the good, the discourse itself is infrequently examined (Carnevale 1998 p.511).

The political, social and moral ideology inherent in the discourse and the cultural construction of the debate or phenomena significantly influence the orientation of the discourse and methodology of any research. This construction and pursuit of good concurs with previously raised criticisms of normative theory; that is, it theorises about the problem, issue and dilemma without acknowledging the significance of context and role, of virtues, power and expertise, or the question of interpretation. Research by Robertson (1996) showed that both doctors and nurses highly valued a utility-based conception of beneficence, but that interpretation alone was not always adequate. Often the emphasis was on 'being' a benevolent practitioner more than on good 'outcomes'.

Midwives in the present analysis also emphasise the 'being with' role of practitioners and the 'being' experience of birthing women rather than utility-like 'outcomes'. Describing the environment in which a teenaged mother birthed her baby, Bev says:

They [hospital midwives] were brilliant. They were very quiet. They were present but not pushy. They weren't telling her 'push, push, push'. They were just there letting her do it the way she wanted. And attentive, present. They were just very quiet. They hardly spoke and that was what we needed. The focus was on the mother. All the attention was on her. We were all creating a supportive environment for her.

Diane, another midwife, describes one ethical facet of her practice in relation to information-giving, epidural pain relief and the birthing woman's self-determination.

You see I think women make the decision that is best for them, and if it's not something that I would do, who's to say that it would still not be the right decision for them? Because they know where they're at now and I don't. If a woman is in transition and I'm sure she's in transition, I will tell her that and say look, if you can just hold out for a few minutes I think that things will change and you'll probably birth and so I'll try and encourage her and get her past that sticky point, but ultimately the decision is hers and I may feel a little disappointed but I have no right to do that because [for instance] maybe I'm looking at my professional reputation. For her, yeah, have I failed this woman? If I'd done such and such would it be different, but what's right to her at the time? I don't know what her history is. I know what she's told me ... she's entitled to feel that need and to express that need and go that way and it's not for me to say that her position is wrong.

When the subject is depersonalised

When the subject is disembodied, s/he is depersonalised. Disembodiment (depersonalisation) of the subject occurs with the abstract principles of autonomy and justice, especially as they are viewed by utilitarianism. When the mind is made superior over the body and feeling, the subject is disembodied. The principle of autonomy requires 'rational' self-determination. On that basis, if one is deemed 'irrational', presumably autonomy is denied. Firstly, this treats 'rational' not only as an absolute and static state, but also as a dualism, the dichotomy of 'irrational'. However, many childbearing women describe moments when they 'go into themselves' as they are birthing their baby, when they become subordinate to the bodily and spiritual experience, but few would describe themselves as irrational women who should justifiably be denied autonomy during that part of the birthing process.

Stephen Toulmin distinguishes the ethics of intimates from the ethics of strangers ... the boundaries of ethics are about these [face-to-face] interactions... The ethics of strangers appeals to formalised principles of justice, rights, and rules. Such rights and rules develop adversarial relations that include malpractice suits. We thereby give up the trust we once had in health professionals (Bandman & Bandman 1995 p.93).

Bodily experience and feelings are consciously ignored in normative bioethics, and the midwife is faced with rational-irrational dualism. Another example of this during childbirth is that the 'scientific' proof of the presence (or not) of physical uterine contractions dominates labour and birth decisions, and the 'irrational' anxiety of the woman and her support person, for which there is no 'scientific' evidence, is essentially excluded from the decision-making. Midwife Ann's narrative illustrates how this occurred with the young couple who wanted something 'done' but were sent home because mother had no uterine contractions or cervical dilation and the hospital protocol was to induce labour 10-12 days after the 'due' mathematically calculated date. 'Rational' science is revered and 'irrational' subjective data is treated as a separate 'issue', perhaps even relegated to the private sphere along with human relationships.

Aristotle emphasises that ethics is concerned both with power and the conditions for human flourishing

... because they enable us to achieve our personal goals and fulfilment as human beings (Thompson, Melia & Boyd 1994 pp.61,44).

Conditions that either enable or constrain human flourishing are values, power, power-relationships and power-sharing.

In his attempt to uncover the ideological debate in the 'futility' of cardio-pulmonary-resuscitation discourse, Carnevale says that

... life derives its value from the projects and endeavours that a person can perform; and when a person is elderly and institutionalized, we can universally declare that this is not a life worth maintaining [this argument can also be adopted for the baby who is born with abnormalities] ... this framework is congruent with the dominant modern western ideal of life as a project of individual pursuits, centred on rational experience (Carnevale 1998 p.514).

Carnevale analysed the struggles of people caring for ill children and found that their struggles were

over differing conceptions of a 'good enough life', as well as tensions over trust, respect and power among many agents (Carnevale 1998 p.515).

Futility discourse seems to disregard this by inferring that their one view is the most good.

The abstract nature of principles

Intellectualist principles are abstracted from practice and motivation.

Jonsen & Toulmin [1988] argue that neglect of practical and applied ethics, of training in ethical decision-making and problem-solving skills and practice in dealing with real cases has opened the way to what they call 'the tyranny of principles'. Pretending that all moral issues can be settled at the level of theoretical discussion of principles has encouraged debate to become polarised between antithetical and dogmatically held view points, or dismissed as simply a matter of personal 'taste in morals' (Thompson, Melia & Boyd 1994 p.86).

Reiterating an earlier comment, Western moral philosophy and normative principles tend to present moral issues in an adversarial way. Principles-based ethics is presented as though moral understanding simply requires a commitment to a code of potentially authoritative rules.

Philosophy concentrates on defining specifically moral rules, and normative principles do not allow for different interpretations of the rules or facts according to variations in context.

Locke's practical principles (now called natural laws) are ideas that originate, either directly or indirectly, in experience, and because these practical principles are to be 'discovered by moral sense or reason rather than through the ordinary senses they may be described as a priori principles' (Langford 1985 p.27). Thus they and values are presented as objective. This implies a faculty of moral sense or reason, just as there are senses of hearing and seeing. If this were so, we would all agree to the same principles of practice, but it is not possible to identify such a set of practical principles about which people universally agree. Furthermore, when the way of seeing is divorced from practice, practical principles become intellectualist. The mere perception of injustice, for example, without the desire for justice, may not lead the person to 'do' anything about it. The perception without a response produces a gap between the principles of practice and the practice itself. The strictly objective argument does not account for how one comes to have such desires and motivation. Finally, if the practitioner acts merely on self-interest, as individualism argues, there is no obvious need for practical principles-based action guides. Practical principles by themselves will not effect social change because

a practice has no reality independently of its practitioners: the two are interdependent. Those who engage in a practice are guided by the way of doing which a tradition provides and the way of doing in turn exists only in the values and purposes of those guided by it. Thus practical principles are abstract but only in the sense that they are abstracted from practice [external to the practice they purport to guide] (Langford 1985 p.35).

The next point of contention is with the principle of utility or greatest happiness. There is no way of measuring and comparing happiness as defined by different people: for example, between fast cars and high-fibre diet and fresh air (Langford 1985). Discussion cannot be confined to how given ends are achieved (the means) without needing to discuss the ends themselves. This leads to a further objection. The contrast between means and ends is always relative to situations and never absolute. For example, is hanging the 'neutral' means to the execution or is the intention of hanging the 'end', and not simply that the person be executed? Is the medicalisation of birth and reduction in the mortality-morbidity statistics the 'neutral' means to 'good' birth for mother and baby, or is the intention of medicalising childbirth and reducing the mortality-morbidity the 'end' and not simply that the mother and baby experience a good birth?

Principles-based ethics claims that its universal principles (beneficence, non-maleficence, justice and freedom of choice/autonomy) are true for all time and people, but critics say that they are atemporal, ahistorical and acultural. They do not take account of changes over time, events and influences in the past or cultural differences (Clouser & Gert 1990; May 1994; Winkler 1993). The present discussion argues that far from being a single event, issue or problem, solvable by using a mathematical equation to produce a just and 'good' outcome, a moral dilemma in midwifery practice is frequently a narrative of relationships that extend over time (Gilligan 1982).

What is ethically 'good'?

What is ethically 'good' is medically defined, decided by experts and acts as a mechanism for social control. Three assumptions of normative bioethics are particularly relevant to midwifery and childbirth practices. The meaning of 'good' is defined by the dominant medical profession, frequently on the basis of mortality and morbidity. Decisions are based on the single 'objective' truth arrived at by intellectual reason. Lay knowledge is denounced and the dominant discourse's assessment of good more accurately reflects social acceptance. In other words, the person making decisions is the professional. Power does not flow equally to and from other key stake-holders such as the woman who is growing, birthing and mothering the baby, the baby's father, and the midwife.

The first of these taken-for-granted assumptions embraced by biomedical ethics is that the dominant medicalised 'way of seeing' is the only legitimate interpretation of the practice of childbirth. Within that orientation, beneficence or 'doing good' is interpreted as saving lives and non-maleficence is interpreted as not actively or intentionally doing (physical) harm, that is, threatening life. Non-maleficence is probably seen as the more important of the two. Codes of practice and legislation support this interpretation as the one truth, and this truth is given to midwives as their mandate. The 'goods' and 'harms' as interpreted by the 'other' – the childbearing woman and midwife – are given lesser value than the interpretations of the dominant cultures of medicine and moral philosophy. The questions of 'good' for whom, and in which way, are not open for debate.

The second and related taken-for-granted assumption is the supremacy of deductive logic, intellectual reason, and medical science in the hierarchical ways of knowing. Science and technology are superior because they are based on deductive logic and reason. Knowledge derived from experience, intuition and shared ethical understanding of a community (Durgahee 1997) is perceived as inferior. Yet Caroline, a mother, illustrates the importance of personal knowledge.

Well I suppose by the time I had fallen pregnant with three of them I wanted things to be, I'd really changed my outlook on life. I'd changed my diet, I'd realised what a healthy, balanced diet can do for a person, and I was determined that I wanted it all natural. I don't like drugs in any way, shape or form and the fact that I actually wasn't offered any drugs in any of those labours is probably – I suppose it's not really an ethical issue, but to me it is important that I wasn't pushed to have an epidural or Pethedine or anything like that.

The pre-modern subject was situated, contextualised, enmeshed, driven by passions that needed to be tamed, and ethically responsible for and to all the people with whom s/he had relationships (MacIntyre 1966). This had to change with the development of capitalism and the state. Being rational was important in order for the subject to know and act in his/her own best interests – emotions were subsumed by reason. Medical science and technology are the domains of doctors. The doctor is credited with a different sort of knowledge, a 'greater' knowledge and expertise, and hence authority. The midwife – and arguably the mother – is subordinate to, but also in alliance with, the doctor when childbirth is medicalised (Donnison 1988; Kirkham 1986; Rothman 1991). The assumption that intellect and science are superior ways of knowing denies the importance of lay knowledge – the subjective lived experience of healthcare and illness. Yet, as research by Durgahee (1998) and narratives in the present analysis demonstrate, the person's unique experience (of, in this instance, childbirth) is an essential part of 'ethical' knowledge.

A third taken-for-granted assumption is the ethical 'goodness' of the dominant discourse. This also relates to both the 'single truth' concept and to the male-oriented construction of the term 'good'. According to this assumption, to act upon the universal principles of beneficence, non-maleficence, autonomy and justice is to be ethical and 'good'. A major criticism of that approach is that it categorises the ethical stance of 'the other'. To assess only actions, and to assess them on the basis of universal principles that are interpreted by the dominant discourse, categorises those who disagree with, or do not act according to, the dominant discourse as 'bad' patients, 'bad' people, or at the very least 'not ethical'. Such an orientation treats inclusiveness merely as social acceptance. The behaviour of those who challenge the dominant discourse is retranslated into ethical evil.

Prior ethical practice, character, virtues and relationships

Dilemma and problem-focused ethics deny prior ethical practice, character, virtues and relationships. According to mothers and midwives, virtues that should exist in the mother-midwife relationship are trust and respect for the birthing woman's wishes. That is, ethical midwifery practice establishes a trusting and respectful relationship between mother and midwife, and the midwife's character is one of

trusted, professional friend. What it means for midwives to practice ethically, therefore, seems to exist in the absence of and prior to or after the resolution of any dilemma or problem.

The problem-solving or applied philosophy approach (Almond 1987) addresses the ethical only when there is a dilemma – a choice between two equally undesirable outcomes (Thompson, Melia & Boyd 1994 p.5). Even if one concedes to addressing problems rather than the unresolvable notion of dilemma, the approach remains inadequate, particularly for the human and 'normal' life process of childbirth. Beginning ethical deliberation at the point of a problem assumes that there is no ethical nature to practice prior to that stage. For this reason, the discourses of bioethics and traditional nursing ethics are not inclusive enough. According to these approaches, the picture of what it is to be ethical is guided by a set of principles. This code of steps or rules aims to inform the practitioner as to the right and wrong actions to be taken regarding the problem or dilemma, and that leaves much unsaid.

A dilemmic and problem-solving approach to ethics does not address the importance of the moral character of stakeholders, virtues possessed by them, and the morality of relationships. When virtues are defined as settled habits and dispositions to do what we ought to do, then virtues become subordinate to principles; benevolence to beneficence, respect to autonomy, fairness to justice. However, virtues are not correlates of principles and rules. Virtues are charity and good faith, caution, humility, discipline and bravery, characteristics that supply human strength (May 1994). Courage, lucidity, prudence, discretion and temperance do not neatly correlate with principles of action. Moral life does not conveniently organise itself into deeds that can be performed, issues that can be decided, or problems that can be solved. Character comes from living. It is an ever-evolving and habituated sensitivity. One knows the right thing to do and becomes the kind of person one is according to moral virtues learned from living, from one's lived reality and from powerful role models.

When we are vulnerable, we depend on relationships with others to help us (Isaacs 1998), and the flow of power within those relationships reflects the ethical nature of a practice. In addition, the character and orientation of moral agents and the context of situations determine the nature of relationships in practice. The principle of autonomy with its emphasis on 'rationality' and individualism, and absolute and dichotomous meaning, suggests that vulnerability and self-governance cannot co-exist. The person is either rational, or not, and therefore entitled, or not, to her autonomy. The principle does not inform the practitioner how she should behave when autonomy has or has not been 'granted', or when the birthing woman moves from autonomous to vulnerable.

To illustrate the inadequacy of normative principles for midwifery, it is helpful to consider the period of time surrounding the birth of the baby and the importance of relationship. The childbearing woman may not be able to 'be' autonomous and communicate independent decisions during all stages of childbirth. For example, when she is in labour, in pain, is very anxious and worried, she is vulnerable and experiences levels of altered consciousness. Childbearing women need to communicate their desires and wishes earlier, at a time when they are in a position to use commonly understood language and act in a more interactive way. Midwives need to be cognisant of the particular woman's response to birthing and her 'birthing language'. Some mothers in the present analysis explain that the benefit of having the same midwife from early in labour until the birth, is that the mother can talk with the midwife about her wishes and desires; that the midwife will get to know the mother as she 'normally' is, not see her as someone screaming and 'uncooperative' in pain. When complications occur, earlier communication may indeed mean that the birthing woman can think and act more independently. Ethical practice for us as midwives sometimes means that when the woman's 'independence' is compromised we need to speak and act on her behalf – according to her known and expressed wishes, not a presumed

'good' as defined by the dominant discourse or a normative principle. Furthermore, self-determination ought to be negotiated and renegotiated from time to time rather than be 'set' at one point in time. Women and midwives enter into a moral relationship together, a relationship that is mutually dependent at various stages and in various ways. The mother-midwife relationship with the 'able' woman and 'competent' midwife is mutually dependent in a way that is different from the relationship between a healthcare professional and a sick person. A dilemmic, problem-solving approach to midwifery ethics fails midwives and mothers in their human engagement, a relationship that reflects the ethics of intimates.

SUMMARY

Normative bioethics is rejected for midwifery because it strongly represents the (male) moral philosophical approach which is too abstract from mothers' and midwives' lived reality. It does not take account of context, character or relationship, and allocates the decision-making to the powerful expert. Neither does the dilemmic and problem-solving approach account for ethical practice in the absence of, prior to, or following resolution of such a problem.

On the other hand, feminist and virtue ethics propose an ethical approach that includes deliberation of contextual features including the nature of language, character of moral agents and nature of relationships. This presents a valid and alternative ethical response for midwifery practice. The feminist writer Rosemarie Tong

embrace[s] contextualism because it enables [her] to move between principles, values, ideals, norms, rules, sensibilities, intuitions, and virtues on the one hand, and situations on the other, in some sort of reflective equilibrium (Tong 1994 p.123).

Furthermore, whilst some researchers deny any gender difference in ethical decision-making (Norberg & Uden 1995; Kuhse et al 1997; Franke et al 1997), others indicate that women concentrate on context, detail and relationship more than abstract principle and justice when structuring ethical meaning or faced with ethical dilemmas (Gilligan 1982; Robertson 1996; Lutzen & Nordin 1995; Lutzen et al 1997; Poole & Isaacs 1997).

The question for us, as midwives, is whether or not the ethical nature of the mother-midwife relationship reflects the nature of a distinctive ethical response for midwifery practice. The proposed premise is that what matters ethically to both mothers and midwives about 'being with woman' during childbirth is best achieved through interaction between them, in a woman-centred, contextually sensitive relationship that distributes power equitably between 'able' persons. The individual does matter, as do our responsibilities to particular others and cultural values. Virtues such as character of moral agents do matter and the midwife's ethical response to the mother and her birthing affect the emerging relationship. Objective decision-making and abstract universalism are not adequately responsive to the ethical nature of this mother-midwife relationship because they exclude individual experiences in preference for rationality and generalisability. Alasdair MacIntyre considers that modern moral philosophy

'is in a state of grave disorder' [largely due to] barren armchair philosophy [and] blind reliance on ideas that have claimed false independence from the cultural, social and historical milieus in which they have been generated (MacIntyre 1985 p.11 cited in Johnstone 1994 p.126).

Feminist moral theorists may offer an alternative for an ethic of midwifery. They consider important the values of sharing, empathy, nurture and caring, context and situational demands, one's responsibility to particular others, and the analysis of concrete cases of conscience, as does casuistry (Toulmin 1986; 1992).

REFERENCES

Almond B 1987 Moral concerns. Humanities Press International, Atlantic Highlands, NJ

Almond B 1995 Introduction: ethical theory and ethical practice. In Almond B (ed) Introducing applied ethics, Blackwell Publications, Oxford

Bandman E L, Bandman B 1995 Nursing ethics: Through the life span, 3rd edn. Appleton & Lange, Norwalk, CT

Beauchamp T L, Childress J F 1994 Principles of biomedical ethics, 4th edn. Oxford University Press, New York

Beauchamp T L, Childress J F 2001 Principles of biomedical ethics, 5th edn. Oxford University Press, Oxford

Callahan J C 1988 Ethical issues in professional life. Oxford University Press, Oxford

Carnevale F 1998 The utility of futility: the construction of bioethical problems. Nursing Ethics: An International Journal for Healthcare Professionals 5 (6): 507-517

Clouser K D, Gert B 1990 A critique of principlism. Journal of Medicine and Philosophy 15: 219-236

Denzin N K, Lincoln Y S (eds) 1994 Handbook of qualitative research. Sage, Thousand Oaks, California

Donnison J 1988 Midwives and medical men: a history of the struggle for the control of childbirth, 2nd edn. Historical Publications, London

Durgahee T 1997 Reflective practice: decoding ethical knowledge. Nursing Ethics: An International Journal for Healthcare Professionals 4 (3): 211-217

Franke G R, Crown D F, Spake D F 1997 Gender differences in ethical perceptions of business practices: a social role theory perspective. Journal of Applied Psychiatry 82 (6): 920-934

Gilligan C 1982 In a different voice: psychological theory and women's development. Harvard University Press, Cambridge

Grimshaw J 1986 Feminist philosophers: women's perspectives on philosophical traditions. Wheatsheaf Books, Brighton

Isaacs P 1998 Social practices, medicine and the nature of medical ethics. In: Society for Health and Human Values Spring Regional Meeting, Youngston State University, Youngston, Ohio

Johnstone M J 1994 Bioethics: a nursing perspective, 2nd edn. Saunders, Sydney

Jonsen A 1995 Casuistry: an alternative or complement to principles? Kennedy Institute of Ethics Journal 5 (3): 237-251

Kirkham M 1986 A feminist perspective in midwifery. In: Webb C (ed) Feminist practice in women's healthcare. John Wiley & Sons, Chichester

Kuhse H, Singer P, Rickard M et al 1997 Partial and impartial ethical reasoning in healthcare professionals. Journal of Medical Ethics 23: 226-232

Langford G 1985 Education, persons and society: a philosophical inquiry. Macmillan, London

Lewins F 1996 Bioethics for health professionals: an introduction and critical approach. Macmillan Education Australia Pty Ltd, South Melbourne

Lutzen K 1997 Nursing ethics into the next millennium: a context-sensitive approach for nursing ethics. Nursing Ethics: An International Journal for Healthcare Professionals 4 (3): 218-226

Lutzen K, Everton M, Nordin C 1997 Moral sensitivity in psychiatric practice. Nursing Ethics: An International Journal for Healthcare Professionals 4 (6): 472-482

Lutzen K, Nordin C 1995 The influence of gender, education and experience on moral sensitivity in psychiatric nursing: a pilot study. Nursing Ethics: An International Journal for Healthcare Professionals 2 (1): 41-50

MacIntyre A 1966 A short history of ethics: A history of moral philosophy from the Homeric age to the twentieth century. Routledge & Kegan Paul, London

MacIntyre A 1984 After virtue: a study in moral theory, 2nd edn. University of Notre Dame Press, Notre Dame, Indiana

MacIntyre A 1985 After virtue: a study in moral theory, 3rd edn. Duckworth, London. In: Johnstone M-J 1994 Bioethics: a nursing perspective, 2nd edn. W B Saunders, Sydney

May W F 1994 The virtues in a professional setting. In: Fulford K W M, Gillett G R, Soskice J M (eds) Medicine and moral reasoning. Cambridge University Press, Cambridge

Noddings N 1984 Caring: a feminine approach to ethics and moral education University of California Press, Berkeley, California

Norberg A, Uden G 1995 Gender differences in moral reasoning among physicians, registered nurses and enrolled nurses engaged in geriatric and surgical care. Nursing Ethics: An International Journal for Healthcare Professionals 2 (3): 233-242

Pairman S 2000 Women-centred midwifery: partnerships or professional friendships? In: Kirkman M (ed) The midwife-mother relationship. Macmillan, Basingstoke

Poole M, Isaacs D 1997 Caring: a gendered concept. Women's Studies International Forum 20 (4): 529-536

Robertson D W 1996 Ethical theory, ethonography, and differences between doctors and nurses in approaches to patient care. Journal of Medical Ethics 22: 292-299

Rothman B K 1991 In labour: women and power in the birthplace. W W Norton, New York

Singer P 1993 Applied ethics. In: The new encyclopaedia britannica. Encyclopaedia britannica, Chicago, Illinois

Thompson I E, Melia K M, Boyd K M 1994 Nursing ethics, 3rd edn. Churchill Livingstone, Melbourne

Tong R 1993 Feminine and feminist ethics. Wadsworth Publishing Co, Belmont, California

Tong R 1994 What's distinctive about feminist bioethics? APA Newsletter 94 (1): 122-124

Toulmin S 1986 How medicine saved the life of ethics. In: DeMarco J P, Fox R M (eds) New directions in ethics. Routlege and Kegan Paul, New York

Toulmin S 1992 Cosmopolis: the hidden agenda of modernity. University of Chicago Press, Chicago, Illinois

Winkler E R 1993 From Kantianism to contextualism: the rise and fall of the paradigm theory in applied ethics. In: Winkler E R, Coombs J R (eds) Applied ethics: a reader. Blackwell, Oxford

Woodward V M 1999 The moral metaphors of nursing. Journal of Advanced Nursing 30 (1): 94-99

4

Midwifery's detour through nursing ethics – a critique of professional codes and influences that shape the midwifery ethics discourse

Chapter 2 examined the historical influence that nursing and medicalisation have had on the educational preparation, practice and ethics of midwifery. Chapter 3 discussed the inadequacy of dilemmic and problem-solving biomedical ethics for midwifery practice. Based on those earlier discussions, the traditional orientation of nursing ethics is rejected as inadequate for midwifery practice on two accounts: firstly, it emerged largely from bioethics and secondly, the contextual responsibilities of nursing generally do not parallel those of midwifery. Some of the more recent, feminist nursing ethics pebbles appear similar in shape to midwifery ethics pebbles perhaps, but different contexts require different ethical responses, and the medicalised and hospital-based practice ethics remain ill-fitting for midwifery. One aspect of difference relates to medicalisation and promotion of 'expert' versus the implementation of 'autonomy' expected by 'able' childbearing women. Another is the conflict that practice settings have on the type of relationship between the birthing woman and the practitioner. Both are illustrated in extracts from the present narratives.

Megan, a mother, discusses what she experienced as conflicting and 'campaign-like' rules rather than practical advice and negotiation from hospital midwives and breastfeeding consultants when she was trying to establish breastfeeding for the first time:

For women in that situation, I mean it's not like they're dealing with people who are too sick to make up their own minds or too sick to be unaware of what's going on. They're dealing with women who are basically pretty well.

Kerry-Anne, a midwife, compares the difference in nature of practising midwifery in a birth centre with working in a traditional hospital labour ward, more in the role of an obstetric nurse. In the birth centre, midwives and women get to know each other over the duration of the pregnancy. Women are admitted to hospital labour wards once labour has commenced, or if there is a problem, and are in the presence of strangers for a relatively short period of time.

I think the trust thing is something that is developed over a period of time, rather than right there at the time. So the 'trust' starts early and that's where if someone is going privately to a doctor and they're seeing him every time, I think that's when the trust builds up. Whereas I think the midwives in the labour ward don't have time to build the trust, but they do 'rely' on the midwife to get the doctor there in time. That's the difference. They're 'relying' on the midwife, but they're not really 'trusting' her.

This chapter does not set out to comprehensively review the nursing ethics discourse. Rather, it aims to discuss the traditions of professional practice, the impact of institutionalisation on healthcare, and the application of a code of practice as a recent addition to those traditions. Secondly, the strengths and weaknesses of codes as models for ethical responses are identified. Lastly, the discussion focuses on how the ethical discourse in midwifery has been shaped through educational curricula, the institutional workplace setting, and text books, journals and conference presentations. These influences are examined for their ethical orientation.

TRADITIONS OF A PROFESSIONAL PRACTICE, INSTITUTIONALISATION, AND APPLICATION OF A CODE

Traditions and codes of professional practice develop from what members consider to be the 'goods' or goals of the practice. Whilst the profession influences and alters the individual who enters it, societal practices influence and alter the goals and practice of those professions.

Professional affiliations and concerns shape one's obligations and commitments, and those who enter a certain profession are obliged to take on the ethics and duties of their profession as part of that undertaking. Traditionally, the orientation of the practice of nursing stems from an illness model based on the Nightingale dedication to rules and regulations (Kingston 1975), and is influenced by institutional values and goals. A recent addition to professional traditions is the application of codes of practice, and given the historical influence on nursing of the illness model, nursing ethics developed from biomedical ethics. Traditionally, the orientation of the practice of midwifery has been that childbirth is a healthy, human and 'natural' life experience occurring in a social context and directed by the values and goals of the individual childbearing woman and her midwife (Summers 1997). However, as discussed in Chapter 2, in recent decades childbirth has been medicalised and midwifery subsumed under the umbrella of nursing. Thus, contemporary and explicit midwifery ethics have derived from nursing ethics.

Medicalisation and institutionalisation of healthcare in the Western world has directed not only the skills, techniques and philosophical orientation of practitioners but also the ethics of their practices. In more recent times, with the emphasis on individualism rather than community, our professional roles and commitments have replaced our communal roles and commit-

ments. Institutionalisation of healthcare has impacted on the ethics of professional practice because different rules and constraints operate in different situations and settings. For example, in primary care or community settings the rules that define the practitioner's duties, responsibilities and arbiters are different from those within hospital situations. Even when the principles and values of practices are similar, variation in the exercise of power and responsibility in those different settings defines the problems, constraints, rules and accountability for practitioners (Thompson, Melia & Boyd 1994). In the vast majority of instances, conception and birth can occur quite independently of the values and goals of healthcare institutions, and of sophisticated science and technology. Since the late 1960s in the Western world, with the medicalisation of childbirth, women have been required to birth in hospitals and the institution has dominated both the modality and ethics of childbearing practices (Ehrenreich & English 1973; Donnison 1988).

As discussed in Chapter 3, biomedical ethics evolved through formal codes of medical and nursing ethics, research ethics, and reports by government-sponsored commissions. Historically, caring professions first develop a code of practice and then formulate their ethics around it (Thompson, Melia & Boyd 1994). They do not construct their code on an ethical approach derived directly from membership, and client values and beliefs. Nor do they incorporate the reality of the workplace or the impact of the institution on the individual. They are idealistic. Nevertheless, codes of practice demonstrate a desire on the part of the profession to self-regulate, and thus they afford professional status to a practice. Application of codes is aimed at preventing malpractice such as that which occurred during World War II.

A CRITIQUE OF ETHICAL CODES

Codes draw on principles-based and problem-solving ethics, and act as a set of rules to guide practitioners in their ethical decision making. However, as discussed in Chapter 3, that approach is acontextual, atemporal, does not take account of relationship or human engagement, and does not provide a strategy for response.

One of the problems of a monistic deductive approach is that it does not recognise that different ethical approaches are suited to differing circumstances ...While a rights-based approach is appropriate at the policy level it is not as useful in guiding concrete intervention strategies (Jordan 1996 p.53).

Perceived strengths of codes

Codes are intended to act as a set of rules-of-thumb to guide practitioners in their decision making. They make explicit the perceived 'goods' or goals of the practice and thereby provide a forum for debate and confirmation within the profession.

For example, discussions continue on the role and purpose of a professional code of practice. On the positive side, a code may seek to prevent a decline in standards by responding to a particular ethical debate, as happened with the Nuremberg Code of 1947, or to cases in practice that have gone wrong. Secondly, codes are seen as part of the process of claiming professional status for the practice and this has been claimed as both a strength and a criticism (Thompson, Melia & Boyd 1994; Pritchard 1996).

Furthermore, disagreement centres around whether ethical codes are rules of conduct or guidelines for responsible professional behaviour (Veatch 1989). Perhaps rights-based ethics such as those expressed by codes are best applied at the policy level, within the ethics of strangers. That is, codes may be more than an expression of professional consensus. They can have legal standing or be the basis of disciplinary action by the professional regulatory body. Put to that purpose, codes play a significant role in the self-regulation of a profession. Codes have also been divided into three categories; 'codes of ethics', 'codes of conduct', and 'codes of practice' (Pritchard 1996). According to those categories, a code of ethics contains broad principles without practice-specific meaning. On the other hand, a code of conduct specifically guides the behaviour of members of a particular

profession, and is most effective when combined with training in ethical decision making. A code of practice resembles a customer charter because it is the professional body's warrantee of certain standards of care or service to clients.

Codes convey the rules and requirements of the profession to its members and their most useful function is to advise, encourage and support members to behave morally over and above any legal obligations practitioners might have (Pritchard 1996). They are usually prescriptive in that they spell out the moral standards for professional conduct, and members are expected to carry out their duties in the best interests of clients (Thompson, Melia & Boyd 1994; Clarke 1996). The integrity of the practitioner is assumed.

Codes tend to justify crisis interventions by carers in terms of their duty to care for the vulnerable and incompetent and to protect them from harm ... to prevent malpractice and protect carers from unfair claims or demands being made on them by those for whom they have provided care (Thompson, Melia & Boyd 1994 p.50).

Some take endorsement of the benefits of codes a step further, claiming that a single code for healthcare is desirable. In an attempt to update medical ethics, the Tavistock Group is developing a shared code of ethics for everybody in healthcare, which they say would be more conducive to cooperative behaviour and mutual respect (Smith, Hiatt & Berwick 1999). The group's draft document is primarily constructed around universal principles which all stakeholders in healthcare can recognise and accept as guides to correct action. They argue that separate moral frameworks are inferior because each discipline seeks to gain the moral high ground. Yet, this again reduces ethics to right and wrong 'action', and positions different disciplines as adversaries. It is not inclusive of difference.

Perceived weaknesses of codes

Firstly, codes that are meant to reinforce professional and societal values often highlight the lack of agreement about those same values. For example, pregnant women and midwives have felt for some time that the medical profession has undermined women's ability to give birth without technology and intervention, and this is illustrated in practice when professional judgements take precedence over the individual's rights and moral values (Siddiqui 1997 p.98).

The assumption is that codes represent the collective wisdom of the group that authored and endorsed them: that is, they express and promote generally accepted ethical norms (Veatch 1989). However, usually a code is not constructed directly from the grassroots values and beliefs of the profession's membership or clients (Thompson, Melia & Boyd 1994). Constructing codes on a 'top-down', theoretical basis follows the intellectualist tradition and tends to distance the document from the practice, even though the individual practitioner can ratify it within her/his own practice, and the membership can endorse it via a formal voting system. Further, whilst a code can give coherence to professional behaviour by disclosing the profession's values and duties to the public and distinguishing its boundaries of practice, no code provides moral sensibility or practitioners who will act ethically.

[E]thical reflection is morally superior to ethical theories ... ethical reasoning cannot be reduced to the application of norms ... morality requires also personal experience, habits of virtue and moral sensibility (Sala & Manara 1999 p.461).

These are features of the ethics of intimates.

Another criticism is that historically, nursing and therefore midwifery codes have been based on biomedical ethics, and medical codes have focused on non-maleficence and confidentiality to the exclusion of other principles such as veracity, respect for autonomy and justice (Beauchamp & Childress 1994). Although these other principles have now been included, professional codes still place most emphasis on beneficence and non-maleficence. As Toulmin (1986) points out in relation to the ethics of strangers and intimates, problems arise at the level of applying principles, not with the 'universal' principles themselves, and moral obligations are not universal, as our relationships

with friends and relatives demonstrate. In addition, emerging in response to malpractice, codes have tended to be more reactive than proactive (Pritchard 1996).

Recent criticism has been levelled at codes for their idealism and prescriptiveness. Codes that are idealistic and prescriptive without explaining how the concepts relate to actual practice do not adequately guide the practitioner in ethical practice. Codes often do not state how nurses (or midwives) ought to fulfil their moral responsibilities during day-by-day encounters (Johnstone 2000). Another criticism is that 'prescriptive' supposes that there is a definite response to a situation. If that is the intention, then the code standardises behaviour with rules (Clarke 1996). Prescriptiveness in codes also leads to deceptive simplicity which gives rise to dangerously simplistic interpretations, especially by those who are morally and politically naive. Certain types of questions are hidden; for example, 'how are the interests of any client to be defined and identified', 'what would happen if the midwife's interpretation of interest clashed with the obstetrician's interpretation', and 'whose definition of interests would have priority in the care of the client' (Clarke 1996). Basing the expected standard for professional practice on idealism means the individual's real life practice is compared with the ideal. That does not acknowledge the real life constraints which make it impossible to achieve the standard; and worse, the individual is punished for failing to meet the expectation. As discussed in Chapter 3, May (1994) argues that principles and ideals should be respected but we should only aim to approximate them and thereby also respect the difficulties of realising them in an imperfect world. This criticism links the abstraction of contemporary applied ethics and principles with the abstraction of right and wrong 'action' oriented codes. That is, just as radical individualism overlooks the interaction of mediating structures and intermediate institutions (Toulmin 1986), an idealistic code overlooks the interaction and impact of structures and institutions on the individual's practice.

A final criticism of ethical codes for healthcarers has to do with prescribed positions of power. The carer is always referred to as the one in control, relative to the client's vulnerability. Codes emphasise that ethical practice demands the carer accept responsibility for the client.

... few have stressed the importance of the commitment the carer must make to return control to the client as soon as she is again capable of being independent. None of the existing medical codes stresses that the doctor has a primary moral duty to assist (where possible) the rehabilitation of the patient. [The ICN and RCN identify the nurse's responsibility to restore autonomy to the individual, thus] emphasise a value fundamental to nursing ethics which appears to arise out of reflection on the distinctive nature of nursing care (Thompson, Melia & Boyd 1994 p.75).

Nevertheless, whilst codes ought to focus more on how the carer can return control to the client/patient as soon as possible, codes also need to reposition control and power more equitably between carer and client throughout their entire relationship, on a more fluid basis. Since the focus of the present discussion is on midwifery, this is particularly pertinent: the able childbearing woman ought to 'retain' control, not lose it in the first place. In what is a healthy, human and 'natural' process, the midwife ought to be working with the woman to 'retain' and 'maintain' the woman's self-determination rather than 'returning' control to her. An adequate ethical response is one that is distinct to the context of different practices and settings. Sometimes, the childbearing woman needs to be 'looked after', cared 'for' and have things done for her by someone else, but mostly she does not. Sometimes the unwell or injured patient does need to at least try to be self-sufficient and independent, but mostly s/he cannot 'fix' the health problem without help from science, technology and/or medicine – Western or Eastern medicines. The person with a health 'problem' is less likely to be able to 'fix' the health problem her/himself than the childbearing woman is able to birth her baby herself. An intention of the present analysis is to examine taken-for-granted assumptions in the conceptual frameworks of healthcare, and to critically question our patterns of thinking: to

investigate whether or not there is coherence when they are transposed across practices. The problem-based orientation of medicalisation does not seem to be a good 'fit' for childbirth, a 'natural' and creative life process. Some values and principles, such as respect for life and justice, might be universal to the human condition, and others, such as beneficence and non-maleficence, might be commonly shared, for instance between medicine, nursing and midwifery (Robertson 1996; Woodward 1998). The interpretation and application of those such as 'autonomy' and informed choice, however, reflect the different practice contexts and the distinctiveness required for adequate ethical responses in them.

There is a fragile element within the notion we call 'informed choice' ... Embracing uncertainty sometimes brings a sense of calm ... This is not about engendering a passive fatalism but more about enabling [childbearing] women to learn to trust that they will cope with whatever comes their way. Working through these issues is particularly important in a culture that privileges the notions of 'choice' and 'control' (Leap 2000 p.5).

The unwell patient's ability to self-determine may be compromised by the illness or disease itself, quite separately from the institutional influence. The unwell patient arrives at the situation with reduced 'autonomy'. Unlike the unwell 'patient', the 'well'/'able' childbearing woman's ability to self-determine is not reduced because of her altered condition – that of pregnancy. She arrives at the childbirth situation as an able, albeit awkward and tired, independent person. In most instances, she remains capable of making decisions about her birthing. The brief but intense periods of time during the actual birth when she is less able to linguistically interact with those around her, reduce her ability to verbalise her wishes through common language. Women agree that they are vulnerable and susceptible to suggestions during the second stage of labour.

The women did not equate entering an altered state of consciousness with being out of control: on the contrary, it was a powerful coping strategy that increased their sense of being 'in control' (Anderson 2000 p.96).

The birthing woman does not indicate an inability to know and carry out what she wants to do with her own body, and often what she knows her body needs to do. It is less likely that the unwell 'patient' knows in the same way, what her/his body needs to do in relation to the illness or injury, the health 'problem'. Mostly, the birthing woman is also able to position and 'do with' her own body that which she feels she can and is 'right for her'. It seems that it is when others require her to do otherwise, when others 'take over', the birthing woman surrenders her self-determination to institutional influence. She cannot deal with the huge job of birthing her baby and at the same time debate strategies and ward off the assault of powerful experts.

Rather than 'restoring' independence to the individual mother, therefore, after the so-called high-risk event of birth, ethical midwifery practice and codes of ethics for midwives need to emphasise the 'retention' and 'maintenance' of self-determination for the 'able' childbearing woman – the sustainability of her independence throughout the birthing process.

Pritchard (1996) defines the internal goods of a profession as the unchanging ends whereas the means to those ends alter with scientific and medical advancement. She identifies the intrinsic 'good' of the midwife's role as 'skilled mediation' in childbirth and argues that if mediation through client choice is the central value to midwifery, then 'good' action is decided by how much a particular circumstance promotes that value. This is surely also true for practices other than midwifery. Nevertheless, it may be especially applicable to midwifery, given that the majority of childbearing women are healthy and able to make certain choices. So:

in this sense it is argued that client choice is an ethical option for midwifery and on that basis skilled mediation is an intrinsic good that helps women have a fulfilling experience of childbirth (Pritchard 1996 p.192).

Strategies of skilled mediation and client choice do appear to constitute at least a part of the concept of an adequate ethical response in midwifery practice.

Examination of the Australian College of Midwives Incorporated (ACMI) Code of Ethics, for example, shows that the profession does value relationship, and the Code does begin to offer strategies for response. Section III advises midwives to support women in their right to participate actively in decisions, to empower women to speak for themselves, to work with and liaise with women and the various personnel, and to support and sustain each other. Its weaknesses, however, are similar to those of the UKCC Code of Professional Conduct (Clarke 1996); that the midwife is expected to be accountable, an advocate and an autonomous practitioner when the employment conditions do not permit her to be all those things. Section IIIB of the ACMI Code of Ethics refers to supporting and empowering women. The brief analysis offered in that document says that the principles and concepts inherent in the section are accountability, advocacy and autonomy. Firstly, the hospital midwife does not have a client, a sentiment reflected in midwife Kerry-Anne's comparison of birth centre and traditional hospital midwifery practice quoted earlier. The client belongs to the consultant, and the consultant has the ultimate authority regarding practice decisions. Secondly, the Code assigns midwives a moral responsibility for clients, but if the midwife tells the woman what happened during certain situations, she risks being charged with gross professional misconduct.

There is little evidence that the code of ethics for midwives in the United Kingdom (i.e. the UKCC Code of Professional Conduct) is a source of empowerment to practitioners (Clarke 1996). This is also true for Australia, in that neither codes of practice nor legislation give midwives the right to practice decisions or mothers the right to procedural and treatment choices within the medically dominant power differential of an institutional workplace. Furthermore, it is unjust for midwifery's governing bodies (for example, the Australian College of Midwives Incorporated or the State Nursing Councils) to impose the code's principles on midwives in an environment where the employer prohibits their freedom to act on them.

Authentic midwifery has become invisible within

obstetrics and she is permitted only to provide midwifery care as it is defined by obstetrics, that is, carry out those routine observations and monitoring tasks that do not require, and indeed prevent, the establishment of professional intimacy and responsibility ... The evidence also casts doubt on the assumption of the UKCC that midwives have the professional, clinical and moral autonomy necessary to practise as directed by the Code of Professional Conduct (Clarke 1996 pp.216-17).

In summary, the ethical validity of individual principles such as beneficence, non-maleficence, autonomy and justice, or the caring aspect of medical and nursing ethics, is not rejected. Rather, the disagreement is firstly with the abstraction of principles because of their inadequacy to address context, historical changes, culture, character and relationship. Secondly, it is inappropriate to apply the orientation of an institutional context of practice to midwifery because it sits dysfunctionally with the intensely personal experience of well-woman-centred midwifery practice. The ethics of strangers is not helpful for a practice whose members and consumers express the need for an ethic of intimates. The aim, and in some instances the lived reality, of midwifery at the micro level, according to current literature (see Chapter 9), is that of partnership not patient, friendship not unknown expert within the hospital system, and individual persons 'within' relationship, not the powerful professional body with elite knowledge practising on the respectful powerless. It is on these grounds, therefore, that this analysis sets out to examine what women and midwives identify as their ethical concerns and goals, based on their personal experience. If midwifery is a shared tradition of woman and midwife, then the ethic of midwifery practice ought to be one based on a consensus of their beliefs and goals rather than the beliefs and goals of institutions such as science, medicine and moral philosophy. The latter are not inclusive enough of women and other ways of seeing.

How ethical discourse in midwifery is shaped

Ethical discourse in midwifery is shaped by more than the formal code. It is shaped through educational programmes, workplace settings and professional meetings. Let us now examine the relevant literature for ethical orientation, looking at whether or not the discourse is based on the contemporary Western applied ethics framework, and noting the inclusion or absence of women's voices.

Chapter 2 discussed the first assumption drawn for this analysis; that is, that a distinctive midwifery ethic is not explicitly available. The second assumption is that frameworks of bioethics and traditional nursing ethics are inappropriate guides for midwifery practice because they are not adequately responsive to the ethical nature of the mother-midwife relationship – to the concerns of mothers and midwives in the context of their lived reality. The people who have shaped the healthcare ethical agenda are those with elite knowledge and power. Often they have been from outside the particular practice. Traditionally, bioethics have been determined by practitioners from moral philosophy and medicine. Because, after the Second World War, nursing ethics and thus midwifery ethics emerged from bioethics, some of the first formally documented approaches and codes for ethics in midwifery were also shaped by those outside the practice and not by midwives or childbearing women (Thompson & Thompson 1986; Thompson & Thompson 1991; see also Chapter 2). Presenting 'the ethical', based on moral philosophical reason, masks the crucial influence of power and renders the voices of the disempowered inaudible. When the ethical is defined by 'so-called' objective acts, relationships, and in particular power relationships, are ignored and obscured.

Accessing the lived experiences of mothers and midwives is critical to repositioning the ethical response of midwifery. Until recently, the discourse on ethics in midwifery (curriculae, texts, journals and conference presentations) has excluded the voices of some key stakeholders. By excluding the voices of mothers and midwives, the discourse does not speak to them as one might expect it would if it were reflecting midwifery practice as a partnership built on relationship.

Studies specifically investigating the ethical nature of the mother-midwife relationship from the point of view of these two groups were not located in midwifery or nursing journals at the time of writing. Instead, literature on midwifery and ethics focuses around three main areas: educational curriculae and their ethical components (what and how to teach and learn ethics), the role and function of Institutional Ethics Committees (IECs), and healthcare practitioners' decision-making, including the conflict that exists between the workplace, ethical principles and personal-professional ethics.

The next part of the discussion concentrates on (i) educational curriculae and their ethical orientation, (ii) the workplace setting and institutional influence on midwifery practice, and (iii) the ethical orientation of textbooks, journals and conference presentations.

Educational curricula and their ethical orientation

When midwifery is seen as an extension of nursing, nursing ethics are presented as equally applicable to midwifery. This is evident in many graduate diploma midwifery programmes conducted within nursing faculties. Such programmes frequently do not devote time to the area of ethics and those that do, do not present ethics in any midwifery-specific way. Ignoring the distinctiveness of ethical responses in different practices and contexts, and omitting ethics from postgraduate programmes assumes not only that nursing ethics are equally applicable to midwifery but also that the only 'legitimate' ethics which midwifery practitioners use are those from their undergraduate nursing orientation.

Research indicates that post-basic nursing education, experience and the practice setting do influence the ethical response of nurses (Lutzen & Nordin 1995). Firstly, those nurses who had undertaken a post-basic psychiatric nursing course focused on patients' feelings and reflected on values underpinning actions. Secondly,

nurses who had not specialised in psychiatric care were more dependent on the knowledge and advice of the physician (Lutzen & Nordin 1995 p.48).

Conclusions drawn from that study, therefore, were that (i) education increased self-confidence and independent decision-making, (ii) experience as mental care workers appeared to increase awareness of the moral implications of one's actions, and (iii) the influence of the setting was not unexpected in that nurses who cared for patients in a hospital setting needed more help from the medical staff (for example, medication issues) than nurses in community clinics where they made more independent decisions.

Later Lutzen, Everton and Nordin (1997) compared the results of their survey of psychiatrists with nurses' responses from the earlier study. They relate Gilligan's theory to the results of their own study; that when faced with a conflict, women are more likely to ask the question, 'How shall I respond?' than 'What is the right action?' There was a significant difference ($p < 0.001$) between males and females when structuring moral meaning. Females saw that rational thought was

aimed at making sense of seemingly contradictory moral principles and the need to justify the actions taken by means of objective facts (Lutzen, Everton & Nordin 1997 p.479).

Their research indicates that (i) the question of right or wrong 'action' depends on the situation within a specific context, and (ii) whilst context does influence moral sensitivity, 'moral sensitivity' itself is temporal and not constant – it is developed by experience, and increases with age regardless of the type of clinical practice. Such findings lend support to the claims that what we see depends on what we are taught to see, virtues are acquired, and sensibility is habituated from living life. Experience, socialisation and training will increase our sensitivity, especially when the 'measurement' of that response is based on what the practice considers to be its intrinsic 'goods'. Similarly, the context determines the action, because the practice provides the way of seeing, the skills and techniques, and the way of seeing guides the practitioners' use of skills and techniques. This also supports the claim that different contexts require different ethical responses. Just as results from research conducted in nursing contexts cannot be applied in their entirety to midwifery contexts, neither can nursing ethics be transposed in their entirety to midwifery practice. The specificity of a midwifery context requires separate research, as well as a specific ethical response in practice.

The workplace setting and institutional influence

I was concerned about her and I wanted her to be seen by a doctor. According to her, her dates and my calculation, she was 37 weeks pregnant. So we went to the antenatal clinic and we were seen by a specialist obstetrician. We went into this room and he sat at the desk and faced the wall, she sat at one end of the desk and I sat at the other end of the desk. He turned away from me and towards her. Without looking at her he picked up her notes and went through it, found an ultrasound report and said 'We haven't been seeing much of you' and without waiting for her to respond he said in a fairly shocked voice, 'You're 43 weeks pregnant'. She smiled. 'I'm 37 weeks'. He said 'You're 43'. And she was very insistent, 'No I'm not, I'm 37 weeks pregnant, I'm sure'. He said 'I've got this ultrasound, it was done at 18 weeks, ultrasounds are very accurate, you MUST be 43 weeks pregnant. And this is very dangerous, very dangerous to your baby. Your baby could die'. She's quite a tough little street kid kind of person and she's not easy to intimidate, and again she said, 'I'm not 43 weeks' and he said 'You have to be admitted to hospital today'.

(An extract relating to autonomy, paternalism and institutional dominance, from Bev's narrative; a midwife practising in a community clinic.)

The setting influences the practice, as does the institutionalisation of healthcare, through variation in the exercise of power and responsibility in different settings (Thompson, Melia & Boyd 1994).

The majority of midwives in Australia and a large number in the rest of the Western world today work in a hospital setting and practice under the authority and direction of doctors. The working structure experienced by midwives is rigid and policy-driven (Clarke 1996). From that point of view they have a similar work environment to nurses, and are likely to

experience conflicts of values. Those who claim that the ethics of a practice are influenced by the setting attribute such conflicts to the different intrinsic values or 'goods' of each practice (Pritchard 1996), and to the different conceptions each practice has of ethical decision-making principles (Robertson 1996).

David Robertson's (1996) British study confirmed that doctors and nurses on the psychiatric ward differed in their conceptions of the principles of beneficence and respect for patient autonomy. Nurses shared with doctors a commitment to liberal and utilitarian conceptions of these principles, but also placed much greater weight on relationships and character virtues when expressing the same principles. Nurses also emphasised patient autonomy, while doctors were more likely to advocate beneficence when the two principles conflicted. He found that 'mainstream, principles-based healthcare ethics', when supplemented by both feminist, relationship-orientated, ethical theory and character-orientated virtue theory, were together helpful in describing the ethical talk and actions of the doctors and nurses whom he observed on the ward. Robertson's findings reflect the similarity of nursing and midwifery in that both practices are carried out in the context of relationship. The nature of the mother-midwife relationship, however, differs from the nature of the patient/client-nurse relationship, and therefore the 'adequate' ethical response is different in the different practices.

Robertson's (1996) results demonstrated that the social context of the ward influenced ethical patterns. Whilst doctors emphasise clinical problem-solving, assessing and maximising patients' organic functioning, doing research, and the use of technology and technological explanations, nurses' priorities are daily care, fostering patient normality and independence, and social and psychological alternatives. The ethical case study concluded that in relation to (i) 'justice', day-to-day resource allocation within the ward is discussed exclusively along egalitarian lines and is concerned with the equal worth and entitlement of patients; and (ii) 'beneficence', both doctors and nurses valued this utility-based concept highly, but nurses emphasised being a benevolent practitioner (an idea better described by virtue theory) and fostering good relationships with patients (a concept elaborated in feminist relationship theory) rather than merely achieving the utility of good outcomes.

Virtue and relationship conceptions of beneficence effectively coincided [and] virtue- and relationship-based conceptions of beneficence were far more often voiced amongst nurses than doctors (Robertson 1996 p.295).

Both groups are also highly committed to rights- and rationality-based views of autonomy. However, nurses are strongly committed to patient autonomy as constituted in relationship (doctors were less so). This is

consistent with Susan Sherwin's (1992) assertion that Gilligan's relationship ethics can often be integrated with the principles of more traditional approaches to healthcare ethics (Robertson 1996 p.296).

Robertson further discusses the tension between (i) autonomy and beneficence, (ii) justice and beneficence and (iii) beneficence and respect for patient autonomy. He suggests that nurses' preference for respecting patients' autonomy over beneficence, when these conflicted, might be explained by nurses' closer relationships and greater identification with the patients. Doctors were more likely to support beneficence at the cost of respect for autonomy. Bev's narrative about the obstetrician's dispute over weeks of gestation seems to support this too; however in that obstetric context beneficence clearly only referred to saving life.

Given that the internal 'goods' of the practices differ,

doctors and nurses are likely to have different priorities from midwives and also from the client (Pritchard 1996 pp.195-6).

For example, autonomy, or self-determination as it is referred to in the present discussion, is a central value for midwifery. Medicine, nursing and midwifery may each define it differently. The meaning of autonomy for midwifery needs to be expanded beyond self interest so that it encapsulates the midwife's right to prac-

tice decisions and the mother's right to procedural and treatment choices.

Yet basing the ethical approach on abstract principles leaves much unsaid. Even when different practices share certain values and perceive certain principles to mean similar things, variation in the exercise of power and responsibility in those different settings defines the constraints and conditions of practice; that is, the situations, roles, rules and arbiters (Thompson, Melia & Boyd 1994). Midwives practising independently in primary obstetric care in The Netherlands agreed that the setting influenced their behaviour, which in turn shaped their relational care (van der Hulst 1999). Midwives were more informal and interactive with expectant parents during a home birth than in the hospital, and their relational care was more intense and woman-centred.

Commonly, codes reflect the Kantian theory that the intention behind the act is more important than the outcome. End-oriented, business-like management of institutions conflicts with this 'means' orientation of professional codes and practice.

There are risks in the new corporatist approach to the ethics of organisations, insofar as it may lead simply to reinforcement of corporate self-interest or may be expressed in closed and authoritarian institutions. On the other hand, there is a real potential to rediscover an holistic approach to ethics as an enterprise of the whole organisation, based on equal opportunities policies and fair and equitable power-sharing between people, in a working community that sees itself as a moral community (Thompson, Melia & Boyd 1994 p.154).

Thompson, Melia and Boyd (1994) argue not only that different settings impact on the overall practice of professions, but also that different situations within that practice require different ethical approaches from the practitioner. Codes characterise the duty to care, of advocacy. The relevant paradigm is crisis intervention, wherein the client is very dependent and vulnerable. The professional is in control and acts *parens patriae* with beneficence and non-maleficence as the guiding ethical principles. Contractual ethics concerns mutual rights and duties, and is based on the paradigm of voluntary request for help. The client is independent, competent and ambulant, while the professional offers service and acts in the client's interest. The relationship is between the person-with-the-problem and the person-with-the-power-to-help, and is inherently unequal. Within the relationship, the client entrusts her or himself into the knowledge, skills and resources of the carer and agrees to pay the costs of the commitment. The carer is involved in direct negotiation with the client about the nature and scope of the help required and is guided by the principle of justice (universal fairness). Covenantal ethics promotes an enabling and empowering role. Its paradigm is that of befriending and mutual partnership. The client is self-directed, seeking support, companionship and partnership. The professional promotes the autonomy of the partner and acts *parens inter pares*, guided by the principle of respect for a person's rights. Thompson, Melia and Boyd (1994) recommend this approach during the continuity of care for long-term or chronic illness, particularly where there is no hope of cure but only amelioration of symptoms, a situation that requires a different kind of commitment on both sides. The 'patient' is competent and consultable, and the contract-to-care is renegotiated as necessary. The client has a right to know, accept or refuse the care, and the carer has a duty to clarify what is being offered. Respect for persons means that the rights and dignity of both the client and the carer are protected. Based on this interpretation, the covenantal approach to ethics presents a valid alternative to the abstraction and universalism of normative theories and principles.

The final type of ethics described by Thompson, Melia and Boyd (1994) is that of charter ethics. In this era of corporate ethics, organisational development and citizen's charters, the charter approach promotes being responsive to public services. The paradigm is concerned with guaranteeing service standards, quality assurance, and informing clients who are empowered to claim their rights by proactive professional help. The professional is responsible and accountable, acting as the custodian of public rights. The principle guiding this approach is equity in mutual rights and duties. Such an approach seems compatible with feminist ethics and provides a strategy for making the corporate ethics compatible with those of midwifery practitioners.

In his critique of Robertson's research, Gillon (1996) agrees that the four principles approach is not antagonistic to either virtue ethics or the importance of good relationships. Rather, he suggests that when it comes to differences in the way conflicting principles are prioritised in particular cases, the views of the doctors and nurses themselves on why they gave priority to one rather than to another principle requires far more study than it is currently obtaining, either philosophically or empirically. The present analysis addresses this recommendation in its aim to examine how mothers and midwives give meaning to a concrete situation, why they respond to it through a specific action, and how mothers and midwives give meaning to ethical conflicts and subtle tensions within midwifery practice.

Norberg and Uden (1995) recommend that future research examine how different care workers alternate between and combine different forms (moral development) and content (moral orientation) of moral reasoning for real-life situations within various fields of healthcare. Whilst the present analysis does not compare male and female responses to ethical reasoning, or the longitudinal aspect of moral development, it does investigate real-life episodes, and the ethical meanings and orientations of individual mothers and midwives. It also examines how relationships emerge according to the midwife's approach, moral orientation, and claims that the ethical nature of the mother-midwife relationship emerges as different from that of the nurse-patient relationship. Similarly, in view of the unresolved debate over the influence of setting, differences between the mother's relationship with hospital ward midwives and with birth centre and independent midwifery practitioners are identified. The distinctiveness of ethical midwifery practice, the impact of setting for the human and 'natural' life process of childbirth, and the midwife's moral orientation, role and function during this process, are also demonstrated in mothers' and midwives' personal narratives.

Textbooks, journals and conference presentations: their ethical orientation

As discussed in Chapter 3, the practitioner works and thinks contextually, but due to the dominance of paradigm theory, s/he is surrounded by conferences, classes and programmes that preach autonomy, beneficence and justice (Winkler 1993).

Conversely, the voices of women have been largely excluded from the discourse on midwifery until quite recently. Whilst occasional projects may have addressed midwifery topics from the childbearing woman's point of view, it is only since the mid-1990s that the emphasis in research has been on the importance of women's experiences of childbearing, for them and for midwifery. Recent studies have examined women's experiences in relation to their feelings and participation at the birth, their satisfaction with the care surrounding childbirth and their perceptions of the attending midwives (Berg et al 1996; Halldorsdottir & Karlsdottir 1996; Handler et al 1996; Machin & Scamell 1997; Collington 1998; Hall & Holloway 1998; Leach et al 1998; Ogden, Shaw & Zander 1998; Ryding, Wijma & Wijma 1998; Shields et al 1998; Fleming 1998; Fraser 1999; Hildingsson & Haggstrom 1999; Morison et al 1999; Salmon 1999; Walsh 1999). Later chapters discuss that current literature in detail, and in relation to findings from the present analysis. The latter contributes to the body of knowledge by adding to that discourse the ethical experiences of mothers and midwives during childbirth according to their lived reality.

Major textbooks and discussion papers available in the area of healthcare ethics usually discuss the generic topic of bioethics. Where 'medical ethics' is specified in the literature, it always refers to doctors and the practice of medicine. Where medical ethics also refers to nurses it usually does so as a means of distinguishing between the different roles of the two professions, pointing out the hierarchical responsibility of the doctor in relation to decision-making with, for instance, life-threatening situations or sophisticated scientific technology. An exception to this is Robertson (1996) whose research compared the approaches doctors and nurses take in everyday patient care, relative to ethical theories. Similarly, although some authors refer to midwifery within nursing ethics (Johnstone 1994; Webb & Warwick 1999), and some only to the extent of using the word 'midwifery' in the title (Scheilliing & Drury 1994; Rich & Parker 1995), much that has been written on nursing ethics is specific to nursing and does not infer or refer to the characteristics of midwifery practice. Midwifery practice and childbearing are subsumed under the problem-solving, dilemma orientation of bioethics and moral philosophy.

There is very little written on ethics and midwifery practice, with the exception of Thompson & Thompson (1986; 1987; 1991), Jones (1994) and Frith (1996). Even so, such texts tend to differentiate midwifery ethics from those of nursing and medical ethics on the basis of the ethics of science, technology and reproduction – on ethical 'issues'. The mother-midwife relationship is not identified as an integral aspect of midwifery ethics. Often when text and reference books discuss childbirth, issues are raised merely by way of an exemplar for the application of principlism or problem-solving dilemmic ethics. For example, the case of a mother and unborn baby, and a meaningless choice between two lesser evils in a life-threatening situation, serves to illustrate the mother's (or baby's) right to autonomy and the midwife's duty towards beneficence and non-maleficence for the baby (or mother). This dualistic approach fails us as midwives, when we seek a sensitive ethical response to the mother (or to the partner, if the mother's life is threatened) who is vulnerable and reliant upon her relationship with us for that very autonomy. It fails us for a sensitive response to the fact that ethical deliberations have context, extend over time, and are influenced by events of the past. How do we include factors such as what to say and do next day when mother and midwife meet again, and the mother's conversation seeks or requires genetic counselling; and again, next year, when the mother returns pregnant with her next child? It is also inadequate in an everyday practice and practical sense. How does the midwife promote and facilitate the other's self-determination and empowerment during childbearing? Context and relationships do matter.

Even those books specifically devoted to midwifery address ethical issues from the logico-reason basis of moral philosophy. Examples are: the implications of human reproductive technology and the changing labour markets for midwives and mothers (Sutton 1996); maternal versus fetal rights (dualism rather than relationship); resource allocation (comodification of healthcare); utilitarianism, deontology and principlism as the basis for objective decision-making; and the use of case studies to demonstrate that a principle such as confidentiality, accountability, autonomy or consent legitimises action (Jones 1994). The focus of ethical decision-making in those texts is on the rightness and wrongness of 'acts'. Debate does not include the significance of virtues, the character of the moral agent, the nature of human relationships or the context of lived reality. Neither is the ethical appropriateness of the midwife's 'inaction' discussed.

Whilst Frith focuses on acts and abstract principles to some extent too, she does emphasise that

the main ethical issues and dilemmas that midwives face in practice have received relatively little coverage in mainstream ethical literature. Midwives have had to use textbooks written for other healthcare professionals (1996 p.1).

The chapter by Heather Lewison (1996) is unique in that it explores ethical issues from the woman's point of view and from outside the profession, as a user and representative for maternity services. She focuses on the principle of autonomy but also points to the importance of empowering the woman, of greater openness between the professional and the consumer, and of the midwife knowing the labouring woman and being ideally placed to check that the woman has understood what is happening and why.

It is important that childbearing women are afforded informed choice, not merely asked to give consent. This suggests that context, character and relationship are important. Lewison (1996) gives two everyday examples of conflict during childbirth. They are (i) where a woman is in labour in hospital and her preferred way of coping with the pain of labour is to have the constant physical and emotional support of a midwife (context-specific, case-specific, and relationship-oriented) but that is not possible for various reasons, and (ii) if a labour ward protocol such as routine artificial rupture of membranes is inconsistent with research findings which the woman knows from her reading and attendance at antenatal classes (requiring a partnership response not a paternalistic reaction). Neither of these examples constitutes a life-threatening ethical dilemma. Both typify the less glamorous, everyday situation in which the childbearing woman can be rendered invisible and powerless by institutional influence. Again, the ethically sensitive response to a woman's concerns during childbirth involves more than choosing the right or wrong 'acts' as proposed by contemporary Western applied ethics and bioethics. It involves the ethics of intimates, not those of strangers. The latter approach offers choices that exclude the voice of the woman's lived reality, and its use of problem-solving only recognises the ethical in the presence of a dilemma or problem.

Although contemporary midwifery literature discusses the experiential needs of childbearing women and the importance of the midwife's approach to those women, the ethical orientation of the preparation for, and ongoing discourse on, midwifery practice remains attached to traditional nursing ethics and therefore, Western (male) moral philosophy and bioethics. Other orientations such as feminist ethics, virtue ethics or postmodern ethics go largely unnoticed in relation to childbirth and midwifery practice. With the exception of Kirkham (1986) who discusses the appropriateness of feminism for midwifery and childbearing women, and Pinch (1996) who discusses feminist ethics and bioethics in relation to nurses' outlook on reproductive health, the need to apply feminist ethics to childbirth and midwifery practice is ignored by most of the literature.

To the extent that nursing and midwifery are practised in the context of relationship, albeit that the nature of the relationship may differ in the different settings, a similar criticism can be made of the nursing ethics discourse. There is a need to include context, values and culture, virtues and caring in nursing ethics (Scott 1995; Lutzen 1997; van Hooft 1999), and to utilise multiple approaches to ethics. For example, postmodern ethics claims to accept not condemn difference, and unlike the normative bioethics principles, to recognise that many moral issues in nursing are unsolvable, sometimes requiring the nurse to live with the moral dichotomies that exist between responsibility to others and personal desires (White 1993). Bowman recommends that nursing students be exposed to both traditional rules and justice-based ethics, and a feminist care perspective because

Contextual constraints, professional and organisational expectations or protocols, and perceived powerlessness often determine how, and to what extent nurses respond to ethical situations (Bowman 1995 p.33).

In relation to nursing, Holmes (1999) adds to this. Rationality needs to be displaced with 'non-rational' constructs; elements of human experience such as compassion, love, empathy, sentiment and friendship. Despite the relevance of feminist and virtue ethics to nursing, and except for Johnstone (1994)

feminist views go unmentioned [in nursing literature] ... most contributors assume a privileged position for those versed in moral philosophy (a masculinist enterprise for many centuries), and explicitly dismiss the moral knowledge and insight of the ordinary individual ... this could be viewed as reflecting masculine notions of 'expertise' (Holmes 1999 p.13).

Nevertheless, it is doubtful that simply redressing this absence of feminist and postmodern ethics within the current discourse would make nursing ethics appropriate for the non-institutional, contextual responsibilities of midwifery practice. Because the natures of the practices and settings are different, so too is the nature of an adequate ethical response within them. Practices are settings defined by power and relationships, and the practitioner's role is articulated around certain notions of power (Thompson, Melia & Boyd 1994). The normative, universal theory approach appears inadequate.

For example, the nurse is entitled to do 'x' and s/he has obligations to certain others according to the nature of the practice itself. Role can only be understood in the context of power. For the unwell or injured (incompetent) patient, power relationships with the practitioner vary between power 'over' in a crisis intervention or emergency situation, to power 'for' in a therapeutic-consulting contract when nursing care aims to restore health and autonomy to the individual (Thompson, Melia & Boyd 1994). Outside of such situations, and especially in a community practice setting, the childbearing woman's relationship with the midwife is more appropriately one of power 'with' (of partnership) as both mother and midwife work together to 'retain' and 'maintain' the childbearing woman's self-determination, albeit that she experiences periods of great vulnerability. Often, the less the midwife 'does' during childbirth, the more we give.

Putting our faith in women gives them powerful messages, especially during labour where the quiet 'midwifery muttering' – 'You can do it' – when a woman is saying words to the contrary is often all it takes to get women through the aptly named 'transition' phase of labour (Leap 2000 p.8).

The ethical appropriateness of this type of 'inaction' from the midwife is, I believe, one of the distinctive features of the mother-midwife relationship.

SUMMARY

Discussion in this chapter focused on the impact of institutionalisation on healthcare, the strengths and weaknesses of codes, and how midwifery's ethical discourse has been shaped through education, workplace setting, literature and conferences.

Institutionalisation of healthcare altered the setting of midwifery practice and redefined its rules and constraints. Practitioners' duties, responsibilities and arbiters are different in hospital situations from those in primary care and community contexts. Even when practices share similar principles and values, power and responsibility are exercised differently, problems are defined differently, and constraints, rules and accountability for practitioners differ in different contexts. Ethical responses need to be inclusive of difference.

Codes make explicit the perceived 'goods' or goals of the practice. They draw on ethical principles and problem-solving, and guide practitioners' decision making. However, that approach is not adequate for midwifery because it does not take account of relationship, recognise that different ethical approaches are suited to differing circumstances, or provide a strategy for response.

In educational curricula, midwifery is seen as an extension of nursing, and nursing ethics are presented as equally applicable to midwifery.

Programmes that do devote time to ethics subsume midwifery ethics under nursing ethics, and much of the related literature only nominally includes midwifery. The distinctiveness of ethical responses in different practices and contexts is ignored. The work environment for many midwives in the Western world today is a hospital setting under medical authority and direction; an environment governed by acontextual, 'strangers' bioethics. Furthermore, like other healthcare practitioners, their conferences, classes and programmes espouse the ethics of abstract principles. Yet it seems that midwives work and think contextually, and require the ethics of intimates.

Finally, it is suggested that although nursing and midwifery may similarly practice in a context of relationship, the nature of the mother-midwife relationship differs from the nature of the patient/client-nurse relationship, and if this is so then the 'adequate' ethical response will be different in the different practices.

REFERENCES

Anderson T 2000 Feeling safe enough to let go: the relationship between a woman and her midwife during the second stage of labour. In: Kirkham M (ed) The midwife-mother relationship. Macmillan, Basingstoke

Beauchamp T L, Childress J F 1994 Principles of biomedical Ethics. Oxford University Press, New York

Berg M, Lundgren I, Hermansson E, Wahlberg V 1996 Women's experience of the encounter with the midwife during childbirth. Midwifery 12 (1): 11-15

Bowman A 1995 Teaching ethics: telling stories. Nurse Education Today 15: 33-38

Clarke R 1996 Midwifery autonomy and the code of professional conduct: an unethical combination. In: Frith L (ed) Ethics and midwifery: issues in contemporary practice. Butterworth Heinemann, Oxford

Collington V 1998 Do women share midwives' views of their educational role? British Journal of Midwifery 6 (9): 556-563

Donnison J 1988 Midwives and medical men: a history of the struggle for the control of childbirth, 2nd edn. Historical Publications, London

Ehrenreich B, English D 1973 Witches, midwives and nurses: a history of women healers. Feminist Press, New York

Fleming V E M 1998 Women-with-midwives-with-women: a model of interdependence. Midwifery 14: 137-143

Fraser D M 1999 Women's perceptions of midwifery care: a longitudinal study to shape curriculum development. Birth 26 (2 June): 99-107

Frith L (ed) 1996 Ethics and midwifery: issues in contemporary practice. Butterworth-Heinemann, Oxford

Gillon R 1996 Editorial: ethnography, medical practice and moral reflective equilibrium. Journal of Medical Ethics 22: 259-260

Hall S M, Holloway I M 1998 Staying in control: women's experiences of labour in water. Midwifery 14: 30-36

Halldorsdottir S, Karlsdottir S I 1996 Empowerment or discouragement: women's experience of caring and uncaring encounters during childbirth. Healthcare for Women International 17 (4): 361-379

Handler A, Raube K et al 1996 Women's satisfaction with prenatal care settings: a focus group study. Birth 23 (1): 31-39

Hildingsson I, Haggstrom T 1999 Midwives' lived experiences of being supportive to prospective mothers/parents during pregnancy. Midwifery 15: 82-91

Holmes C A 1999 Editorial: virtue ethics and feminist ethics. Collegian-Ethics Society 6 (1). Royal College of Nursing Australia, Deakin ACT

Johnstone M J 1994 Bioethics: a nursing perspective, 2nd edn. Saunders, Sydney

Johnstone M J 2000 Deficiencies of codes. In: Daly J, Speedy S, Jackson D (eds) Contexts of nursing: an introduction. Maclennan & Petty, Sydney

Jones S R 1994 Ethics in midwifery. Mosby-Year Book Europe Ltd, London

Jordan T 1996 Applied ethics and action research methods. Second Annual Conference September 1995, Australian Association for Professional and Applied Ethics/Keon Publications, Brisbane

Kingston B 1975 My wife, my daughter, and poor Mary Ann: women and work in Australia. Thomas Nelson (Australia) Ltd, Melbourne

Kirkham M 1986 A feminist perspective in midwifery. In: Webb C (ed) Feminist practice in women's healthcare. John Wiley & Sons, Chichester

Leach J, Dowswell T, Hewison J et al 1998 Women's perceptions of maternity carers. Midwifery 14: 48-53

Leap N 2000 The less we do, the more we give. In: Kirkham M (ed) The midwife-mother relationship. Macmillan, Basingstoke

Lewison H 1996 Choices in childbirth: areas of conflict. In: Frith L (ed) Ethics and midwifery: issues in contemporary practice. Butterworth-Heinemann, Oxford

Lutzen K 1997 Nursing ethics into the next millennium: a context-sensitive approach for nursing ethics. Nursing Ethics: An International Journal for Healthcare Professionals 4: 218-226

Lutzen K, Everton M, Nordin C 1997 Moral sensitivity in psychiatric practice. Nursing Ethics: An International Journal for Healthcare Professionals 4 (6): 472-482

Lutzen K, Nordin C 1995 The influence of gender, education and experience on moral sensitivity in psychiatric nursing: a pilot study. Nursing Ethics: An International Journal for Healthcare Professionals 2 (1): 41-50

Machin D, Scamell M 1997 The experience of labour: using ethnography to explore the irresistable nature of the bio-medical metaphor during labour. Midwifery 13: 78-84

May W F 1994 The virtues in a professional setting. In: Fulford K W M, Gillett G R, Soskice J M (eds) Medicine and moral reasoning. Cambridge University Press, Cambridge

Morison S, Percival P, Huack Y, McMurray A 1999 Birthing at home: the resolution of expectations. Midwifery 15: 32-39

Norberg A, Uden G 1995 Gender differences in moral reasoning among physicians, registered nurses and enrolled nurses engaged in geriatric and surgical care. Nursing Ethics: An International Journal for Healthcare Professionals 2 (3): 233-242

Ogden J, Shaw A, Zander L 1998 Women's experience of having a hospital birth. British Journal of Midwifery 6 (5): 339-345

Pinch W J E 1996 Feminism and bioethics. Medical Surgical Nursing 5 (1): 53

Pritchard J 1996 Ethical decision-making and the positive use of codes. In: Frith L (ed) Ethics and midwifery: issues in contemporary practice. Butterworth-Heinemann, Oxford

Rich A, Parker D L 1995 Reflection and critical incident analysis: ethical and moral implications of their use within nursing and midwifery education. Journal of Advanced Nursing 22: 1050-1057

Robertson D W 1996 Ethical theory, ethnography, and differences between doctors and nurses in approaches to patient care. Journal of Medical Ethics 22: 292-299

Ryding E L, Wijma K, Wijma B 1998 Experiences of emergency cesarean section: a phenomenological study of 53 women. MIDIRS Midwifery Digest 9 (1): 67-72

Sala R, Manara D 1999 The regulation of autonomy in nursing: the Italian situation. Nursing Ethics: An International Journal for Healthcare Professionals 6 (6): 451-467

Salmon D 1999 A feminist analysis of women's experiences of perineal trauma in the immediate post-delivery period. Midwifery 15: 247-256

Scheilling S M, Drury E 1994 Everyday ethics and nurse/midwifery education. Nurse Education Today 14: 203-208

Scott P A 1995 Aristotle, nursing and healthcare ethics. Nursing Ethics: An International Journal for Healthcare Professionals 2 (4): 279-285

Sherwin S 1992 No longer patient: feminist ethics and healthcare. Temple University Press, Philadelphia

Shields N, Turnbull D, Reid M et al 1998 Satisfaction with midwife-managed care in different time periods: a randomised controlled trial of 1299 women. Midwifery 14: 85-93

Siddiqui J 1997 Midwifery values: part two'. British Journal of Midwifery 5 (2): 97-99

Smith R, Hiatt H, Berwick D 1999 Education and debate: shared ethical principles for everybody in healthcare: a working draft from the Tavistock Group. British Medical Journal 318 (7178): 248

Summers A 1997 Sairey Gamp: generating fact from fiction. Nursing Inquiry 4: 14-18

Sutton H 1996 Childbearing and the ethics of technology: a feminist approach. In: Barclay L, Jones L (eds) Midwifery: trends and practice in Australia. Churchill Livingstone, Melbourne

Thompson H O, Thompson J E 1986 Code of ethics for nurse-midwives. Journal of Nurse-Midwifery 31 (2): 99-102

Thompson I K, Melia K M, Boyd K M 1994 Nursing ethics. Churchill Livingstone, Melbourne

Thompson J E, Thompson H O 1987 Ethical dilemmas in women's health. In: Sonstegard L J, Kowalski K M, Jennings B (eds). Women's health: crisis and illness in childbearing, 3. Saunders

Thompson J E, Thompson H O 1991 Ethical decision making skills for midwives. Birthday, Birthways: 7th Biennial Conference of the Australian College of Midwives Incorporated, Australian College of Midwives Inc., Perth

Toulmin S 1986 How medicine saved the life of ethics. In: DeMarco J P, Fox R M (eds) New directions in ethics. Routledge and Kegan Paul, New York

van der Hulst L A M 1999 Dutch midwives: relational care and birth location. Health & Social Care in the Community 7 (4): 242-247

van Hooft S 1999 Acting from the virtue of caring in nursing. Nursing Ethics: An International Journal for Healthcare Professionals 6 (3): 189-201

Veatch R M 1989 Medical ethics. Jones and Bartlett Publishers, Boston

Walsh D 1999 An ethnographic study of women's experience of partnership caseload midwifery practice: the professional as a friend. Midwifery 15: 165-176

Webb J, Warwick C 1999 Getting it right: The teaching of philosophical healthcare ethics. Nursing Ethics: An International Journal for Healthcare Professionals 6 (2): 150-156

White F 1993 Bioethics, postmodernism and nursing. Shaping nursing theory and practice: 2nd National Conference, Department of Nursing, La Trobe University, Melbourne

Winkler E R 1993 From Kantianism to contextualism: the rise and fall of the paradigm theory in applied ethics. In: Winkler E R, Coombs J R (eds) Applied ethics: a reader. Blackwell, Oxford

Woodward V M 1998 Caring, patient autonomy and the stigma of paternalism. Journal of Advanced Nursing 28 (5): 1046-1052

5

Off the beaten track – feminist virtue ethics and midwifery

As a feminist midwife I do not seek to confront the system, but to help women to beat their own paths around and through that system (Kirkham 1986 p.48).

This chapter discusses the values and assumptions of feminist theory, and feminist virtue ethics. Adopting a feminist approach for midwifery ethics is proposed as an appropriate alternative to Western (male-oriented) moral philosophical thought, as presented in positivism and principles-based ethics. Unlike the latter, a feminist approach claims that the personal is political, renders visible the ways in which power is exercised to this end, rejects the notion of 'one truth', and gives priority to the ethical and value-laden dimensions of feminist research. Insight from feminist constructivist theory provides the theoretical perspective, and feminist ethics resonate with mothers' and midwives' personal narratives (Thompson 2001).

The epistemology and ontology of feminism and constructivism represent an appropriate philosophy for midwifery practice – woman-centred partnership. The way we see or interpret our social world determines the way we see our practice (whether that practice is midwifery, philosophy or accounting) and how we practice it. Furthermore, feminists and constructivists agree that language and discourse – including metaphors – not only reflect social organisation but also construct our identity and subjectivity (Wurzbach 1999). Linguistic features of mothers' and midwives' narratives such as metaphors and dichotomies demonstrate such identity and subjectivity. Dualisms or dichotomies frequently position woman opposite to man; woman is a defective version of man and lacks the superior characteristics of the male. In Western thinking, reason is frequently characterised as a distinctive male capacity whilst emotions, sense perception and the body are typically coded as female capacities. Associating birth with 'the primitive' and 'the animal' further subordinates the achievement of childbirth to intellectual pursuits. The bodily or 'primary' attributes are seen as more basic and place the female comparatively closer to the animal world (Thiele 1989; Bordo 1992).

The binary terms which organize western thought about bodies are those which organize the differences between the 'animal' and the 'truly human' ... [it is] reproduction which feminists most often sacrifice in their rush to describe women's bodies as social construction [therefore] it is surely not surprising that when a midwife turns academic, she should theorize about reproduction and body in a way that feminist theorists before and after her have not managed to do (Thiele 1989 pp.7,10).

The way a midwife identifies with childbirth affects her/his practice and relationship with the childbearing woman. Does the midwife's theorising about reproduction assign the process of childbirth a privileged status of female achievement, or the lesser one of an apparently 'unintellectual', defective and base activity which requires medicalising? Do midwives describe women's bodies in terms of social construction, endeavouring to demonstrate how 'equal' women are to men (an exercise that tends to perpetuate dualism), or do they celebrate the uniqueness of female bodies and birth?

Reproduction has a cultural meaning and significance beyond the biological; there are multiple bodies, not only one. Seeing reproduction as a holistic experience rather than merely an event includes social construction, cultural meaning and historical variability without making 'biology' redundant.

To the extent that feminist constructivist inquiry requires public scrutiny of the researcher's history, values and assumptions, the following self-reflection adds to the discussion in Chapter 2. It situates me and my social construction. What is now known as structuralist feminism (Wearing 1996) first offered me a different 'gaze' from that of the 'biological systems and procedures', the formal nursing and midwifery education of the 1970s. However, this meant that my new 'way of seeing' midwifery practice, as needing to be woman-centred, contextualised and relationship-based, conflicted with the lived reality of childbirth for the woman and the role of the midwife within medicalised and disembodied childbirth. In the latter, one is a passive dependent 'patient', and in the other one is the doctor's subordinate assistant, distanced from the embodied childbearing woman.

Whilst structuralist feminist theories such as liberal feminism, Marxist feminism and radical feminism raise consciousness of women's oppression, it is post-structuralist feminism that offers strategies of resistance (Diamond & Quinby 1988), celebration of difference (Bacchi 1990; Wearing 1996), and deconstruction of dichotomies such as sex/gender, mind/body, sameness/difference, natural/cultural, good/ bad (Thiele 1989; Green 1993). Our old ways of seeing are not discarded completely; rather, the old and the new merge to form a different way of seeing, a different orientation.

VALUES AND ASSUMPTIONS OF FEMINIST THEORY – EPISTEMOLOGY AND ONTOLOGY

Traditional philosophical discourse in bioethics delineates roles according to gender (Pinch 1996) and sex. Women's roles are determined by biology and function (sexual, procreative, and child-rearing) and men's roles are those of political and economic power and authority. Oppression of women, imbalance of power and positioning of male as the normal and ideal in healthcare are practices rejected by feminists. These practices are pivotal to the analysis of bioethical issues because the healthcare arena is a microcosm of society. Winifred Ellenchild Pinch asks

What assumptions about gender, biases, or possible discrimination are brought to the ethical dilemma, its accompanying analysis, and solutions? (Pinch 1996 p.56).

This imbalance of power in a patriarchal society, of men over women, is based on socially constructed gender differences (Firestone 1970 & Millett 1971 cited in Wearing 1996). Through culturally constituted gender roles, men are ascribed the power to define women's roles and traits, to place less value on these than on their own, and to assign domestic service and infant care to the underclass of women. Woman as 'a sex' (not only 'a gender') is a class. Human interest, achievement and ambition is then the province of the male.

Within such a patriarchal society, the woman's body is a receptacle for the male's sperm, and carriage for the developing child. Women are not supposed to enjoy sex. Sexual pleasure is solely the male's domain. As Anne Summers (1994) writes, women in the colony of Australia fell into two categories – dammed whores or God's police. The double standards categorised women into either sex objects or asexual mothers of children. Remnants of this attitude can be seen in current obstetric practice, when the importance of the woman's intact perineum and surrounding nerves and muscles, is generally ignored. Episiotomy is an agent of social control and its increased use coincided with the medicalisation of childbirth (Tew 1990; Way 1998). Sometimes large episiotomies may be performed (often without the woman's consent) and cobbled together (rather than skilfully repaired) (Salmon 1999) to heal (often with extensive scaring and loss of integrity of feeling, and sometimes with medical injury/illness complications). The woman's pelvic floor and its sensation seem far less important in Western cultural thought than the cosmetic appearance and sexual allure of her face and 'figure'. Diane, a midwife in the present research, describes such a circumstance. Her narrative demonstrates what she perceived as a more sinister exertion of power over childbearing women: that which occurred when disruption and damage to the perineum was used as punishment, to maintain the subservient and passive role of the 'patient' and midwife (the status quo), and to teach the otherwise autonomous adult woman her place in relation to the expert (male, in that particular instance) healthcare practitioner. To question medical authority is unacceptable. When the 'able', birthing woman dares to exercise self-determination for her birthing process she risks being perceived as troublesome, ignorant, aggressive or arrogant – insulting to the doctor's superior knowledge and intellect (Kirkham 1986).

Stanley and Wise (1993) argue that rather than 'going beyond the personal', which is to talk of the institution again, feminists need to 'go back into' the personal. Everyday experience is lost in the desire to generalise about things, but everyday experience needs to be questioned because 'the system' exists in the personal, everyday experiences of individuals. For example, does the concrete experience of oppression vary for women, or is it the same all the time, or some of the time? When, and why? These are relevant questions to explore in the context of midwifery and ethics. Women's experiences of childbirth, their relationships with people surrounding childbirth and indeed their relationship with their newborn baby seem to go unrecognised in medicalised birth, when experts take over and assume prime responsibility for the mother's body and baby.

Feminism exists because women are, and have been everywhere oppressed at every level of exchange from the simplest social intercourse to the most elaborate discourse ... whether or not we can in fact escape from the structuring imposed by language is one of the major questions facing feminist and nonfeminist thinkers today (Marks & de Courtivron 1981 p.4).

Three characteristics that are distinctive to feminist research are (i) issues considered important are derived from women's experiences, (ii) the research design provides explanations of social phenomena that women want and need, and (iii) the researcher is located in the same 'critical plane' (Harding 1987).

The most central and common belief shared by all feminists, whatever our 'type', is the presupposition that women are oppressed [and] 'the personal is the political'. This argues that power and its use can be examined within personal life and, indeed, in some sense that the political *must* be examined in this way. It also emphasises that 'the system' is experienced in everyday life, and isn't separate from it ... [thus feminism argues] systems and social structures can best be examined and understood through an exploration of relationships and experiences within everyday life (Stanley & Wise 1993 pp.61,63).

For Sheila Rowbotham (cited in Stanley & Wise 1993), theory is not some fixed and removed universal 'truth' but rather it is more like a map, providing pathways and footholds for women's liberation. Feminists identify (i) the body as the site of power and subjectivity, (ii) the significance of local and intimate power ('the personal is political'), and (iii) the capacity of discourse to produce and sustain hegemonic power. The intellectual dominance of heterogeneity obscures the dualistic nature of power in Western culture. Feminism recognises that we do not participate equally, with individual diversity, in our culture. We are located within structures of dominance and subordination, some of which are organised around gender. One of the most important of these is the social construct of male/female duality, and by exposing the 'gendered' nature of Western thought, feminism has

contributed to intellectually dismantling the Enlightenment mythology of abstract, universal man and its epistemological corollary of an abstract, universal reason (Bordo 1992 p.159).

Feminists also criticise the hierarchical modes that dominate Western society and the privileged position of the Western masculine elite

as it proclaims universals about truth, freedom, and human nature (Diamond & Quinby 1988 p.x).

Martha Saunders (1996) argues that whether 'privilege' comes from maleness, whiteness, class position, sexuality, age, or any combination of privileged locations, it is difficult for those who are advantaged to see how taken-for-granted patterns of discourse and behaviour silence or oppress some members. It is the privileged who benefit from the protection of individual rights. It is difficult for those who believe in liberal democratic values and enjoy their benefits to recognise that legitimate practices and social structures/institutions, for example, actively promote the advantages for some members of society at the expense of others. For that reason, the discourses of these mothers and midwives are examined for indications of oppression or 'silencing', referring to language to assist in the deconstruction of dichotomies and dissolving of dualisms.

Reproduction is a bio-social process rather than a quintessential biological event (Thiele 1989). Western (male) thought about bodies is binary in the same way that differences between 'animal' and the 'truly human' are. According to that type of dualism, our mind (consciousness, intellect, capacity to communicate) is the 'truly human' part of us while our body is mundane, burdensome and a barrier to achievement with its tiredness, toilet needs, headaches, chronic pain, sickness and ageing. Its pleasures, such as eating, drinking, having sex, exercising are 'functional' and doing any of these things to excess is seen as animal-like rather than human. Along with this mind-body split, Western thought associates women with bodies and men with minds (Thiele 1989). Another consequence of this mind-body split is that women are seen to be more biological because women's bodies are more involved in reproduction. This biological-only gender division fragments the body, privileging some relations and dismissing others. Reproduction is defined as 'natural' in the dichotomy of nature/culture. Women are biological and 'reproductive' and thus by virtue of the dualism, are not cultural; men are cultural. Yet women are not more biological than men, who also have to eat, sleep, defaecate and die (Thiele 1989 p.8).

According to Betsy Wearing (1996), the structuralist feminist theories have presented women as universally oppressed whereas post-structuralist feminists such as Irigaray (1986), Lloyd (1989), Pateman (1986), Grosz (1986) and Thiele (1989) emphasise resistance and difference, and deconstruct dichotomies. They resist male domination at the theoretical level by arguing for 'sexual subversions' of male-stream theory. Male theories they say, are remote from women's actual experiences of life. Patriarchal systems, methods and presumptions are recognised but their dominance and power is resisted, and they are ultimately transformed ... ['feminist' autonomy is] the right to choose and define the world for oneself (Grosz 1986 p.195 cited in Wearing 1996). A major tenet of post-structuralist feminism is that there are differences not only between men and women but also within and between women.

All women may currently occupy the position 'woman' ... but they do not occupy it in the same way. Women of colour in a white ruled society face different obstacles than do white women ... By deconstructing the term 'woman' into a set of independent variables, this strategy can show how consolidating all women into a falsely unified 'woman' has helped mask the operations of power that actually divide women's interests as much as unite them (Poovey 1988 p.59 cited in Wearing 1996 p.39).

Structuralist feminists argued for equality via sexual neutrality and an implied passivity of the body, but that approach reduces politics to gender difference

as if women's bodies and the representation and control of women's bodies were not a crucial stake in these struggles (Gatens 1983 p.156).

Thiele (1989) places even more emphasis on biology and women's reproduction as a complex process, not just an event: it involves menstruation, conception, pregnancy, parturition, lactation and menopause because these differences are socially interpreted and normatively organised in each society in the discursive frameworks we use to speak about them.

In a patriarchal society, both equality and difference are problematic for women (Pateman 1992 cited in Wearing 1996 p.49). On the one hand, equality with men can be seen as extending the rights of men and citizens to women, making women like men. On the other hand, equality that encompasses difference is incompatible with patriarchal citizenship because the latter excludes difference; for example, motherhood excludes women from employment and war but requires them to bear future citizens as a political duty. Pateman concludes, therefore, that women's subordination is the central issue. While equality can include difference it cannot encompass subordination. Indeed, on the topic of difference, Scott (1995) rejects the binary opposition of equality and difference, pointing out that if individuals or groups were identical there would be no need to ask for equality.

Flax also endorses the importance of difference but she argues from the stance of social justice:

In contemporary Western culture, differences appear to generate and are used to justify hierarchies and relationships of domination including gender-based ones (Flax 1992 cited in Wearing 1996 p.50).

Domination occurs because of the inability to recognise, appreciate and nurture differences not sameness. For Flax, the concept of justice recognises differences and, unlike equality, it does not have a finite set of rules instituted once and for all: it bridges the gap between self and other, between connectedness/dependency and the integrity of each person.

One of Sara Ruddick's claims to difference is that reason is

socially constructed by those people living at a particular time and that the projects in which people engage are partly defined by, and in turn demand, distinctive ways of thinking ... There is no ahistorical, asocial privileged vantage from which to assess either the projects or the constructions of reason that arise from them (Ruddick 1987 p.241).

For example, if women and men engage in different work then they can be expected to think differently. However, when culturally dominant and pervasive explanations of reason are inappropriate to women's lives and when objectivity selects for and rewards 'manliness', women's thinking appears not as reason, but as a deficiency of reason. This supports a main

argument of the current discussion, that our ways of 'seeing' determine to a great extent our ways of acting. When we enter a practice we are taught our ways of seeing within the practice and take on the ethics of the practice as part of the commitment of entering that practice. Therefore, our ways of 'seeing' determine our ways of practice, of 'doing'. Moral reasoning is connected to conceptions of self and since we understand our selves through our relationships with others, moral reasoning also connects us with others – it is relational and contextual.

The implications for methodology, of the tension between applied ethics and ethical practices are the embedded nature of relationships and the significance of philosophy beyond the moral; that is, of both empirical and historical social inquiry. The conceptual theoretical frameworks implicit in research questions reflect our ways of seeing.

Stanley and Wise claim that there is a direct and necessary relationship between theory and experience. They use 'practice' and 'experience' interchangeably because they see them as standing for

all things that we say, do, and feel, and have said to us or done to us, in our everyday lives. [Theory] should be a set of understandings or conceptual frameworks which are directly related to, and derive from, particular facets of everyday relationships, experiences and behaviours (p. 57) [whereas grand theory] presupposes that [the individual and the society, the personal and the structural] are separate ... it is inevitable that the researcher's own experiences and consciousness will be involved in the research process as much as they are in life, and [argue that] all research must be concerned with the experiences and consciousness of the researcher as an integral part of the research process (Stanley & Wise 1993 pp.56,58).

Language is never gender-free. The socially constructed duality of male/female is a discursive formation (Bordo 1992) which has profound consequences for the experiences of those who live them. As Thiele (1989) points out, the binary terms of Western thought about bodies are those which hierarchically organise the differences between the 'animal' and the 'truly human', our minds and our bodies, and Western culture associates men with minds and women with bodies.

Women have been subsumed by the generic masculine, trivialised and degraded through derogatory metaphors, deprived of access to sacred languages, or silenced altogether (Diamond & Quinby 1988 p.xv).

From the post-structuralist feminist perspective, therefore, metaphors and discourse may demonstrate not only the differences between women and their experiences but also women's resistance (or not) to such oppression during childbirth. If this is so, a deconstruction of dichotomies may be a strategy for resistance to that dominance: to celebrate difference as 'distinction' rather than create oppositional and hierarchical dichotomies and contradictory dualisms.

A FEMINIST APPROACH TO ETHICS IN MIDWIFERY

'Cause I wasn't just a body coming in to deliver. I already had ideas about what I wanted (Judy, mother).

I feel really good about the work I'm doing now, but I still have some feelings about the way classes may need to be conducted in other areas where women's experiences may well be different ... It's difficult isn't it because you want to give women the confidence to be able to give birth but you don't want to see them completely traumatised when their own dream is just not realised (Diane, midwife, referring to the potential punishment of women for challenging the status quo of medicalised childbirth).

Instead of approaching the interviews and analysis as a site of empirical findings that correlate with some pre-existing problem in the literature, considering the actual life experience of mothers and midwives opens us to the ethicality of that reality. Hearing these women's experiences and reflecting on their meanings gives insight into what it ethically means for mothers to engage with midwives during childbirth and for midwives to be 'with woman' in their practice of midwifery. Sharing some deep structures of that lived reality through narrative inquiry shows the ethics surrounding childbirth practices to be gendered (Thompson 2001). Why is it

that despite the outcome being a live healthy mother and baby, some births leave either the mother, the midwife, or both, with feelings of conflict? Midwives conceptually understand the principles of beneficence, non-maleficence, autonomy and justice, yet either struggle with the tension of which one to apply or are left feeling powerless to improve a situation in which those principles have been acted upon. Mothers, too, relay that although midwives heeded all four principles they felt disempowered during their childbearing. Why does the topic of ethics seem remote and unfamiliar to many midwives? Perhaps the current explicit midwifery ethics are those of strangers and are not consistent with the implicit ethics of the practice. The explicit ethics focus on 'public' issues and do not address the special engagement required during what is a very intense and intimate human experience for the mother. The implicit ethics, however, look more like the ethics of intimates, more like feminist ethics. Feminist ethics provide strategies that take into account context, relationship and the flow of power during human engagement.

Western (male) moral philosophy offers normative, universal ethics that 'fit' everyone and every practice. The problem-solving approach of bioethics claims to produce an objective 'single truth' which is reliable across cases. Yet, neither appears adequate for midwifery and childbirth. Feminist writers, on the other hand, have presented several alternative ethical approaches. They have shown that even within Western culture and thinking there is indeed a pool of ethics – where those who are marginalised in hegemonic societies explore their contexts and what the human condition means for them.

Each ethical approach within feminism is distinct in its argument, but collectively they share a criticism of power and oppression, characteristics which they claim are central to the universal truth ethic of Western male-moral philosophy (Pinch 1996). Feminist approaches to ethics emphasise that the personal is political, and examine the ways in which power is exercised to this end. Writers of feminist ethics argue that what Western moral philosophy ignores and excludes is the personal: the context, the concrete circumstances of life, and the voices of women.

By definition, midwifery is the practice of 'being with woman' during childbearing, a creative, 'natural' life process for both the mother (including but not restricted to her biological body) and the baby. The process is never the same experience, either between women or for the same woman with subsequent birthing. Midwifery practice, therefore, is temporal in nature and very much concerned with particularity, context and relationship – especially those with women. Its ethics are concerned primarily with ordinary everyday practices and less frequently with life-threatening or end-of-life dilemmas, as is usually the concern of normative bioethics. Traditional Western-world ethics is based on utilitarian and deontological theories, and principles which are supposedly universal and impartial, and that govern everyone irrespective of race, class and gender (Tong 1993; Pinch 1996). Yet these theories do not address women's values, and relationship and the particularity of context are excluded for objectivity and dilemma resolution. It follows, then, that if gender, context and relationship are important influences in constructing ethical meaning for feminine and feminist consciousness, and if midwifery relationships are the kind which are, in particular, 'with woman', midwifery may need a different ethic from the reductionist, dilemmic and problem-solving types.

Feminine/feminist and virtue ethics offer alternative approaches. They argue for analysis of specific, concrete cases of conscience (Fry 1989), for seeking the good in particular situations and the development of virtues of character (Tong 1998), for paying attention to context, detail and relationship (Gilligan 1982; 1993), and for one's responsibility to particular others (Noddings 1984). Concrete diversity, context and temporal elements are integral to ethics and decision-making.

Rosemarie Tong (1993) asks if it ultimately makes sense to speak of ethics in gendered terms and decides that only when we understand women's different approaches to ethics will we know whether or not these new approaches offer better ways to be moral than the old, traditional ones. Inherent in arguments coming out of feminism are both the 'feminine' and 'feminist' approaches to ethics: a feminine approach to ethics

at present refers to the search for women's unique voice and most often, the advocacy of an ethic of care that includes nurturance, care, compassion, and networks of communications (Sichel 1991, p.90 cited in Tong 1993)

[and]

consists of observations of how the traditional approaches to ethics fail to fit the moral experiences and intuitions of women (Sherwin 1992 p.42).

A feminist approach to ethics

argues against patriarchal domination, for equal rights, a just and fair distribution of scarce resources, etcetera. (Sichel 1991, p.90 cited in Tong 1993);

it applies a specifically political perspective and offers suggestions for how ethics must be revised if it is to get at the patterns of dominance and oppression as they affect women (Sherwin 1992 p.42).

Feminine approaches are generally interested in care and connectedness whereas feminist approaches examine the ethical implications of allegedly masculine concepts such as justice and autonomy (Tong 1993). This current analysis is influenced by both the notion of connectedness or relationship, and self-determination ('autonomy'). In addition, the critical and post-structuralist strategies of resistance, celebration of difference, and deconstruction of dichotomies are incorporated. It examines taken-for-granted assumptions and metaphors within ethical discourses, and the use of power, including language, to maintain the status quo in hegemonic systems.

Virtue ethics – context, character and relationship

Although Aristotle's virtue ethic from the fifth century BC is one of the traditional ethics, it differs from utilitarianism and deontology because it focuses on the goodness or badness of people's characters, not the rightness or wrongness of people's actions (Tong 1993). Sara Ruddick (1987) distinguishes two kinds of morality; the morality of justice for which the primary virtue of individuals and institutions is fairness, and the morality of love in which the primary virtues for individuals and institutions are care and the realistic perception of needs.

Michael Stocker (1987) also draws upon the work of Aristotle in relation to duty and friendship. A practitioner uses the values of the practice. One's training, education and moral criticism become integral to one's desires and motivations. These things are not mere rote copying. They are part of our learning to be 'good'. One may still want to be well thought of and to do well but as a midwife one now wants to be well thought of for one's midwifery values and standards, and to do well at midwifery specifically.

It is also useful to refer to Aristotle with regard to self-determination. The difficult thing about human activities is prioritising and coordinating them. Aristotle suggests that there are two types of virtues: intellectual and moral. Practical wisdom refers to intelligence and the ability to discern, while a moral virtue such as courage or justice, activities which one can perform almost spontaneously, results merely from habit. Through practical wisdom, intelligence and knowing the right thing to do, we are able to prioritise and coordinate human activities. We know the means to the desired ends and we exercise those virtues needed to attain specific internal and general goods, the 'ends' of worthy practices. Without practical reason the person exhibits not virtue but either its excess or its defect; for example, rashness, cowardice, stingyness or vulgarity (Tong 1993). Aristotle's moral virtues include courage, temperance, liberality, magnificence, pride, ambition, good temper, friendliness, truthfulness, ready wit, shame and justice. On the other hand, contemporary ethicists reserve the term 'virtue' for moral virtues only, restricting them to character traits, such as honesty, benevolence, non-malevolence and fairness. Optimism, rationality, self-control, patience, endurance, industry, cleanliness and wit are non-moral virtues and as such are gendered psychological traits in contrast to moral virtues which are ungendered (Tong 1993). The mothers and midwives quoted in the present analysis consider character of person to be an integral feature of the mother-midwife relationship.

Tong (1998) proposes that there are four kinds of virtue ethics:

1. masculinist virtue ethics
2. male or masculine virtue ethics
3. female or feminine virtue ethics, and
4. feminist virtue ethics.

The first distinguishes between the virtues attributed to men and those attributed to women; temperance, justice and fortitude are appropriate for men, and patience, docility, and good humour are the virtues of women. This produces an harmonious whole.

The second is derived from Friedrich Nietzsche's master and slave morality in which the 'slave values' are those that Western culture associates with women – kindness, humility and sympathy. MacIntyre's (1984) virtue ethics are also classified as masculine because care, benevolence and compassion are noticeably missing from his list of fundamental virtues.

Although Tong agrees that practices and civilised society cannot survive or thrive unless people are just, courageous, and honest, she criticises MacIntyre for failing to note

that unless people 'feel' something positive towards each other – unless they genuinely care about each other – they will have little or no motivation to be co-operative with each other (Tong 1998 p.146).

Nel Noddings' (1984) relational ethic of care represents the third type, feminine virtue ethics. It is an interpretive style of reasoning typical of the humanities and social sciences. The one-caring consults feelings, needs, impressions and a sense of personal ideal in their motivation to attend to the cared-for in deeds as well as in thoughts.

[It] is not about serving one's own interests. Rather, morality is about serving one's own and others' interests simultaneously (Tong 1998 p.148).

Critics of 'care' ethics say it is a gendered concept because as long as caring continues to be associated with women it is implicated in the division of labour, in both the home and public arena (Poole & Isaacs 1997). Other criticisms are

1. the current conceptualisation of caring is too vague to support any substantial theory of nursing or the foundation for an ethic of care (see too Allmark 1995; 1996)
2. caring leads to exploitation of the caregiver
3. an ethic of care does not solve ethical conflicts
4. caring as the sole basis for a moral decision leads to relativism
5. a relational ethic of caring is not just; it is based on partiality or favouritism
6. the intensity of caring described by nurse and feminist theorists may not be desired by the patient nor practical for the nurse
7. caring may focus too much on the nurse and not enough on the patient, and
8. if caring is an emotional response, it may hinder healthcare professionals' ability to 'care for' their patients (Crigger 1997).

Rosemarie Tong's fourth type of virtue ethics, feminist virtue ethics, endorses the relational ethic of care but adds that fully authentic caring can only occur in the absence of domination and subordination,

conditions that increasingly characterise the world of medicine (Tong 1998 p.150).

Furthermore, a feminist virtue ethic of care requires that healthcare practitioners do more than their 'duty' – when duty means to work hard to fulfil responsibilities, and adhere strictly to principles – because morality consists of more than conscientiousness. Practitioners ought to

at least try to develop caring feelings as well as conscientious desires and empathetic skills (Tong 1998 p.151).

Not everyone agrees with the suggestion that feminist approaches to ethics should adopt Aristotle's virtue ethics. For example, some argue that he positions women unfavourably (Johnstone 1994). Furthermore, it is debatable that 'living well' as Aristotle puts it, depends on the full use of one's limbs and one's senses of sight, hearing, smell, taste, and touch.

Aristotle had argued that health is a necessary condition of a completely happy life. Aristotle also held that the good life for humans, which consists in 'living well,' depends on the full use of one's limbs and one's senses of sight, hearing, smell, taste, and touch. One appreciates this insight if left with broken or missing limbs, or if one becomes blind or deaf (Bandman & Bandman 1995 p.7).

An argument can be made for the specific attributes of a life that does not have the full use of limbs and senses.

Notwithstanding these criticisms, virtue ethics does seem to offer a more adequate ethical response to the human condition than that of abstract universalism and decontextualised principlism. For MacIntyre

ethics is the science which is to enable men to understand how they make the transition from the former state to the latter ... [virtues of character] instruct us how to move from potentiality to act, how to realize our true nature and to reach our true end (MacIntyre 1984 p.54).

Instructed by such virtues, each human life ought to be seen as a whole, but social and philosophical obstacles prevent that concept of unity. The social obstacles are the partitions established by modernity: work is divided from leisure, private life from public, the corporate from the personal, and human life itself has been placed on a continuum resulting in childhood and old age being separated from the rest of human life. The philosophical obstacles are (i) the tendency to analyse complex actions and transactions in terms of simple components, and (ii) the tendency to separate the individual and his or her roles so that life becomes nothing but a series of unconnected episodes. Yet, the whole is different from the parts. Aristotelian virtues function within social relationships and when this kind of separation occurs the self no longer has that arena within which its virtues can function. Neither is there scope for exercising dispositions, and this is important because a virtue is not a disposition that is successful only in one particular type of situation, in the same way as a professional skill is effective.

Someone who genuinely possesses a virtue can be expected to manifest it in very different types of situation (MacIntyre 1984 p.205).

Secondly, MacIntyre (1984) argues that it is very natural to think of the self in a narrative mode and that to understand behaviour (the intelligibility of action) it is crucial to know the agent's short- and long-term intention. For example, if the primary intention in relation to childbirth (that is, the practice orientation or ways of 'seeing') is to deliver live, healthy babies, reduce perinatal mortality/morbidity statistics and maintain the professional status of healthcare practices (all of which would be applauded by both Western moral philosophers and feminists) and it is only incidentally the case that, in so doing, the childbearing woman is enriched and empowered by the experience, then we have one type of behaviour to be explained; but if the agent's primary intention is to empower a healthy mother to maintain her integrity of self and body, and support her in achieving her potential, whatever that may be, through birthing a live, healthy baby, we have quite another type of behaviour to be explained, and we will have to look in a different direction for understanding and explanation. Both intentions have been situated in narrative histories, but within particular settings. Behaviour cannot be characterised independently of intentions, and intentions cannot be characterised independently of settings, because settings have a history and individuals with their histories are situated within those settings. Midwife Anne's personal narrative of parents wanting to be heard amidst changing hospital protocol illustrates this point. Moreover, changes that occur through time, to both the individual and the setting, are only intelligible within the context of the setting and with knowledge of what the shorter and longer term intentions are – thus this kind of narrative history is

the basic and essential genre for the characterization of human actions (MacIntyre 1984 p.208).

This complex sequence of individual actions runs counter to the analytical philosophers' accounts of human actions as 'a' human action.

Narratives, identity and traditions

MacIntyre also discusses conversation, and says that both purposes and speech-acts require contexts. Linking action with narrative and history involves intelligibility and each requires the other. He disagrees that narratives falsify human life, that there are not and cannot be any true stories. Although

the story-teller imposes on human events retrospectively an order which they did not have while they were lived (MacIntyre 1984 p.214)

to describe actions allegedly outside any narrative is to present disjointed parts of some possible narrative. Much like travel notes, 'an' action is always an episode in a possible history (MacIntyre 1984). What Aristotle, MacIntyre, Bruner (1986) and constructivists appear to have in common is the notion that we are only ever co-authors of our own narratives. We are always under certain constraints. There is more than one 'truth' or 'reality' which also changes with time, and both participants and researcher construct reality through their interpretation of the situation. That is, to talk about experience is to talk temporally (Clandinin & Connelly 1994).

Narrative, intelligibility, accountability, personal identity and the nature of human action are all inter-related. 'What is good for me' and 'what is good for persons' are questions that lead to understanding the purpose and content of virtues, and the place of integrity and constancy in life. Or, as Marilyn Friedman says:

The 'You' dilemma [considering yourself as the person in the situation] confronts us with the gap between moral reasoning and moral behavior (Friedman 1987 p.199).

Virtues are dispositions which sustain the relationships required for practices, and the relationships from the past, present and future. They enable us to achieve the 'goods' that are internal to practices as well as overcoming harm, danger, temptation and distraction. However, traditions that transmit and reshape practices are also influenced by larger social traditions. Traditions of a practice develop around the pursuit of those 'goods' which the practice deems as its purpose or intention. These traditions are passed on historically and are socially embodied as the reason or basis for the 'goods' that constitute the tradition. Traditions are relationship based; therefore, the only way that tradition could be embraced within the individualism of modernity is as an adversarial notion because in individualism 'I am what I myself choose to be'. There is not the commitment to relationship, context and history. Virtues, then, strengthen traditions because they sustain the 'good' of the individual life. They sustain relationships necessary for achieving the internal 'goods' of practices and they sustain those traditions that give historical context to practice and individual. A benefit of having a sense of tradition, itself a virtue, is that tradition indicates future possibilities derived from the past and results in a capacity for judgment (MacIntyre 1984).

The public and private

As outlined earlier, an ethic of care is proposed by some as being more representative of women's moral experiences than Western male, moral philosophical theories (Gilligan 1982; Gilligan 1993; Noddings 1984). According to Joan Tronto (1993) our current moral boundaries were set in place at the end of the eighteenth century, when women's arguments were contained within a lesser, private, moral sphere through the Kantian distinction of 'public' and 'private'. Such an ethic separates morality from personal interest. Whilst agreeing with the values of caring and nurturance, and the importance of human relationships, Tronto argues:

we need to stop talking about 'women's morality' and start talking instead about a care ethic that includes the values traditionally associated with women [values such as attentiveness, responsibility, nurturance, compassion, meeting others' needs] ... both Kohlberg's original argument and Gilligan's version of an ethic of care basically leave intact the boundary between public and private life, and between justice and caring. But as many feminists have noted, the division of public and private life is not a case of separate but equal spheres; indeed, the public is of considerable more importance than the private. And since political life is identified with public life, the relegation of caring to private life means that it is beyond (or beneath) political concern. Hence the radical potential of Gilligan's ideas have

been contained within current moral boundaries (Tronto 1993 pp.3,96).

Sharon Welch (1985 cited in Saunders 1996 p.21) uses the nuclear arms race to critique dominant and privileged practices and describes the basis of such practices as an ethic of control and an ethic of risk. Her ethic of control refers to an immoral balance of power that ensures absolute invulnerability and security. In such an ethic responsibility means 'doing something'; to act means to determine what will happen through that single action and to ensure that a given course of events comes to pass.

According to actual life experience, mothers and midwives describe the midwife in an ethically adequate mother-midwife relationship, as a professional friend (Thompson 2001). Diamond and Quinby (1988) suggest that friendship provides a model for non-hierarchical, reciprocal relations, and draw on Foucault's proposal that ethics should be grounded in resistance to whatever form totalitarian power might take, rejecting the notion of a single ethic. Feminist analysis of power highlights masculinist power over women and Foucauldian analysis exposes the effects of normalising power on human subjects.

Combining both the feminist analysis and the Foucauldian analysis allows a better understanding of power and strategies for resistance. An ethics of activism, for instance, would confront domination without the smashing and terror so characteristic of masculinist revolutionary action. It would foster empowerment as well as an awareness of the limits to human agency.

Privilege

Why is the labour of childbirth – the hard work of producing a person (not a product) – not valued highly by our Western medicalised childbirth system? Moira Gatens (1996) argues that Western thought is governed by the dualisms of nature and culture, body and mind, passion and reason which she says are transposed onto reproduction and production, the family and the state, the individual body and the body politic. These political representations of life have constructed some individuals as social agents and others as passive objects. As a consequence, political right and privilege are accorded to, and monopolised by, members of the political body that has the status of rational rights and virtues (Gatens 1996; MacIntyre 1984).

[M]oral philosophies, however they may aspire to achieve more than this, always do articulate the morality of some particular social and cultural standpoint: Aristotle is the spokesman for one class of fourth century Athenians, Kant ... provides a rational voice for the emerging social forces of liberal individualism (MacIntyre 1984 p.268).

Martha Saunders also draws on the notion of privilege (unearned advantage) within power and ethics, and argues that

the value of the work goes back to the value of the one traditionally performing the work (Saunders 1996 p.20).

Privilege produces value in both an economic sense and in a social/emotional sense. The argument of the dominant privileged, however, is circular. Work that the advantaged prefer to do (for example, technological intervention by those who practice medicalised childbirth) is work that is socially valued (medical science as opposed to humanist relationships) and therefore remunerated accordingly, but 'professional' work has been done only by the privileged. In a capitalist society, value always has economic connotations (Saunders 1996). To eradicate the unjust effects of privilege, therefore, the advantaged people (obstetricians and those in the science-technology world in this instance) need to scrutinise the ways in which their advantages depend upon the disadvantaged situations of other groups. For example, white privilege is based on a racist social system, 'elite' medical authority privilege is based on medicalised childbirth. In other words, Saunders recommends using privilege to dismantle the structures of privilege.

If childbirth were considered socially valuable work, and if midwifery were a valued profession, both mothers and midwives would be in privileged positions and therefore would be in a position to dismantle the privileged institutional

structures which disadvantage childbearing women. However, it is the medical profession that is privileged in the Western healthcare system, and thus to use privilege to dismantle such structures would require that privileged medical practitioners and institutional workers do the dismantling. This is unlikely for two reasons. Firstly, social change means change for the privileged as well as for the oppressed. Secondly, under the guise of 'hearing women's voices', the words of childbearing women are often used to further the work of the medicalised system/institution rather than to demonstrate that women's work in childbirth is valued in itself. Women said that they wanted more control of their own reproduction – new medically owned and operated technologies were presented for this purpose. Women said they wanted more control during childbirth – they have been encouraged to utilise medical and surgical inductions, and operative births, so that the baby can be born on the couple's planned date within a shorter period of time and with no or minimal maternal pain during the intrapartum. Routinely, women are now discharged from hospital within two days of birth so that they can relax at home and get to know their baby, but the midwifery assistance once provided in hospital during the first seven to ten days has not been transferred to a community-based infrastructure. These changes have not transformed women's work in childbirth to being valued for itself. They have furthered the work of the economically-oriented healthcare industry and the medicalisation of childbirth. Such attempts at inclusion – to 'bring in' the outsiders – actually reinforce existing power relations, as the language reflects. Those doing the including retain the power of gatekeepers.

So far, the discussion has outlined some of the alternative ethical frameworks proposed by feminist writers, and argued that injustices are related to privilege in a patriarchal society wherein particular advantages depend upon particular oppressions.

[P]rivilege gets in the way of the achievement of justice, which is not quite the same as saying that privilege causes injustice (Saunders 1996 p.20).

Difference

Caroline Whitbeck (1989 cited in Tong 1993) believes that we need a non-oppositional, non-dualistic, non-hierarchical ontology because we understand ourselves and reality 'through' others rather than 'against' others. Rosemarie Tong further connects this relational ethic with Confucian ethics describing how a person is not a self 'first' and 'then' a mother, husband (etcetera) – s/he

becomes a self to the degree that he is good at relating to the other people who together define him (Tong 1993 p.52).

Unlike in the economic contractarian ethics, rights then become secondary, seen merely as claims on society and others if a person meets the relationship responsibilities.

Men and women are differentiated on the basis of gender. Biological differences do exist between men and women and differences also exist within and between women. Difference though, is insufficient justification for subordination. Rather than continuing solely with the victim-of-oppression argument therefore, this analysis proposes that to 'make visible' the discourse – documents, language and metaphors – surrounding childbirth contributes another pathway and more footholds for women to go around and through the system while maintaining their integrity and distinctiveness.

Normal/abnormal – the impact of linguistics

The dichotomies of 'normal' and 'abnormal', 'natural' and 'cultural' are pertinent to midwifery. To continue to defend childbirth as 'normal, abnormal and potentially abnormal' – in particular, 'normal' only in retrospect (Kirkham 1986) – is to construct its social meaning within the medical model and constrict it to the biological only. There is no such thing as 'normal' vomitus. Likewise, childbirth is 'natural' or 'medically assisted': it is not 'normal' or 'abnormal'. A socially constructed meaning of 'normal/abnormal' places childbirth along the disease/illness continuum, with its associated high risk, fear and need for expert control and

intervention. It obscures the power relations 'over' the woman which separate her from the process and experience.

She is separated as a person, as effectively as she can be, from the part of her that is giving birth (Rothman 1991 p.165).

The woman is 'relieved' of the last week or two of discomfort (or of getting to know her body's changes and preparation for birth) with elective induction of birth. She is 'relieved' of painful contractions (or of the deep 'connection' with her body to actively birth – as Taylor (1995) would say, her 'altered conscious state') with medication that blocks all sensation in the lower body including the urge to push, or with surgical birth. Finally, she is psychologically and sociologically separated from her birthing body with the 'clinical' medicalisation of birth through hospital procedures and practices – of vaginal examinations, medical assessment criteria and standardised time lines for 'normal' progress in labour, the expert's control.

Neither is it accurate to assign women to the 'natural' and men to the 'cultural', bodies and minds. Virginia Held (1993) distinguishes between natural and human, claiming that experiences of choice, consciousness and imaginative representation are distinctly human, whereas calcium, as a component of bones, is not. She argues that the language of 'natural' in that dichotomy is misleading. Women are distinctively human and therefore they should insist that childbirth be controlled by those who give birth; that nature should be respected rather than conquered. The emphasis ought not to be on the differences between human and natural. Rather, what needs stressing is the humanness of choice, consciousness and imaginative representation and the fact that women can experience these at least as fully as men can.

Metaphors in childbirth reveal practice orientation

In structuralist terms, childbirth is an event. However, it is common to hear mothers and midwives who are woman-centred in their approach refer to childbirth as a journey, and to labour as being hard work. Mothers' and midwives' conversations and stories are based on relationship and particularity. Childbirth is a time when 'you go into yourself' or when you do not want others touching you in private places, when you want them to help you to do what is right for you, to let you do it how you want to and need to do it. These metaphors are not expressed in abstract theories or institutional belief systems. The latter seem to concentrate on 'relieving' the woman/'patient' of the various aspects of childbirth, and on tangible, quantifiable 'product' outcomes such as live baby and mother, with mortality statistics being the guiding principle of practice. In contrast, woman-centred metaphors are relational, reflecting context, history and connection with self and body.

We don't just 'fall' pregnant or 'give' birth or 'have' children, we do so in a process that is multifaceted and complex [biological, cultural and historical aspects are integrated and mutually transforming] (Thiele 1989 p.10).

Feminists have presented not only a sound critique of normative, Western (male) moral philosophy and principle-based ethics but also an alternative ethic that takes into account both the individual and the socio-political frameworks and structures. They are wanting to acknowledge difference, give voice to the disempowered, pay attention to history, context and character, and include responsibility to 'particular others' in the public discourse. Feminists oppose subverting these concerns and relegating them to a socially constructed private sphere.

SUMMARY

This chapter addressed the values and assumptions of feminist theory and feminist ethics – the philosophical foundations of this analysis. A more detailed discussion of the research method is available in Thompson (2001). The values and assumptions of feminist theory are seen as an alternative to those of Western (male-oriented) moral philosophical thought, for midwifery, and feminist virtue ethics are said to provide a more appropriate strategy for guiding midwifery ethics.

Midwives practise in a context of intimate professional relationship with childbearing women. Childbirth is a creative, emotional, unique and human life experience, not a dilemma. Western (male-oriented) moral philosophical thought, contemporary applied ethics and biomedical ethics recognise only 'so-called' objective science and problem-solving, and normative ethical principles. Conversely, feminist theory rejects the notion of 'one truth' and feminist ethics acknowledge the importance of relationship, our responsibility to particular others, the character of moral agents in the social construction of human engagement, and the exercise of power as a means of subordination and exclusion. Feminists and constructivists agree that language including metaphors reflects social organisation and constructs our identity and subjectivity.

REFERENCES

Allmark P 1995 Can there be an ethics of care? Journal of Medical Ethics 21: 19-24

Allmark P 1996 Reply to Ann Bradshaw. Journal of Medical Ethics 22: 13-15

Bacchi C L 1990 Same difference: feminism and sexual difference. Allen & Unwin Australia Pty Ltd, Sydney

Bandman E L, Bandman B 1995 Nursing ethics: through the life span. Appleton & Lange, Norwalk CT

Bordo S 1992 Feminist scepticism and the 'maleness' of philosophy. In: Harvey E D, Okruhlik K (eds) Women and reason. The University of Michigan Press, Ann Arbor

Bruner J 1986 Actual minds, possible worlds. Harvard University Press, Cambridge MA

Clandinin D J, Connelly F M 1994 Personal experience methods. In: Denzin N K, Lincoln Y S (eds) Handbook of Qualitative Research. Sage, Thousand Oaks, California

Crigger N J 1997 The trouble with caring: A review of eight arguments against an ethic of care. Journal of Professional Nursing 13 (4): 217-221

Diamond I, Quinby L (eds) 1988 Feminism and Foucault: reflections on resistance. Northeastern University Press, Boston

Friedman M 1987 Care and context in moral reasoning. In: Kittay E F, Meyers D T (eds) Women and moral theory. Rowman & Littlefield, Totowa NJ

Fry S T 1989 The role of caring in a theory of nursing ethics. Hypatia 4 (2): 93-112

Gatens M 1983 A critique of the sex/gender distinction. In: Allen J, Patton P (eds) Beyond Marxism? Interventions after Marx. Intervention Publications, Sydney

Gatens M 1996 Imaginary bodies: ethics, power and corporeality. Routledge, London

Gilligan C 1982 In a different voice: psychological theory and women's development. Harvard University Press, Cambridge

Gilligan C 1993 Reply to critics. In: Larrabee M J (ed) An ethic of care: feminist interdisciplinary perspectives. Routledge, New York

Green K 1993 Reason and feeling: resisting the dichotomy. Australasian Journal of Philosophy 71 (4): 385-399

Harding S 1987 Introduction: is there a feminist method?. In: Harding S (ed) Feminism and methodology: social science issues. Open University Press, Milton Keynes

Held V 1993 Feminist morality: transforming culture, society, and politics. The University of Chicago Press, Chicago

Johnstone M J 1994 Bioethics: a nursing perspective. Saunders, Sydney

Kirkham M 1986 A feminist perspective in midwifery. In: Webb C (ed) Feminist practice in women's healthcare. John Wiley & Sons, Chichester

MacIntyre A 1984 After virtue: a study in moral theory. University of Notre Dame Press, Notre Dame, Indiana

Marks E, de Courtivron I (eds) 1981 New French feminisms. The Harvester Press Ltd, Brighton

Noddings N 1984 Caring: a feminine approach to ethics and moral education. University of California Press, Berkeley

Pinch W J E 1996 Feminism and bioethics. Medical Surgical Nursing 5 (1): 53

Poole M, Isaacs D 1997 Caring: a gendered concept. Women's Studies International Forum 20 (4): 529-536

Rothman B K 1991 In labor: women and power in the birthplace. W W Norton, New York

Ruddick S 1987 Remarks on the sexual politics of reason. In: Kittay E F, Meyers D T (eds) Women and moral theory. Rowman & Littlefield, Totowa NJ

Salmon D 1999 A feminist analysis of women's experiences of perineal trauma in the immediate post-delivery period. Midwifery 15: 247-256

Saunders M J 1997 Feminist ethics and 'privilege'. Resources for feminist research/Documentation sur la recherche feministé 25 (3&4): 18-25

Scott P A 1995 Aristotle, nursing and health care ethics. Nursing ethics, an International Journal for Health Care Professionals 2 (4): 279-285

Sherwin S 1992 No longer patient: feminist ethics and healthcare. Temple University Press, Philadelphia

Stanley L, Wise S 1993 Breaking out again: feminist ontology and epistemology. Routledge and Kegan Paul, London

Stocker M 1987 Duty and friendship: towards a synthesis of Gilligan's contrastive moral concepts. In: Kittay E F, Meyers D T (eds) Women and moral theory. Rowman & Littlefield, Totowa NJ

Summers A 1994 Damned whores and God's police: the colonization of women in Australia. Penguin Books Ltd, Ringwood, Victoria

Taylor K 1995 The ethics of caring: honoring the web of life in our professional healing relationships. Hanford Mead Publishers, Santa Cruz CA

Tew M 1990 Safer childbirth? A critical history of maternity care. Chapman and Hall, London

Thiele B 1989 Dissolving dualisms: O'Brien, embodiment and social construction. Resources for feminist research/Documentation sur la recherche feministé 18 (3): 7-12

Thompson F E 2001 The ethical nature of the mother-midwife relationship: a feminist perspective [unpublished PhD dissertation]. University of Southern Queensland

Tong R 1993 Feminine and feminist ethics. Wadsworth Publishing Co, Belmont CA

Tong R 1998 The ethics of care: a feminist virtue ethics of care for healthcare practitioners. Journal of Medicine and Philosophy 23 (2): 131-152

Tronto J C 1993 Moral boundaries: a political argument for an ethic of care. Routledge, New York

Way S 1998 Social construction of episiotomy. Journal of Clinical Nursing 7 (2): 113-117

Wearing B 1996 Gender: the pain and pleasure of difference. Addison Wesley Longman Australia Pty Limited, Melbourne

Wurzbach M E 1999 The moral metaphors of nursing. Journal of Advanced Nursing 30 (1): 94-99

6

A conducted tour or independent travel?
Examining underlying assumptions and values

I am saying that the study of women calls attention to the different way of constituting the self and morality; [my critics] are focusing on the issue of sex difference [and] take the ideas of self and morality for granted as these ideas have been defined in the patriarchal or male-dominated traditions. I call these concepts in question by giving examples of women who constitute these ideas differently and hence tell a different story about human experience (Gilligan 1993 p.207).

This chapter represents what some particular mothers and midwives say about ethical midwifery practice, and my interpretation of interview transcripts as validated by the women – constructed consensual meanings.

OWNERS OF THE ORIGINAL KNOWLEDGE

Profiles of those women telling their experiences

Informants are eight mothers and eight female midwives: six of the eight midwives are mothers themselves. For confidentiality, pseudonyms are used throughout.

Brenda, Ellie and Maree are mothers for the first time. Arline, Judy, Kay and Megan are mothers for the second time, and Caroline has three children. They have experienced childbirth within the public and private healthcare sectors, and their birth settings range from large regional hospital wards to a room in a birth centre attached to a large urban hospital.

Those women who are not first-time mothers have experienced different modes of care with subsequent births. In the mothers' narratives, their carers also vary from hospital-employed midwives to midwives practising independently and on the margin of mainstream (Western) maternity services.

Ann, Bev, Diane, Gemma, Katie, Kerry-Anne, Madonna and Ruth are all endorsed to practice midwifery within their specific Australian state, and are also registered nurses who have been educated through the Western-medicine hospital system. Their narratives derive from a range of experience-status, over 15-38 years. All of them have worked as a midwife in a large urban hospital, but their current working positions vary from clinical practitioner in a traditional hospital ward to independent midwifery practitioner in the community.

The informant-researcher relationship

I have written the women's stories of their childbearing experiences as I understand my own midwifery experiences. That is, that childbirth is an intensely personal time for the mother and her support people, an emotionally and physically exhausting achievement for her, and a special privilege for the midwife to be sharing. I have great respect for all childbearing women and continue to marvel at the adaptation of the woman and her body during the birthing-borning process. My understanding of these women's experiences is embedded in my own emotional experience as a practitioner and educator, and this involves my beliefs and values of midwifery practice.

Some informants seemed empowered by reliving their experiences; others seemed to have had their personal values and ethics simply affirmed or reaffirmed. I myself have reflected on some of my earlier beliefs and practices as a newly-registered midwife and 'system worker', and with new insight regret having actively perpetuated the medicalisation of birth, the hegemonic status quo of healthcare services for childbearing women. Regardless of how this narrative inquiry has influenced us, I propose that we have all undergone some degree of transformation from the telling of these stories, and to some extent have addressed the feminist research goal of facilitating social change and empowering participants. Finally, it is necessary to situate this within the scope of the analysis, and to reiterate that egalitarianism in research ought not to be mistaken for egalitarianism in the real world (Glucksmann 1994).

CONSTRUCTING CONSENSUAL MEANINGS

Their personal narratives portray a group of mothers and midwives who are very homogenous in their ethical values and beliefs about the mother-midwife relationship.

Three major themes are identified across both mothers and midwives: institutional dominance over childbirth, values conflict between workplace or service provider ethics and personal ethics, and 'being with' women during childbirth. A central theme that links all other themes and sub-themes is 'power in relationships'.

It is helpful, at this stage, to reiterate the underlying assumptions of this analysis. One is that the nature of midwifery practice is different from the practices of moral philosophy, medicine and nursing, and thus the currently dominant mainstream ethical frameworks from those other practices are not adequately responsive to midwifery practice. Another is that a distinctive midwifery ethic is implicitly available in the lived realities and shared engagement of mothers and midwives, and that listening to their voices provides an initial mapping strategy for the development of this distinctive midwifery ethic. In other words, mothers' and midwives' narratives reveal that which exists and has not previously been made explicit in ethics.

Birthing is an occurrence that impresses itself upon the woman and one that is unique to that woman. The manner in which the woman is affected by the experience is subject to individual interpretation based upon a shared commonality of meaning. The way we interpret our social world determines the way we act or behave in that world, and for midwives this translates into the way we see our practice and how we practice it. If this shared common meaning is to be rendered explicit, stipulation of a thematic framework is essential: this analysis is guided by feminist ethics which are discussed in the previous chapter. Feminists and constructivists agree that language and discourse not only reflect social organisation but they also construct our identity and subjectivity (Wurzbach 1999). Hermeneutical analysis describes a process of comparative sieving of data for the purpose of discovery and presentation of context and meanings (Benner & Wrubel 1989). Furthermore, regardless of research method, an underlying tenet of feminist research is that women's lives are important (Reinharz 1992). Women can be empowered by giving voice to their experiences.

Gilligan explored the dissonance between psychological theory and women's experience. She did not ask how much women are like men; rather she sought to discover

whether something had been missed by the practice of leaving out girls and women at the theory-building stage (Gilligan 1993 p.208).

Similarly, this current analysis sought to discover whether something was missed by the practice of leaving out mothers and midwives (women) at the (male-philosophy) theory-building stage of bioethics, for ethics surrounding childbirth. Perhaps some social, historical and cultural phenomena are missing from the bioethics theories. Giving voice to the perspective of mothers and midwives has identified women's ethical meanings and experiences from their particular position in the hierarchy of healthcare and maternity services. Relationship, context and virtues are recurring features of what mothers and midwives consider adequate ethical responses surrounding childbirth – features which are absent in the abstract universalism of normative bioethics. To this extent, these mothers' and midwives' narratives have provided insight into the ethical nature of the mother-midwife relationship and the suggested gap in knowledge between normative ethical theories and midwifery practice.

Mothers' and midwives' shared values

Good and bad ethical aspects surrounding childbirth are important in understanding the mother-midwife relationship. For mothers, their narratives are about their own birthing experiences and for midwives, their narratives are of their professional practice.

Mothers tend to begin with the contextual and historical detail of their early labour experience. Midwives more commonly begin with an experience that was distressing for the mother, themselves, or both, and which involved another healthcare practitioner. All give 'factual' information and the context of events, followed by an expression of their related emotions and feelings, finishing with a description of their subsequent 'good' experience or preferred approach to birthing. As discussed earlier, intentions inform behaviour, and are situated in narrative histories within particular settings. These narratives tell us that mothers and midwives alike identify the practitioner's intention, and how intentions differ in particular settings.

Good experience is often accompanied by transformative comments such as 'it opened my mind', 'I've changed my practice since then', 'I know a lot more about it now' – sentiments which support the earlier claim that our ways of seeing determine our ways of behaving and practising, and that personal experience is legit-

imate knowledge. Being aware of the need for confidentiality, quotes are deliberately general, with few identifying factors.

POWER IN RELATIONSHIPS

Use and abuse of power in relationships is the central and frequently recurring theme in mothers' and midwives' narratives. Different types of power are identified as power 'over', power 'for', and power 'with'; that is, exploitative, manipulative, competitive, nutrient and integrative power (May 1972).

All beings have power, but May (1972) distinguishes between potential and actual power, when power is defined as the ability to cause or prevent change. He places status, authority and prestige as central to the problem of power, and likens coercive power to the middle ground between power as energy and power as violence. Exploitative power is the simplest yet most destructive type. It occurs when one person has power over the bodies of many persons; for example, slavery. It identifies power with force and presupposes violence or threat of violence. Victims have no choice. Manipulative power may originally stem from the person's own desperation or anxiety, because of her own hopelessness and inability to do anything else, but after that there is little or no spontaneity or choice left. The apprehensive primigravida woman might request induction of labour or pain relief in labour but having entered the world of medicalisation and 'handed herself over to the doctor to look after' as one participant said, she may be left with little or no spontaneity or choice. The critic is forcefully silenced. In humans it is seen as the need or passion to control the other, a need which the individual often has not consciously confronted. Both of these types of power are referred to in the present analysis as power 'over'.

Power 'for' is based on nutrient power. This is a form of power that is often necessary and valuable with friends and loved ones, such as the normal care and attention of the parent for the growth and flourishing of the child. As humans we derive pleasure from exerting ourselves from time to time for the sake of the other (May 1972 p.109).

It also comes out of the statesperson's concern for the welfare of the group (for example, the midwife for childbearing women), and is constructive in its political and diplomatic nature as when the midwife acts as the woman's advocate.

Power 'with' refers to integrative power. This power is not merely cooperative power (because the latter can slide back into manipulative power which silences the critic), or competitive power (which makes the critic look silly). Nor is it nutrient power which, if misused, can patronise the critic by implying she is confused and needs our care. Rather, integrative power leads to growth by a dialectic process of thesis, antithesis and synthesis: a new 'truth' results. Integrative power is seen as an appropriate interpretation of concepts identified in 'being with' woman in childbirth because participants are critical of the standardised, power 'over' approaches to childbirth within mainstream hospital services. When they refer to an adequate ethical response they speak of the particularity of each birth experience and themselves as persons, as if these latter concepts are the antithesis of standardised practices. Unlike the power 'over' approaches, childbirth practices that are oriented towards 'being with' woman construct new, collaborative meanings throughout each childbirth process, between the mother and the midwife. It is a shared, negotiated experience resulting in a commonality of meaning – a dialectic process of thesis, antithesis and synthesis. Two midwives say in their narratives that they have learnt a lot from the mothers. Typical comments from mothers refer to 'getting to know me and what I wanted and needed' and to 'letting me do what was right for me but if there was a problem the midwives would not just let you go on, they would say I think it's better if you do this or that', and the woman then chooses again. Her second choice may not always be the same as the midwife's. This negotiated or power 'with' approach most commonly occurs in narratives involving birth centre or independently practising midwives.

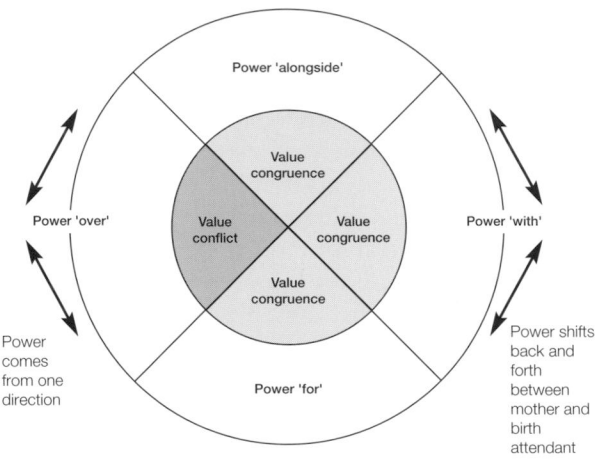

Figure 6.1 The use of power in mother-birth attendant relationships, and the effect on personal/professional values of these mothers and midwives.

Power 'alongside' is not identified frequently, but this might be explained by the fact that the analysis focuses on the mother-midwife relationship rather than the midwife-colleague relationship. Similarly, the features of 'competitive' power in the midwife-colleague relationship are not discussed separately but are identified in relation to exerting power 'over' the other and thereby disrupting the mother-midwife relationship.

Whilst all of these types of power can be present in the same person at different times, the moral goal for practitioners and service providers is to use them in ways that make relationships ethically appropriate for the given situation. A power 'with' approach is predominantly the most adequate for mothers and midwives, during the process and experience of childbirth.

Figure 6.1 illustrates the use of power in mother-birth attendant relationships according to mothers' and midwives' narratives (Thompson 2001). Mothers and midwives experience a conflict of personal and professional values when institutional values dominate the relationship with the mother and when practitioners use power 'over' others. On the other hand, most of these mothers and midwives express a congruence of personal and professional values when relationships are oriented towards 'being with' the woman during childbirth, and when practitioners utilise their power 'with' the childbearing woman.

Power 'over' – exploitative, manipulative

Power 'over' refers to the exploitative, manipulative and competitive use of power within the mother-birth attendant relationship. This use of power often includes paternalism and institutional dominance. Gemma, a midwife, was working within an aboriginal community in a remote area of Australia. All pregnant women in that community, indigenous and non-indigenous, were required to fly to the nearest capital city and spend the last weeks of their pregnancy there. For the aboriginal women it meant that they did not 'birth on their homelands', 'in their country'.

They were allowed to have one support person with them but often the support person didn't stay because they didn't like being away from home either. When they did go into hospital they were often put into a room with other aboriginal women because it was perceived that they should be able to communicate with them. Whereas in fact, it was an area where there were very different languages. It was really purely because they had the same colour skin that they were put together and expected to communicate and to support each other, and it often didn't work at all because they were just from completely different communities ... At times I felt angry because I thought the system was so paternalistic and so much set up for the white fellows and so much medically oriented, that there wasn't any room for these women, for anything they felt or wanted, or there was no taking into account their needs, their own personal needs. It was almost like they didn't have any. Yeah, so I guess it was just paternalistic. They'd been having babies on the island for many, many years before the health services started and 'what should and shouldn't be'. (Gemma)

The paternalistic and power 'over' approach reflects what Rothman (1991) describes, in her social construction of birth, as the 'active-passive' relationship in which the doctor makes all decisions, and the patient is 'worked on', much

the same way as mechanical repairs are done. It is typified by the doctor using forceps or surgery to pull the baby out of an unconscious or anaesthetised mother. The doctor has the authority to define normal, variations from normal, and the 'state' of the patient. An example of this is seen in the comments from a mother receiving private healthcare from an obstetrician for her first birth.

Oh it was just really like I was [pause] to be operated on. I don't feel like I was being consulted or anything. I felt like I was just there and I was the thing that had to be worked on. This is the task, she's the task and that's how it kind of felt yeah. (Brenda)

Diane, a midwife practising in a mainstream hospital setting at the time of her narrative, witnessed paternalism and a power 'over' approach from an obstetrician when he spoke to a pregnant woman prior to entering the operating room for a trial of Kielland's forceps. The woman had expressed her wish, based on the research and information she had read, to tear naturally and to not have an episiotomy unless it was necessary – even though the midwife had told her that it would probably be necessary with a Kielland's forceps birth. After speaking to the woman, the obstetrician performed an excessively large episiotomy on the woman who subsequently had faecal incontinence and required extensive physiotherapy during the immediate postnatal period.

It was just totally traumatic. It was an invasion, it was an abuse of her body, her psyche, it was totally not what she wanted and there was no respect for her as a woman, none at all. He treated her like a bit of dirt. He told her she was wrong, that she was misinformed, that she really had no 'right' to have any view on what should happen to her, it was like 'I know best'. And he told her that – that he was the doctor and he knew best ... To me it was just, the whole thing was to do with power. His authority was challenged and he didn't like it [pause] that anyone would have a birth plan and would tell him how to conduct his professional practice. I think that was how he saw it. That this woman who knew nothing about obstetrics would have the gall to write on her birth plan that she didn't want an episiotomy and in his judgement that was wrong. (Diane)

Diane's ethical dilemma is, does she as a midwife and antenatal educator make it worse for some women by giving them information and encouraging them to make decisions about their own birthing process? For example, did the fact that the woman had written a birth plan and had expressed a preference to not have a certain procedure lead to the woman's traumatic experience? If the woman had not been perceived as challenging the doctor's authority, perhaps she would not have been abused and would not have suffered to the extent that she did. In promoting a power 'with' relationship between mother and birth attendant, had Diane contributed to the woman's suffering? That is this midwife's ethical concern.

Both mothers' and midwives' narratives illustrate a combination of power 'over', lack of self-determination for the woman and midwife ('silenced', punished and restricted from exercising professional midwifery judgment), and 'doing to' the woman. For mothers, lack of self-determination is the result of being 'silenced', and Brenda's story demonstrates this.

I was just feeling like I was constantly being belittled and to the stage where I was complacent to what they wanted me to do ...

and the anaesthetist has come in and has gone WELL GIRLIE, and I've gone 'girlie'?! [questioning and indignant]. Do whatever you like then, but leave me alone I'm not talking to you, do you know what I mean? Girlie!! Oh! I was shocked. I was really shocked. Even in my drug induced state that I was in, to be called 'girlie' I just like went 'I don't like him'. Like that.

[and]

With this other lady [the second midwife] just walked in and I feel like she took over and she was the one that said 'we're going to have to talk pain relief now', and I didn't feel like I had any option after that. I just felt like it was totally her. Whatever she wanted was fine. I wasn't going to argue with her. She had that kind of – I'm not going to argue with this woman, whatever she wants she knows best, and instead of being like a mother figure and being really encouraging [like the 1st midwife], it was more like being a school teacher and being told what to do. Does that kind of explain it? (Brenda)

Anderson reports similar research findings.

Difficulties arise when midwives abuse their position, undermining the woman's sense of being in control rather than reinforcing it. Six women in the study talked unprompted of feeling like a naughty little schoolgirl, with the midwife that well-known authority figure, the harsh and unkind schoolmistress ... Several women were called a 'good girl' when they did well. More often, though, they talked of a sense of 'not doing it right'. They were sure that there was a 'right' way to do it and that they were inadequate or deficient in some way (Anderson 2000 pp.104-105).

For the practitioner, being 'silenced' means being unable to exercise professional midwifery judgment, a lack of self-determination professionally, or being kept in a subordinate role. It is often accompanied by real or threatened punishment. A midwife of extensive experience, Kerry-Anne, told of how she did not carry out a 'private' obstetrician's written standing orders which were for all primigravida women under his care to have an episiotomy. The woman birthed her baby vaginally with no tears to the perineum and was 'over the moon' according to Kerry Anne.

I couldn't bring myself to actually cut this woman unnecessarily ... And soon after delivering the placenta the doctor actually walked into the room and greeted us both and immediately said 'Give me a tray Sis and I'll stitch her,' because he presumed that I had done an episiotomy. And I said 'She doesn't need any stitches doctor, I didn't do an episiotomy and she's got an intact perineum'. And he showed his anger by more or less pushing me aside and pushing her legs apart and saying 'Let me have a look.' And he looked at her perineum and said 'I'll put a stitch in her, there is a tear here.' And I felt really embarrassed because I'd actually told her there was nothing and I'd told him there's nothing and then I had to get a tray out of the cupboard and go out of the room to get some catgut. So while I was out of the room I calmed down and calmly walked back in to the room and gave him the catgut and stood by him while he sutured her. I never confronted him. I just felt so bad about it. And he was a very senior obstetrician in this hospital, and I was a labour ward CNC [Clinical Nurse Consultant] but I still didn't have the power that he had.

... Well she was just a body wasn't she? To him. She was just a body. She wasn't someone who had any rights. She was having something done to her without her really knowing what was being done. I felt at the time I would have liked to have got a mirror and shown her.

The relationship between Kerry-Anne and the birthing woman resembles what Rothman (1991) describes as a 'mutual participation' relationship (and what I and informants in this analysis identify as 'being with' woman) in which the practitioner and woman work together toward a common goal. This relationship denies the patient role and medical control but the institutionalisation of childbirth works against the development of such a relationship. The hospital patient is outnumbered and overpowered. She may be allowed to act as if she were an equal participant, bringing an advocate such as her husband or coach with her, but if she becomes disagreeable, difficult or disruptive, as defined by the birth attendants, her true powerlessness is made clear. Her advocate is there only as long as the hospital attendants choose to allow him/her to be there, only as long as s/he continues to coach the woman in accord with institutional rules.

As she was actually birthing she screamed very loudly and this doctor got extremely angry and told her to shut up and then he turned to the husband and said 'You, get out of the room until she behaves herself' were his words ...

and then after the baby was born I wrapped it up and she was holding it and she wasn't even taking any, very much notice of her baby because she kept apologising to him for screaming. And he kept on saying to her 'That's OK girlie, you just needed to be controlled girlie'. And then he said to me 'Her husband can come in after I've stitched her'. (Kerry-Anne, midwife, second narrative)

For mothers, being 'silenced' occurs via the 'system workers' and their own support person. Caroline's husband coached her according to the hospital's 'rules':

[The doctor] said 'Oh well, we're going to have to put her on a drip'. As soon as they said drip I just [pause] I was ready to go home. I said I want out of here. I want to go. I don't want to have the drip. And then [husband's name] said 'Look, you've got to have the drip. Just, you know, calm down, you've got to have the drip'. I said 'Well if I'm having the drip I want an epidural right now' 'cause I didn't want, you know, going through that sort of that thing.

Part of Brenda's narrative is another example of this. She told of how her husband agreed to

her having an epidural anaesthesia against the couple's pre-arranged plan to have only gas unless mother or baby was distressed. This is due partly to his powerlessness within the hospital hierarchy but also because he was distressed by what he perceived as her extreme suffering:

I couldn't have any more gas, I'd had too much gas. Would you like to have an epidural? And [husband's name] was going Yes! and just stop the pain, and I don't know what I said about it, but [husband's name] said yes and that was fine by me, whatever he said went, I was too busy rocking and I had my eyes shut ... And I've gone oh well I'll have it then. And I was strong, like I wasn't going to have it, I was going to do it just on gas, and he's gone 'Give her the epidural' [spoken in a gasping, 'urgent' voice], he's my support partner and he's going 'Just stop the pain, give her an epidural', so I've curled up and they've done it.

He also coached her during the actual birth, in accord with staff wishes and 'rules':

I'm thinking everyone can see me and I'm over this bar and I want my clothes on and I, and I don't really like this ... so I wrapped my leg around it so that they couldn't make me stand up, and [husband's name] untangled my legs for me and made me stand up [spoken with exasperation]. So as a support person he was doing all the right things for the staff but not for me, sort of thing (Brenda).

Power 'for' – nutritive

Power 'for' occurs when the midwife uses her power for nutritive purposes (that is, parental, protective, for growth and flourishing of the mother) within the mother-midwife relationship.

Power 'for' is nutritive when the mother receives help and assistance that she determines either then or on a previously negotiated understanding, and because she is unable to meet her own needs at the time. It is temporal in nature. Doing 'for' the woman is relative to, and lasts only as long as is necessary to meet, the particular immediate needs or desires of the childbearing woman. It does not disempower the woman and usually aims at returning the locus of power to the woman.

An example of midwives using their power 'for' the mother is when hospital midwives performed reflexology on Caroline without her full understanding or consent. Caroline expressed strong objection to medical augmentation of labour. The midwives asked her if she knew about reflexology and she implied that she was not interested in it. Caroline became aware of the midwives doing something to her feet, a particularly sensitive area for her, and asked what they were doing. At the same time, the midwives carried out the doctor's orders to set up for an intravenous infusion to medically augment labour. Caroline interpreted the latter as the midwives' betrayal of her wishes. The midwives, however, did not commence the infusion. Rather they continued applying reflexology, thereby avoiding the need for the 'drip':

But, because of that – they knew I didn't want the drip and because of that they didn't have to put the drip in, and I just sort of felt [pause] well I felt like I wanted to kiss 'em, 'cause it was, it was [pause] far preferable to me to have something natural than a drug and well I suppose reflexology is quite natural. And I suppose I felt quite relieved after that betrayal. (Caroline)

Another situation of power 'for' is when the midwife is being an advocate for the birthing woman. This nutritive power does not occur in narratives when the mother-midwife relationship is one of not 'being with' the woman; that is, when it is one of separateness, and disparate relationships. When the mother-midwife relationship is one of being with woman, the power 'for' and the 'being with' woman ethical responses are identified in the same narrative. To be a defender of the woman the midwife

must really concentrate on the woman and her needs (Kirkham 1986 p.40).

Comments from Maree, a primigravid woman birthing her first baby, illustrate the second situation in which the midwife acted as an advocate and used her power 'for' the woman, within a 'being with' woman relationship.

And I always remember that visit because I was in so much pain and he stood at the end of the bed and I had a lot of respect for the doctor, I felt he was very capable, but what he did was stood at the end of the bed while I was in tremendous pain and started talking to me, saying 'Well we're going to have to

speed up the drip' and dah, dah, dah. Now I could barely hear him over this pain. What I was very impressed about is the midwife turned to the doctor and said 'You'll just have to wait', and walked up to me, dropped everything again and just talked me through this pain and said to me 'Just ignore the doctor. Let's get through this'.

Without the midwife's advocacy, the doctor's hasty approach excludes the woman from any meaningful decision-making and increases her vulnerability. Such haste teaches that the doctor's time is more important than the birthing woman or her understanding and experience (Kirkham 1986). The 'expert' role demeans and patronises the woman. Maree validated this when she reviewed the interview transcript.

Practitioners' narratives reveal values and beliefs similar to those of mothers. Katie, an independent midwifery practitioner with extensive experience and advanced qualifications, illustrates the use of power 'for', within the mother-midwife relationship. Her comment further links the centrality of relationship with that of supporting the woman – and colleagues in this instance – which demonstrates the use of power 'alongside'. She identifies the inadequacy of an institutionalised approach by midwives to childbearing women:

There are certainly midwives in the hospital that are good women. And they say just the right thing at the right time. You know, the doctor's saying I do want a clip on this baby's scalp and the midwife will say 'Look it's not a busy night, I'll be more than happy to listen. I can listen in more frequently. I'll be here' and she'll just intervene. She knows what the woman wants, she knows what we're advocating for the woman and she'll just deflect and diffuse the situation by saying 'Look I'm a hospital person and I'm sort of just softening this for you doctor. I'm helping you save face here'. You know, and she's actually protecting the woman's interests and rights, and us, and him, and you know, she's on fire. But most of them, 60-70% most [pause and sighs] are just completely institutionalised. They approach people in institutionalised ways and they provide care which is devoid of relationship, proper relationship.

Power 'with' – integrative

An ethical mother-midwife relationship demonstrates the use of integrative power. The midwife uses her power 'with' the mother, and the mother uses hers 'with' the midwife. There is mutual participation of mother and midwife, and whilst the locus of power shifts back and forth between the mother and midwife, it predominantly rests with the mother. Both parties have a common goal, a shared philosophy and orientation or 'way of seeing'. The mother-baby relationship is not an adversarial one. The midwife's role is portrayed more as 'be with' not 'do to'; she is present, she is 'there'. 'Not doing' is not seen as uncaring, rather it is described positively by mothers – 'being there for me', 'didn't get in my way', 'she let me do what was right for me'. The participants use terms such as 'confidence', 'empowered', 'proud of my/herself' when they speak of the influence such a mother-midwife relationship has on the woman's birthing ability and process. They consider the character of the practitioner as ethically important too and refer to concepts such as trust, respect, empathy and honesty – virtues displayed by the individual for the individual. This indicates the importance of particularity in an adequate ethical response for midwifery practice. Communication and informed choice for childbearing women maintain their self-determination, and mothers and midwives alike emphasise the essential nature of these for ethical practice.

For midwifery practice, a major component of the power 'with', or 'being with' relationship is that the midwife's prime relationship is with the childbearing woman, and the mother's prime relationship is with her baby (Guilliland & Pairman 1995). Unlike a procedure-oriented practitioner, the midwife who uses integrative power with the mother does not have disparate relationships. By focusing on mother as her/his primary orientation, the midwife ensures that the birthing woman has 'freedom of space' to do what is right for herself and her baby.

The use of power 'with' is most evident in narratives from mothers and midwives whose experiences were in birth centres or with independent midwifery practice. Arline, a woman receiving care from midwives in a birth centre and who was birthing her second baby in that environment by choice, says:

They don't ever make a decision without consulting you or your partner and that's really important too because you want to be able to, I like to be able to feel like I was the one that was in control because it's my birth, you know? I mean it's my experience. She's there to facilitate and make sure that everything goes safely and she's largely there to support me to make sure that I do it the way I want to do it, and in our case the midwife, she was fantastic. So that was really good.

Kay, a mother who had a caesarean birth for her first baby, employed an independent midwife to attend her next birth. She wanted the opportunity of trying to birth her second baby 'naturally' (vaginally) despite the previous surgical scar to her uterus. Given the associated risks, the midwife obtained visiting practising rights in a major hospital, they occupied a single room, and only the two independent midwives and Kay's husband were in attendance. The second experience contrasted with the first and Kay describes the mother-midwife relationship during that second pregnancy-birth as follows:

[thoughtful] Because I was really this time being given the opportunity of having a totally natural childbirth, drug free, thank you [midwife's name], for creating that environment for me and stepping I guess from that care of the obstetrician where you do hand yourself over to them to a point. Like you, 'I want to have this baby, I know I'm a bit frightened but I know you'll look after me, solve it all for me'. Whereas with an independent midwife I had to take full responsibility for choosing to go that way and I did want to try it with no drugs but I had no idea how to deal with labour and that was another really important thing, and what [midwife's name] was able to do for me, was that she was able to discuss in detail, ways of dealing with labour and actually talk about it!

Three other main themes emerge in both mothers' and midwives' narratives: institutional dominance, values conflict and 'being with' woman. A congruence of personal/professional (midwifery) values is portrayed in relation to the 'being with' woman childbirth practices.

SUMMARY

Personal narratives of mothers and midwives were analysed, interpreted and validated, for insight into the ethical nature of the mother-midwife relationship and, therefore, the nature of a distinctive ethical response for midwifery practice.

The use of power within relationships is a central theme throughout. These mothers and midwives reject as unethical, power 'over' approaches by individual practitioners and institutional dominance over childbirth practices, especially when they render the individual woman invisible.

Trust and talking with the practitioner appear to be an indication of a 'power with' or 'power for' relationship. When the childbearing woman withholds information from and is not 'cooperating' with health professionals it indicates that the individual mother/client is attempting to prevent or minimise a 'power over' relationship.

People give or withhold information about themselves in communication with health professionals depending on whether they trust the people involved, because they are aware that possession of sensitive and private information about themselves gives health professionals further power over them ... to be kept in a state of ignorance is to be kept in a state of impotence, to be infantilised and controlled (Thompson, Melia & Boyd 1994 p.79).

When the midwife acts 'for' the woman, the balance of power reverts back to the woman quite quickly, as soon as the woman's vulnerability is reduced. Power 'for' is used to negotiate for the birthing woman according to her wishes rather than being paternalistic or authoritative. Values-conflict is not identified within the themes of power 'with' and 'for'; mothers and midwives in the present narratives express a congruence of values with those approaches.

REFERENCES

Anderson T 2000 Feeling safe enough to let go: the relationship between a woman and her midwife during the second stage of labour. In: Kirkham M The midwife-mother relationship. Macmillan, Basingstoke, pp. 92-119

Benner P, Wrubel J 1989 The primacy of caring. Addison-Wesley, Sydney

Gilligan C 1993 Reply to critics. In: Larrabee M J (ed) An ethic of care: feminist interdisciplinary perspectives. Routledge, New York, pp. 207-214

Glucksmann M 1994 The work of knowledge and the knowledge of women's work. In: Maynard M, Purvis J (eds) Researching women's lives from a feminist perspective. Taylor & Francis, London

Guilliland K, Pairman S 1995 The midwifery partnership: a model for practice. Victoria University of Wellington, Wellington, NZ

Kirkham M 1986 A feminist perspective in midwifery. In

Webb C (ed) Feminist practice in women's healthcare. John Wiley & Sons, Chichester

May R 1972 The meaning of power. In: Power and innocence. Souvenir Press, New York

Reinharz S 1992 Feminist methods in social research. Oxford University Press, New York

Rothman B K 1991 In labor: women and power in the birthplace. W W Norton, New York

Thompson F E 2001 The ethical nature of the mother-midwife relationship: a feminist perspective [unpublished PhD dissertation]. University of Southern Queensland, Toowoomba, Queensland, Australia

Thompson I M, Melia K M, Boyd K M 1994 Nursing ethics. Churchill Livingstone, Melbourne

Wurzbach M E 1999 The moral metaphors of nursing. Journal of Advanced Nursing 30 (1): 94-99

7

Facing obstacles along the way – mothers' and midwives' narratives of unethical childbirth practices

These mothers and midwives are very homogenous in their ethical values. They have similar beliefs about the mother-midwife relationship and the ethically inadequate or inappropriate aspects of mainstream maternity services. They reject practices that fail to respect the individual, and dominate the birth process, birthing woman, or midwife. They express the often enduring, emotional impact such practices have on them.

INSTITUTIONAL DOMINANCE

Both mothers and midwives are critical of institutional dominance over childbirth, especially noted in medically-oriented care. Institutional dominance refers to dominance by doctors, nurses, allied healthcare practitioners and midwives, over the individual childbearing woman or midwife, or birthing/borning process. Strategies to exert such dominance include paternalism, a lack of self-determination for the mother and often the midwife, an emphasis on safety, fear and mortality (negativity of attitude) to the exclusion of supporting the woman, and a procedure-oriented approach that manifests itself as 'doing to' the childbearing woman.

Paternalism

The paternalism of medicalised healthcare towards childbearing women and midwives occurs when the explicit or implicit wishes of the birthing woman or the professional judgment of the midwife are overruled or disregarded, choosing a course of action that is directed at the good of the mother (Beauchamp & Childress 1994). That is, when the principle of beneficence, as defined by experts, dominates over the principle of autonomy (Brown, Kitson & McKnight 1992). Paternalism, therefore, is a construct within the power 'over' relationship. In addition, paternalism is characterised by 'labelling' and 'dismissing the other'.

Kay is a primigravida woman who chose a female obstetrician and private healthcare, believing that such a choice would improve her chance of having a 'natural' birth. She received care in a mainstream hospital ward, and has no real memory of the midwives in attendance during her birthing process. Kay describes her experience of early labour prior to caesarean as follows:

And she [the obstetrician] went to go out of the room again from one of these quick visits and I called her back and I asked her, 'What are we doing, where am I at, can you give me some rough idea?' Communicate with me in some way ... and with that she stopped at the doorway, put her head back round the door and said to me 'Well from here on in it just gets worse. If I were you I'd have an epidural'.

This comment also illustrates the strategy of 'dismissing the woman', identified in other narratives about paternalism and the abuse of power in relationships.

Brenda, the primigravida woman previously mentioned, also received care from midwives in a mainstream hospital ward and birthed her baby vaginally. Yet she describes similar feelings to Kay's in relation to power 'over', paternalism and lack of respect for persons:

Brenda: And apparently the anaesthetist had come in and I said to him I don't want an epidural ... and this guy has walked in and said 'Well girlie,' (GIRLIE!) 'you better decide now otherwise I'm leaving' ...

Faye: How did you feel, what was the issue there?

Brenda: Girlie?! You don't, you know, a bit of respect here buddy! I'm not just a girlie, even though I've told you that I don't want an epidural and they've gone to find you and everything, I think I should have been treated with a little bit more respect than girlie! You know it just, I saw red. Just that total, yeah, she's the task again.

Another insight from these narratives is how the medical belief in an adversarial relationship between mother and baby accompanies practices of paternalism and 'doing to' the woman.

Madonna, a mainstream hospital midwife with many years of experience, discusses the mother-midwife relationship at birth:

The person doing the delivery is really calling the shots aren't they, to an extent? ... And this is why I think you need to have a bit of relationship with the mother so that if you're the one giving the commands, that she will listen to you and she will follow you and you've got to get that relationship going and you've got to listen to me and I will tell you when to push, I will tell you not to push, I will tell you when, you know, what to do, and please listen to me because I can see what's happening here sort of thing. And you can't. In that situation I think yes there's somebody handing out the commands. To save the child from being strangled by its own cord or from mother being ripped from fore to aft.

Rothman also describes these features of obstetric and medicalised midwifery practice:

The baby must be stopped from ripping its mother apart, and the surgical scissors are considered to be more gentle than the baby's head. At the same time, the mother must be stopped from crushing her baby, and the obstetrical forceps are seen as being more gentle than the mother's vagina (Rothman 1991 p.277).

An example of paternalism, procedure-orientation, and power 'over' in the postnatal period is seen in Maree's narrative about learning to breastfeed.

One of the midwives in particular, I sat in the chair and I put a pillow on my lap, because I wanted her on the pillow and that way I could relax my shoulders more and she straight away whipped the pillow away and said 'What do you want that for?' and I said 'Well I'm more comfortable if she's on a pillow' and she said 'Well you don't need that and it's not the way to do it' she said, and I said 'Look I've got an epidural in my back', I still had the drip in my arm and I said 'I really feel much more comfortable if I can do that, it doesn't hurt my back so much', and she said 'Well you can do it this way but you know you don't do it in the future' ... So I just waited for her to leave the room and I did how I felt comfortable.

Lack of self-determination

Mothers and midwives are critical of the lack of self-determination for either mother or midwife, when medicalised healthcare dominates childbirth. Given her unsuccessful attempt at communication earlier in her labour, Kay describes her lack of self-determination and informed choice, the feeling of being overpowered by the carers, and of their 'doing to' her, the birthing woman:

and from then when [obstetrician's first name] came back and looked at the monitor and we still had the fluctuating heart beat and I think it was fairly quick then. [obstetrician's first name] said to me that we have an emergency here, we've got 10 minutes to get that baby out. So a caesarean was necessary, and all the while I was still on this bed and had an internal monitor of course, so I was wheeled into the operating theatre and [pause] they touched probably my abdominal area and asked me if I could feel it and I said yes, so they then gave me a general anaesthetic. So, it all is a lousy experience, so 'managed' and yes I had a general anaesthetic and had a caesarean.

Women having emergency caesarean births and instrumental deliveries feel they have not been afforded the same control, the same active participation in decisions about type of delivery as women having 'natural' vaginal deliveries.

Organizational, structural or experiential factors affect women's perceptions of having an active role in the decision-making process more than the healthcare personnel involved (Churchill & Benbow 2000 p.41).

Caroline, a mother for the third time, gives

another example of the individual being dominated by the institution. Her story tells of when she was in early labour with her second baby. She says that a labour with a 'drip' (medicalised birth) resulted in contractions of a different character and increased pain from 'naturally' occurring contractions, and that leads to a lack of self-determination for the woman.

It's very [pause] well you don't get a break, it's just one contraction after another and the contractions are so different to a natural contraction in the fact that they grip you like a vice and you just, you don't even have the – I don't know, what's the word? You just don't know what's going on around you, you're just so consumed by this contraction that nothing else matters. [sighs] You haven't got I suppose the thought process to say, 'Oh give me some pain relief' [spoken in a weaker voice] or something like that. I know I didn't [pause] sort of thing. And just to contemplate having a drip again was really, really scary at this stage, and then disappointing because I wanted this to be a natural labour in every sense of the word.

Ellie has this to say about the lack of informed choice and self-determination for childbearing women and in particular 'newborn' mothers:

... to assume in a modern society that every woman will breastfeed the baby. I don't think that this is an assumption which should be made on the part of a hospital which has a long tradition in birthing practices ... there was absolutely no proposition that a mature woman like me might be offered a choice whether to breastfeed or formula feed. And of course, the second issue is there was absolutely no information concerning what the breastfeeding would be like [Ellie's experience was particularly painful physically and emotionally. She changed to formula feed after six days] and frankly the more I've thought about this, the more preposterous I find it ... I think every person should be afforded the dignity of being informed of what might their experience be so that they've got some framework by which to judge the degree of difficulty they experience and don't have the consequent onset of that deep and abiding guilt that I certainly experienced when ever I was confronted with her hungry mouth.

As a mother birthing her first baby and a health professional though not a midwife, Maree confirmed the following interpretation as 'very accurate': the midwife is 'silenced' and the institutional hierarchy places the status of both mother and midwife as inferior to and with less power than the doctor's. Maree describes not only her own sense of vulnerability, powerlessness, and lack of self-determination as the birthing woman, but also what she perceives as similar constraints for that second group of midwives in attendance at her birthing.

I felt once the doctor entered the room and said 'Well we're going to have to do this' – well it all just, everyone just fell into place. OK you've got to get your legs up, you've got to do this, you've got to do that, and at that point I felt that I was quite capable of making decisions, yes. And I know at times I said to them 'Look if that's not comfortable for me someone's going to have to, you know, pull me up, and I was assertive enough at that time to say 'Look I know you want me like that, but that's not comfortable. You've got to try this or that, which my husband did. But I felt there wasn't a lot of choice given to me at that point, and I can see the doctor-midwife relationship as it occurred then; he comes in, he hasn't been there all day, he said 'We're going to have to get this baby out' and they all 'do their bit'. Everyone has a cue and this is what they all have to do: this one does this and this one does that. You don't ask any questions, you just get it done and you could see the total change. No more decision making going on here thanks; we've got to get the baby out and my job is to do this, my job's that, my job's this and everyone off they went and did all their jobs.

The midwife's 'autonomy' is restricted in mainstream maternity services. This is identified in Kerry-Anne's narrative concerning whether or not an episiotomy is necessary and the appropriateness of 'standing orders' from an obstetrician. Kerry-Anne is not really sure what the main ethical issues in that situation are for her, but says:

I think maybe it was the very fact that this doctor had written standing orders for all primigravids that midwives were supposed to follow. That was one issue. I don't think that's very ethical because it's taking away the midwife's role as a person who is able to assess at the time, what is necessary. So it's instructing somebody to do something [pause] that I don't think they have the right to instruct them about when they're not there.

When the majority of births occur in hospitals, where childbirth is medicalised and medical officers hold the ultimate responsibility of care 'management', midwives are restricted or prevented from exercising professional midwifery clinical judgement. In Britain and New Zealand, midwifery is not an independent, autonomous practice (Clarke 1995; Fleming 1998) but instead is as constrained as the women they attend because of policies, protocols and contractual obligations (Clarke 1995). Workplace conflict is discussed later. With the ascendancy of science (and particularly since specific professional standards for practice were introduced), the degree of autonomy for midwifery practitioners correspondingly fell (Fleming 1998).

Fear, safety, mortality-morbidity (negativity of attitude)

Concepts of safety, fear (as it pertains to the physical) and mortality/morbidity are most commonly discussed by these mothers and midwives in a negative way, but the nature of the concept differs according to the narrator's identity and role. Childbearing women, especially those who have birthed for the first time, express their 'natural concern' due to a fear of the unknown.

Arline, who birthed in a birth centre, says:

Not that my first birth was a bad experience, it was fantastic but there was still that fear of the unknown and I was still very much like 'no, no, no I can't do this'.

Comments from Megan, a mother for the second time, who birthed in a mainstream hospital ward, show that (i) the mother's prime relationship is with her baby, (ii) mainstream maternity practices focus on the safety of the baby to the exclusion of the woman during childbirth, and (iii) mothers are very susceptible to suggestion during the birth of their babies.

Megan: To get the baby delivered safely and that was my option, that was my most important thing. So that, yeah, I can't really comment on that really. 'Cause I guess that's where my focus was I guess, it seems that that's what everybody else was focusing on. Yeah.

Faye: But that was satisfactory for you?

Megan: Yeah. That was fine for me.

Mothers and midwives describe fathers exhibiting concern when they lack knowledge and feel powerless to help their partner and baby. Brenda, a mother who birthed in a mainstream hospital ward said:

And at that stage [husband's name] was a little bit distraught too because I don't think he'd ever seen me scream into a mask before and jibber the way I did and I think he was rather frightened by it.

Katie, an independent midwife, stated:

Oh look we have lots of couples, and this woman that sat at the table and cried about her previous caesarean section and had gone through a very angry stage with her partner because he hadn't protected her from all that went on. And they're not in any capacity to be able to do that. They have no knowledge, they have no knowledge of the system, they're frightened for themselves and for their baby.

Another type of fear is that associated with a belief in the medicalised birth, and a lack of knowledge or specific knowledge. It is linked to the supremacy of technological and medical intervention tenet, and to the belief that women cannot and ought not birth without the help of medical science – the choice of the intelligent person.

Bev, a midwife working in a community clinic, illustrates fear and negativity when she describes a visit to a mainstream hospital antenatal clinic. The young woman from Bev's clinic is sure she is 37 weeks pregnant; the hospital obstetrician is convinced she is 43 weeks pregnant because of ultrasound results.

I doubted myself and believed him and believed the ultrasound and I felt really frightened. I thought 'I've let this person down, her baby might die because of me' so I got really tied up in all of the rhetoric that he was... but I didn't know it was rhetoric then ... And she was still refusing to go to hospital and he was still insisting. And then he said to her, 'If you don't come to hospital today and have an induction your baby could die and you could die, you could get a clot and you could die'.

This was a few years ago before I'd really spent much time thinking about what my role was, I hadn't worked through the issues about what makes childbirth safe ... I didn't feel safe about her because I knew her baby was small for dates. And I knew that she was under weight and under nourished and I suspected that she'd been using IV drugs which also turned out to be true ... Fear. I believed the doctor. Now there isn't any doubt about that. At the time that he was speaking I thought 'Oh my God he's right'. I believed this stuff, you know, I believed him.

Faye: Scientific base?

Bev: Yeah. I believed it. It sounds to me, now, it even sounds naive, but I believed it. And I doubted myself. And so it didn't seem, while it was happening it didn't seem like an ethical issue, it seemed like a safety issue.

Gemma, a midwife who has practised in remote areas as well as major mainstream hospitals, comments on the concept of fear-mongering:

I think that there's still a lot of [pause] fear mongering and all that sort of stuff goes on ... we still have women coming into major public hospitals for inductions and things, that have no idea why they're there, what's going to happen to them, what the implications of the induction are ...[and later, generally] and the belief too these days that women think generally more so I believe, that they can't birth without medical assistance, and we reinforce that every day by our interventions, inductions. I looked at the local hospital recently and their induction rate is 70% – that's totally bizarre to think that only 30% of the women can actually start labour by themselves. Just bizarre. And so we're reinforcing on lots of levels that women need all this intervention. They need our assistance to birth. They can't birth without it. Such garbage.

Mothers, too, identify the dominance of fear and mortality in guiding mainstream birth practices.

Caroline, a mother who birthed in a mainstream hospital ward, said:

With [first baby's name] they did because when the contractions were happening and the heart rate was getting lower. It was going from 160 down to 120 at the start and by the time I was [pause] what, in full blown labour and the change of labour it dropped down to 60 and I was starting to get, I could see they were getting really panicky about it, to get this baby born.

Kay describes her experience of fear, lack of knowledge and a medicalised birth:

Anyhow, I made a comment about the fluctuation in my baby's heart beat [pause] and to that she did show some concern and I just actually wanted her to – I said 'Give me some explanation. Does it mean anything, or what does it mean?' which wasn't forthcoming. I'm not sure how much time lapsed after that but then it was suggested I move onto a bed and have an internal monitor because of this fluctuation in the heart beat. A couple of years down the track, after the birth of my first baby, I then read more widely and I understood then that within a certain range, fluctuation of your baby's heart beat is normal. Now I'll never know whether that was within normal, but she didn't mention that and maybe it wasn't, but I do understand that now. That that's possibly the case – it was within the realms of normality and maybe not have been necessary to pop me up on the bed and give me an internal monitor.

She is also critical of mainstream services in general. Not only is the focus on fear but also the practitioner is unsupportive of the birthing woman and uses haste to exclude her, diminishing her self-determination.

From that moment that your pregnancy is confirmed by a general practitioner, there is no confidence instilled in you that you are well designed to do this, it's a normal, natural function of your body, and there is no reason why you shouldn't have a natural childbirth. There's this [pause and sigh] view of nearly sort of grave resolve that 'Mmm you are about to embark on having a baby, oh dear! What's going to go, what can go wrong?' ...

and yes I had a general anaesthetic and had a caesarean, [name of first baby] was born perfectly healthy, I was perfectly healthy, drugged a lot and it took a long time to recover and deal with then the sharp learning curve of motherhood, and caesarean and leftovers from the drugs and so forth and just going through a certain amount of labour and so, that was a [pause] a very uncomfortable experience, but at that time I was left and [husband's name] probably, left with – we felt that she had saved my baby's life and probably mine as well. It made me feel like I'd just experienced a life-threatening event.

Women and midwives fear punishment if they challenge the purported safety and necessity of medical-science intervention, and the apparent foolishness of not having it; or when medical authority is questioned. May (1972) asserts that exploitative, manipulative and competitive power (power 'over') is usually accompanied by real or perceived threat and real or perceived violence. Commonly it is midwives who depict this induced fear of punishment from those exerting institutional dominance. They see this fear in themselves, junior medical staff and mothers, and disapprove of it in all circumstances.

Diane, a midwife, said:

And he said 'You are totally wrong, you've been misinformed. If you don't have an episiotomy you'll never use your vagina again. And repeated that, and she, lying flat on her back on a trolley, looked very shocked, shot a look at me and then looked back at him and said 'Oh I just thought that it was better'. And he said 'No, you're totally wrong'. So then he walked off and into the theatre to get scrubbed up, and she was really quite scared at this stage ...

She spoke to me actually, the Registrar – and she said 'Wasn't that awful? I didn't know what to sew. There was just a huge hole there and it was so big I didn't know how to sew it up'.

The next morning I contacted the Medical Superintendent's office and asked to see him and I laid it on the line as honestly as I could, and as a consequence of all of that this doctor will have nothing to do with me again ... afterwards if I was caring for a lady and he was involved, if he had to come in to see her for anything, I would actually ask another midwife to be in the room as I was leaving because I felt that he had tried to make a point, to prove a point by abusing women – to prove a point to me – which really upset me a great deal and so it was quite traumatic. I suspect that there is a big gender issue there.

No [spoken definitely] because she was the Registrar in his unit. You know they're pretty vulnerable too aren't they? What kind of report would they get written if they complained about someone?

[Later in narrative]

So that they can have the confidence to say 'I'm planning this and I'm going to have positive views because birth is about getting in and letting go and releasing, not about hanging on in fear, and they won't birth well while they're fearful. They just have to trust their body, trust the process.

Katie gives another perspective; that of an independent community midwifery practitioner. Whilst she encourages self-confidence in the woman for her ability to birth her baby, Katie's personal struggle is to provide informed choice, ensure that the woman owns her choice, and at the same time, as the midwife, to avoid real or perceived coercion:

The notion of fear – I continually struggle with in terms of providing them with informed choice. It's just such a dodgy thing as far as I'm concerned. They're lay people, we're professionals. They've had one or two whether it's the first, second or third birth. They've never been involved with, we've got years of experience, [pause] they have that confidence in our ability to make it right, make it work, we're more aware of the lack of exact science of what we do, the lack of exact art of what we do, the lack of predicability of the outcome, lack of control that anybody has over the whole process and outcome, so ... There is just an enormous sense of frustration that when you feel that, [pause and sigh] you don't want to keep harping on to this person, because that's coercive, but you want them to understand the ramifications of the decisions they're making or their failure to make a decision. And then I say, so that they can live with themselves afterwards, but perhaps it's much more so I can live with myself afterwards, I'm really aware of that as well. 'Cos they're going to have to live with themselves afterwards one way or another. And perhaps they're actually doing all of this so that they don't have to live with themselves afterwards, if you know what I mean. Like, they're just not owning it all ...

They're rare to choose home birth. I think they probably aren't all that rare in the system, in the mainstream system. Because those people have made 'a' decision of sorts to abdicate responsibilities and give it to the hands of experts. So they're different people. And a lot of these people feel betrayed by the system. And they should feel betrayed by the system, but they should also feel that they've let themselves down.

Faye: A lot of the information about birthing regardless of venues, is to do with mortality and morbidity

Katie: And serious disinformation.

Unsupportive of the woman

Childbirth practices that are unsupportive of difference and the individual woman or birthing women generally, are not woman-centred. Impersonal and normative practices which do not support individual women during childbirth maintain the institutional status quo, and mostly, for this to happen conformity is required:

passivity in patients gives us greater control of our working situation (Kirkham 1986 p.40).

The ethical nature of such practices is not based on relationship, but rather on abstract and universal theory or routine.

Narratives from these mothers and midwives frequently illustrate that practitioners working in such an environment and adopting those practices have disparate relationships. That is, they hold a strong allegiance to their employer, to their medical, nursing and midwifery colleagues, and to the infallibility of medical science compared with the subjective experience, desires and birthing ability of the individual woman. It does not mean that those doctors and midwives are uncaring as individuals themselves. Mothers, in particular, refer to them as being 'nice'. It does mean though, that the individual woman is often rendered 'invisible'.

Judy's story depicts how the hospital midwives saw lay and experiential knowledge as not 'legitimate', and how they were supporting medically oriented not woman-centred practices. They have disparate relationships with medical staff, hospital procedures and the patient role. The resultant nurse-patient relationship is confirmed to some extent by Judy's use of the title 'nurse' for the midwife, and her compliance with instruction. It suggests, too, that Judy felt a certain tension between expectations of her own role once she was admitted to hospital (as the patient) and what the doctor and hospital staff were offering, and what she wanted based on her previous experience of birthing.

Yes so I was 40 weeks. [First pregnancy] I started to feel a lot of – well, what I thought was a lot of pain, and the nurse told me that no it wasn't, it was just a reaction to the gel and it wasn't actually contractions, even though they felt like it to me 'cause they were coming and going, so, I just persisted with that.

[Later]

And I said, well I did try to tell him that I had been induced, they'd used the gel twice with the first pregnancy and really it took a long, 24 hours almost,

for it to get going. He said 'No, no, no you will definitely have this baby by 3 o'clock' because he was going on his weekend away at 5 o'clock. So I said 'Look I don't even care if you're not there, just start me off', you know. I don't care which doctor it is. So of course they did that, put the gel in and then I felt more comfortable than ever, just sitting there – nothing's happening. So I hung around the hospital, walking, walking, walking, went for a walk in the park, came back, put the monitor on again, nothing's happening. He came back at 1 o'clock and 3 o'clock and said 'Oh look sorry, go home, come back in again Monday morning and we'll do it again'. And I said 'Oh can't you just put a bit more in? Because I know I'm going to have the baby over the weekend so can't you just, I know that my body just takes a long time to get going'. And he said 'Oh no I couldn't do that to my partner', you know, 'Start you off and have him have to look after you'. And I thought oh God I don't care who it is, just let the midwives do it ...

Brenda's narrative illustrates how she is rendered invisible, how she feels distanced from the hospital midwives in attendance at her birth, and the disparate nature of the hospital midwives' relationships. The midwives' practice seems based on medication for pain relief, and they do not interact to establish with the childbearing woman how they can best assist her to birth her baby.

and I've gone 'Oh, they said I could have a sleep'. So I had a sleep. Within 15 minutes I was saying to someone else 'I can feel contractions again, it's not working, something's happened', and over in the corner, I can remember [husband's name], breakfast had come in, there was [husband's name], his mother and the midwife and they're saying 'I should have given her Pethidine earlier on. If I had have known it was going to be this bad for her I would have given her Pethidine' and [husband's name] said 'Well she seems to be fine now, everything must be OK'. And I'm thinking 'They're talking about me and I can hear everything they're saying'. I'm going, hey I'm having contractions over here and they're having a conversation in the corner and I'm on the bed by myself. Now I was sitting up most of the time when I was having contractions and the gas, I was sitting up on the edge of the bed, and the midwife came over after I said I can feel contractions, she said 'Well you better sit up, you're going to have the baby'.

Ann, a midwife, describes the disparate nature of relationships, the tension of loyalties, and the conflict of values for a hospital midwife, within the normative approach of mainstream maternity services: an environment which is unsupportive of the childbearing woman.

These parents were very anxious and they felt that something should be done immediately: they felt they should be started into labour because they felt this baby – there was something wrong. A lot of those issues weren't addressed at that time – they were merely told there was nothing wrong, go home ...

We had to [pause] look at the full picture and explain to the parents – because the parents wanted to have their baby delivered – but that's not a usual practice, that there has to be a very good reason to have an induction, there has to be a very good reason for interference and that it's not abnormal to go 10 days over or 14 days over. That's not considered abnormal in some circles. And so trying to explain to the parents that all these factors – it's very difficult because they weren't listening, they didn't want to listen to that. So they were looking for someone to blame or they were looking for answers and they were looking to us as being the people they have seen day in day out and who they were getting to know reasonably well, and they were looking to us for the answers and not being directly involved with the obstetrical management it was very hard for us as nursery staff to be able to comment on the delivery and why it took so long and why that had occurred.

In the following comment, the system worker and 'product' orientation of 'we hadn't given them a healthy baby' contrasts with the individual relationship-based support Ann has been suggesting, and thus appears to have resulted in a conflict of values for her: this midwife has disparate relationships within her workplace.

But no [pause] ethically I felt that five years down the track we hadn't really given them the healthy baby they wanted but then no one is guaranteed of having a healthy baby. But perhaps things could have been different if she hadn't been through the meconium, been through the hypoxia.

Diane, a midwife with mainstream experience, describes the unsupportive approach of a particular obstetrician as well as 'the system'. Neither the birthing woman's preferences for birth nor her subsequent malpractice complaints are supported. The midwife's knowledge and expertise are not respected, and she is not supported by her medical superior as a colleague and practitioner in her own right:

I mean she did say to me before that this was to be her only birth and so she wanted it to be a good birth and I feel that that woman is probably still traumatised by it because I don't really feel that [there was] an adequate resolution through the hospital for her, even when she came and spoke to the Medical Superintendent. [pause] In fact what happened when I went to see him, was he said to me 'Sister have you ever seen an episiotomy with a Kiellands' rotation forceps before?' which was more than a little insulting.

Procedure-oriented approach: 'system workers'

The philosophical nature of childbirth practices that are standardised and routine, and which render 'invisible' the individual or birthing women generally, is frequently one of 'product', 'outcome' and 'efficiency' of resources including staff time. This approach accompanies that of 'unsupportive of the birthing woman'. It is commonly associated with medicalised births, when midwives are being 'system workers', when they have disparate relationships, and when they focus on procedures, routines, and their duty to medical authority and their employer, the institution. When the mother-midwife relationship is one of 'distance' or separateness and disparate relationships rather than 'being with' woman, the needs of the very vulnerable person are not met.

And the next midwife was more like no you must be over the bar and I felt like she was, it was her birth then, not my birth. (Brenda)

A procedure-oriented approach frequently manifests itself as 'doing to' the childbearing woman. The approach is impersonal, and often practices are not practical for the individual childbearing woman/mother. They are not woman-centred or partnership-based. Judy's experience refers to that feeling of staff 'doing to' the woman:

And then, I said it got to the point where it was just really, really painful, so they drew up an injection of Pethedine, but I didn't know that they were, I knew that they were going to give me the injection of Pethedine which I agreed to, but I didn't know it was at that exact moment and I was leaning over a sink and the nurse just, the midwife just came up behind me and put the needle in. Because I got a shock, I jumped off the needle back onto the needle and off the needle again and then she said 'Oh no, sorry about that' and I went 'Oh gosh' and you can just see what happened. And so then she put the needle in again, so I had three prongs to get this one injection of Pethedine, but I didn't care, I was in too much pain.

When midwives adopt a procedure-orientation and have disparate relationships, they do not practice woman-centred care within a 'being with' woman relationship. Maree contrasts the approach of midwives involved in the latter stage of birthing of her first baby, with the first midwife she had earlier. She strongly agrees that relationships and procedures which render the birthing woman invisible are 'not good' ethical practice.

Again I found them quite good except they didn't have the same approach as that first lady. And the thing that I remember about that second stage is I went into a tremendous shock and I was shaking, absolutely shaking vigorously and my teeth were going, I couldn't speak and the whole bed was shaking it was such violent shakes, but the thing I remember so clearly was I was trying to say to [husband's name] I can't stop shaking and nobody was really taking any notice and it was one of the midwives said to me, when I actually got her eye contact, I said 'I can't stop shaking' and she said 'That's all right, that's all right' and she just kept going and I just felt that at that point in time I needed somebody to say [explain] ...

Nobody explained to me what was going on at the time it was happening. It was, they were busily getting around ready, getting ready for this delivery and they had to arrange a paediatrician because of the stained liquor and yes they were obviously very busy and intent on what they were doing but they forgot that here is this mother here shaking violently. Because my husband was next to me and he was saying to me 'Yes, yes, you're in shock, you've got some shock from your system' which thank goodness he was there. But again if he wasn't a health professional of any sort he would have been as ignorant as I was.

Ann gives another example of how normative practices and procedures render the woman invisible:

The whole time that they were there it was explained to them about what the effects of meconium and so

on were but these parents were very angry because they felt that maybe if they'd been listened to the week before they would not have got to this stage ...Well when the mother was going through her labour, at about 8 centimetres we got a phone call to say there was some fetal dipping there, that they were calling the medical officer. At the time this girl was very, very frightened, extremely frightened for her baby and the thing that really stands out for me is that I believe she didn't get the reassurance she should have been getting from the midwife. They were too busy looking at the monitors and too busy reporting back what the monitors were saying that they were missing the needs of the people on a one-to-one, basically sitting down talking through the whole situation explaining what the situation was.

Ellie is clearly distressed as she recalls her painful and unsuccessful attempt at breastfeeding, and the midwives' rigid adherence to hospital protocols:

Now, what happened for me is that I used to weep every time they would be bringing her to me, and on some occasions when my fear was so great because the pain was so great they'd get me a nappy – to bite into the nappy as they tried to put her on ... On one occasion I recall a midwife who hadn't had any children, who was pregnant with her first child, she turned to me during one particular occasion, where the pain was so great, when she attached her for about the fifth time, that I actually put my head forward, the tears fell onto my lap. I was in just so much pain. I mean her response was the, the most inelastic in my opinion. She said to me 'Are you sure you've watched the videos?' ... There was one midwife who was clearly struggling with the etiquette of not informing women about the realities of breastfeeding. When I said to her what could I do about my nipples, she said, 'Oh dear, we can't recommend anything'. I distinctly got the impression from her when I pursued it with her that it was about the threat of litigation, breach of interest, that kind of stuff, infecting the hospital regime.

VALUES CONFLICT

Childbearing women and midwives experience a conflict of values when the workplace/service provider ethics differ from their personal/professional ethics, and they express it in terms of emotions and feelings. The conflict most frequently intersects or overlaps with power 'over' relationships, practices that are unsupportive of the childbearing woman, and practices that do not reflect a valuing of the individual, in particular the childbearing woman. The effect of institutional dominance and power 'over' childbirth is most evident amongst the midwives, who all relay a conflict of values between mainstream workplace ethics and their personal/professional midwifery ethics.

Workplace/service provider versus personal/professional midwifery ethics

Conflict between (or congruence with) the ethical response of medicalised healthcare and institutional values surrounding childbirth, and the values of the individual childbearing woman or midwife, is a particularly strong theme amongst this group of midwives, but the mothers too experience similar issues. Judy recalls her first experience of labour, in a traditional hospital birth suite/labour ward, and differentiates 'concern' from 'acknowledgment' or authenticity of the individual experience:

Faye: Did you want more concern from them [midwives]?

Judy: Well no I think they were concerned enough. Except I think you just need to have everything acknowledged: that yes it is painful. Like when I was having [first baby's name] and I had this reaction to the gel and the midwife said 'Oh it's not real contractions it's just a reaction to the gel', and you're thinking 'Oh this is bloody painful you know', [spoken slowly, quietly and in an 'in pain' voice] and I know there was nothing she could do in terms of pain relief at that stage and I wasn't actually in full-on labour yet, but maybe if she'd just said 'I know, it is really painful isn't it? A lot of women find that they have this reaction and then it goes into full blown labour later', and just to be acknowledged, but not say 'Oh you poor thing', that type of thing, but to say 'Yes it is very painful, however these are the facts'.

Mothers and midwives generally consider that the ethical response from mainstream maternity service providers is inadequate when it derives from abstract theory, standardisation and a 'product-efficiency' philosophy, and when it renders the individual woman 'invisible'. Institutionalised approaches that seem to

use the universal principles of justice, beneficence and non-maleficence are ethically adequate only if the practitioner also considers context, individual rights, virtues of personal character, and relationship. Otherwise normative ethical responses are inadequate.

Childbearing women and midwives portray themselves as individuals whose personal and professional ethics focus on relationship and virtues. Midwives commonly deal with their values conflict by becoming 'silenced' or subservient to medical authority, and by 'protecting' the birthing woman by placating the 'system worker'. A quote from Kerry-Anne, discussed earlier in relation to power 'over' and 'silencing', illustrates this intersection between values conflict, emotions and feelings, and the way we see and act, our orientation towards practice.

Ann provides another example of values conflict in the workplace. Her story appeared in Chapter 3, when discussing what constitutes a serious moral concern in its own right and to whom the ethical principles apply.

The sad thing is that at that stage when these parents arrived the obstetric unit was going through a change of management and the belief was that all women should be induced, all women would deliver by a certain time, that they would be assessed regularly, that they would have vaginal examinations regularly, that this was medically driven and the midwives at that time were finding it very hard to accept that they were changing all their principles and the principles were for patient care, using power of observation and not going by the vaginal examinations constantly as to where you were at, and so they had to compromise a lot of their beliefs and a lot of their practices to go with the medically driven model at that time and it was very difficult because the Director was a very strong person.

Further comment from Kerry-Anne again demonstrates the conflict between her values and the ethics of her mainstream hospital workplace with its medicalised childbirth practices:

And from then on I made it my business not to be around when he had a primigravid patient in case I was asked to do the delivery. Because I still felt that in the same circumstances I would not be able to do an episiotomy just because it's written on someone's card – that that is his procedure for primigravids.

Later, in her second narrative about the woman whose husband was sent out of the room because she was screaming during the actual birth, Kerry-Anne says:

Then time went on and within the hour I'd done lots of things for her and talking to her and she cried and said 'I feel really bad that I screamed and that I was a naughty girl'. And I said 'You are not a naughty girl, you are a woman who has the right to scream when you are giving birth and I think doctor was wrong. I'm sorry but I think doctor was wrong in speaking to you like that and if he hadn't been here I would have let you scream as much as you like'.

The above comment also illustrates self-denigration, a frequently used tactic in a male-dominated hierarchy, and the schoolgirl response to a harsh schoolteacher (Anderson 2000). The woman uses self-denigration ('I was a naughty girl') as a way of gaining more information and putting the midwife at ease (Kirkham 1986).

Kerry-Anne tells of her conflict of values with the institutionally dominant approach of her midwifery colleagues in the mainstream hospital postnatal area. The mother-midwife relationship for these 'system worker' midwives is one of separateness, whereas she values a 'being-with-woman' mother-midwife relationship. The midwife's prime relationship is with the woman, while the mother's prime relationship is with her baby. Kerry-Anne is concerned for the mother's feelings about her baby. As a midwife, she is not 'taking over' the baby as if her prime relationship is with the baby. She is not, for instance, intending to feed the baby with a complementary feed or decide what to do for the baby without first consulting the mother.

It was the noise over there and the impersonal things about [the hospital ward] and all the babies crying and nobody even reaching out a hand to pat a baby as they're passing by; or like if a mother had gone to the toilet or the shower and the baby's lying in the cot beside the bed and it's crying, crying, crying and the midwife just walking by. I couldn't do it. I had to stop and pat that baby or pick it up and carry it and just so that when the mother came out of the shower she knew that somebody cared, and it wasn't left to scream. I found it very difficult doing it in that ward because there were so many babies all doing the same thing. But [pause] instead of them saying to the

mother next to them 'Would you mind my baby while I go to the shower' they felt, I can't do that. They're not given that opportunity by the midwives who should say 'When you go to the shower ask the lady in the next bed to mind the baby for you' or pat it or nurse it. It's as though that's not the done thing, you're not allowed to pick up each other's babies. And that still goes on. They're not allowed to, they don't seem to pick up each other's babies as though that's wrong. Well, what's wrong with it? So I had to. I did that.

Katie too, expresses disapproval of mainstream hospital midwifery practice. Again, the main conflict is with the lack of meaningful relationship:

Too many times when the system has been the 'system' as opposed to the support a woman's going to get ... But most of them [midwives], [pause] 60-70% most, [pause and sighs] are just completely institutionalised. They approach people in institutionalised ways and they provide care which is devoid of relationship. Proper relationship ...

I went to a talk the other day for the Special Care Nursery staff ... A few key people, including Head of Special Care Nursery, left, as soon as they knew they were going to have to put in their two cents worth they trotted out the door – bloody wimps – and lots of other people commented you know, 'I'm just not sure about the safety of home birth', dah, dah, but they could say those things. But this one, it got down to this one at the front [a physiotherapist], she said 'Well you see I'm here for the baby'. And I said 'Ah, well actually I consider I'm here for the baby as well. You know I actually think that normal natural labour, drug-free labour, normal non-operative births, you know 94% breastfeeding rate for six months, they're all good for babies. I think they're good for babies, you know.' So I actually think I'm doing the right thing by babies too.

Ruth, a midwife usually working in a birth centre and an avid believer in breastfeeding, experienced conflict with the hospital midwife on duty in the postnatal area to where she transferred the young couple and baby she had just attended in the birthing suite:

We went over to the ward and as we walked into the room where she was going to be for the next couple of days the baby started to grizzle and the midwife who was there said 'I hope you brought the dummy with you, you'll need it if you want any sleep, if you hope to get any sleep'. And I think my mouth must have hit the ground ... Oh my god, I'm leaving this woman and her baby in the care of this midwife whose practices to me are just so out of line. How on earth am I going to deal with this, I just felt angry ... Then I moved into really trying to understand where she [the midwife] was coming from ... We came up with all this stuff like 'Well you just want to be here at night with dummies in all of their rooms and they all use dummies and none of them have got any idea' and the final statement which was to me really most amazing was she said 'Well there's just some people and it doesn't matter what you tell and what you say to them they will not change'. And I thought, she's telling me about herself.

Megan, as a first-time breastfeeding mother in hospital, experienced this:

And the worst part was that the midwives – the conflicting advice that I received from the midwives about breastfeeding. It was just so difficult. And it was for that reason that I couldn't wait to get out of hospital. It was just too difficult.

Ellie describes not only her own conflict of values with those of the service provider but also what she perceives as the midwife's conflict of values within the workplace. Both depictions condemn rendering the woman invisible and 'unable', and support ethical responses that resonate with woman-centred relationship and the particularity of context. Her tone of voice is positive when she speaks of the midwives who tried to counter the system in order to help her. She speaks disparagingly of the rigidity, preoccupation with litigation and impersonal approach of the institution, and lack of informed choice for women.

Anyway, she started to say to me, [Ellie lowers her voice to speak quietly and closely/confidentially] 'I think we'll get her a formula feed at night and give those breasts a really good rest'. So, I don't know if you know this, but one of the little rituals they put you through, is that you have to sign for the formula. You have to authorise that your baby is about to be fed formula. So there you are authorising that the baby is being fed formula and naturally of course, you feel as though, you are an utter failure; I mean the whole process of the private ritual of having to, I mean, it was almost like being, ah I'm being very sarcastic when I say this, but I really feel I must say this because there must be a few points made about this – it really felt like you were authorising dieldrin to be given to your baby or 245T [one of the two active ingredients in 'Agent Orange']. They might as well have been suggesting that you were going to give the baby poison so that they might as well as have had a disclaimer at the bottom, 'We hereby refuse any responsibility for having given this baby perfectly tested formula feed'. I mean, you know, you had to sign off the number of mls, the kind of formula, and this went on for every formula feed that you wanted to give the baby ... So, no doubt if something went wrong with the baby, given our litigious climate, they could then point to this chart as evidence of their fiscal and corporate responsibility ...

And [second midwife's name] brought me the paw paw ointment, snuk down to the pharmacy and got the paw paw ointment irrespective of the fact that there she is saying we're not permitted to. And she was having, her eyes were darting everywhere. She was clearly having the greatest difficulty in looking at me, and saying it; and she was the one of course who brought me the chart and said 'We'll get you a formula feed' and I'm weeping and saying 'the baby', and 'the antibodies' and God knows what. She's patting me on the hand like a mother, and saying 'One little feed doesn't matter', but she's saying it quietly, she's not going to go out in the middle of the hall and say 'Go and get a formula feed immediately!' So I mean, she was struggling and it was evident in her body language. And of course when I announced to her that I had gone onto formula feed, she beamed and said 'Well dear, you gave it your best shot and after all, you know bubby (she always called it bubby) bubby is thriving, you've got a healthy baby. And mumma's milk is lovely but sometimes it can't be done and it's perfectly all right' and with that she said, knowing that she was on safe ground 'My two were bottle fed and they're beautiful – beautifully happy'. So she was released from the mouth guard and permitted to make statements and joining with me as a mother herself.

Not valuing individuals

Valuing the individual means that the person is important, has rights, and deserves respect. S/he needs to be heard, and should be listened to, and actively communicated with by the practitioner. Both mothers and midwives articulate their distress and disapproval whenever childbirth practices do not reflect a valuing of the individual. Often these are procedure-oriented practices and practitioners, or those seen by mothers and midwives to be universal-theory and 'campaign' driven, not practical or based on individual needs.

Megan, a mother, refers to the approach of pro-breastfeeding midwives and lactation specialists working within the hospital. Again, the medicalisation of childbirth is confirmed to some extent by the language Megan uses.

Megan: I think the fact that their opinions and their beliefs overstepped or overshadowed their nursing. They forgot about looking after the patient and perhaps that was because they were just so adamant as to the way it should be done that they forgot to look at the patient as an individual ...

Faye: The individual?

Megan: Yeah, the individual is forgotten in the pursuit of the 'breast is best' campaign.

Much of Brenda's story focuses on the lack of respect and valuing of individuals; the obstetric/medicalised view of birth is that of 'physiological event' and the outcome is defined in terms of neonatal/maternal mortality. The ethically adequate response is that of the midwife who maintained a continuity of relationship from the birth, and showed features of a 'being with' woman approach to practice.

Brenda: Then probably a couple of hours after that we went back to the ward and in my after-care no one even looked at me down there, you know? Like no one, the doctor just poked his head in and said 'Everything OK?' and I've gone 'Yeah' and when that really nice midwife came on, that's the first one that I had, and she came and I said 'Look no one's really had a look. What's wrong? Because I, is it right, is anything wrong?' and she said 'Well, let's have a look'. And she said 'Nope, you're totally fine', but I was really concerned then that the obstetrician even didn't want to see. Before that, everyone wanted to stick their fingers there and now no one wants to even tell me I'm OK! [and later] I haven't actually sat down and thought about it, like I said I haven't really spoken to anyone about it before.

Faye: How do you feel now that you have?

Brenda: I feel really good! [both Brenda and Faye laugh] I'm being a whinger although I just I feel like [pause] yeah, not that you're thinking of me as being really weird, but the things that I've bought up probably only matter to me and to someone else they'd be trivial.

Faye: Did you get the feeling that your wishes were being trivialised?

Brenda: Yeah, yeah, exactly.

Brenda's comments again prompt the question of what something must look like for it to qualify as a serious moral concern while others do not. Ethical concerns as defined by the non-expert appear be of less importance to the professional than ethical 'issues' and dilemmas defined by the 'so-called' experts, theorists and ethicists.

Examples from midwives, of practices and practitioners not valuing individuals, are discussed earlier in relation to paternalism and power 'over'. Narratives from Diane and Kerry-Anne in particular, about not respecting the woman's wishes, and treating the woman like a mere body, typify this criticism.

Emotions/feelings

Conflicts of values are usually expressed as feelings or emotions. These mothers and midwives have a broad range of emotional/feeling responses to values conflict including sad, confronted, awful, bad, relieved, frustration, embarrassed, angry, and betrayed. An implication of this wide range is that an adequate ethical response and theory for midwifery ought to include, not exclude consideration of emotions and feelings as an important part of decision-making and practice. They are essential aspects of ethical deliberation.

Katie, the independently practising midwife, expresses her concern about informed choice for women, and women making responsible decisions:

I just felt enormous frustration because I don't know what the 'right' answer is. I worry that I honour and respect her ability to decide or not to decide, to plot her own course.

Emotions and feelings are in response to an undesirable or ethically inadequate experience and are usually followed by the description of what the desirable or ethically adequate response might have been. A common conflict eliciting such emotions is when workplace or service provider ethics are at variance with their own personal values. This supports the claim that, for these mothers and midwives at least, mainstream childbirth practices which are not inclusive of context and relationship are ethically inadequate for midwifery.

Two narratives from mothers, Kay and Caroline, typify emotions relating to a medical intervention.

Kay: I think the relationship the obstetrician and pregnant women have and their husbands, that can often, can leave it wide open to blame because you hand so much over to them, so much reliance on them.

Faye: Did you therefore feel betrayed by the obstetrician?

Kay: Oh absolutely [spoken spontaneously]. Yes, I was advised a little while later that she had had five caesareans herself. I feel absolutely betrayed especially with during the care that she gave me through my pregnancy, I was communicating to her that I was wanting natural childbirth. I feel as though she never had any intention.

Faye: Did you feel betrayed by the midwives in the hospital?

Kay: Oh I think I saw them as being fairly powerless people.

Faye: Certainly not an ally?

Kay: No [spoken definitely]. No it was not communicated to me at all in hospital.

Faye: Was [midwife's name] an ally?

Kay: Absolutely [spoken spontaneously and definitely]. Absolutely. Loyal, loyal.

Caroline: And I was disappointed because I didn't really want any interference with this labour and you know that to me, I mean it's probably not an ethical issue with regards to midwifery but it [pause] and it's probably not really my choice either I don't know, whether to allow the labour to go naturally or – at that stage there didn't seem to be any risk or harm to the baby in my eyes, I don't know about what the midwives thought, and I just thought well I would have just loved for it to keep going.

Diane, a midwife, talking about the woman expressing a desire to not have a certain intervention and then suffering severe complications from an episiotomy, says:

But afterwards I felt very bad that maybe I hadn't said something

Kerry-Anne, a midwife, describes her feelings in relation to the woman whose obstetrician sutured what Kerry-Anne believed was an intact perineum, and how she was 'silenced':

[The mother-midwife relationship] sort of ended I'd say. I didn't follow through. I didn't visit her in the wards and maybe I should've but I just felt so bad about it that I couldn't bring myself to even go and see her again. And I've never heard from her since. I can't even remember her name. I just remember very much the incident, and the disappointment – for her and myself.

Other examples of conflict expressed as emotions and feelings are:

Bev, midwife: And I felt really terrible [spoken slowly] that first of all that I had doubted myself ... and at the time I think responding very much like a traditional hospital-based midwife, where medical authority just goes ... But that was very, very confronting for me and I know she would NOT have had that induction if I hadn't said do it.

Ruth, midwife: Yes, but that is that conflict thing isn't it, that I spoke about, in terms of the doctor who came in and did the chinning of the baby's head and hurt that woman and I felt like a participant to abuse and that's what spun me off out into the community work. But, I didn't address that at the time. And that to me was a real ethical dilemma: that was all about not being honest and not being authentic and not – I didn't speak to the doctor about that after because I was too disempowered in myself. I didn't feel able to do those things. All I did was feel awful. And felt just so sad for that woman.

Ellie feels angry towards mainstream hospital protocols and practices, about her experience of breastfeeding. Her comments also demonstrate her conflict of values with institutional values, those of the service provider.

Faye: It also leaves you angry obviously.

Ellie: Very angry because this emotion lost in guilt and anguish and terror of my baby's mouth was unnecessary. It was unnecessary! Absolutely unnecessary. I can understand it if giving birth is a new discipline but I mean this is not the latest in HIV therapy and which we're all going to practice on the first group of human guineapigs. I mean this is something that's been going on that they've known about, they know this.

Emotions link personal values to the social construct of justice and, in this way, communicate our conflict and congruence of values. Personal values are composed of cognitive beliefs and emotions. They constitute identity and help build a moral vocabulary for evaluating ourselves and others. A desired state of affairs is relevant to one's moral agency and integrity as well as to one's collective life, therefore personal values both imply and reveal evaluation of the self. Justice as a relational concept refers to social positions that afford privileges to some and not others. Justice originates in the embodied lives of real people, not abstractions, and is not independent of the embedded values at stake. Emotions are a response more than a motivation, thus they are not private subjective states, but responses to social situations. Knowing or being open to the social position and lived-meaning of others seems to be an important requirement for justice. Distributive justice focuses on material goods taking institutions and practices as given, but oppression exists in systematic institutional processes. Those emotions that structure or inform personal values in such a way that one recognizes and acknowledges the social conditions that prevent self-enhancement and that motivate one to work toward their elimination are consistent with justice (Liaschenko 1999).

SUMMARY

Personal narratives resonate with the feminist argument that the powerful and public sphere relegates women's concerns to the disempowered and private sphere.

These mothers and midwives also indicate that normative, values-and-context-free, problem-solving bioethics are inadequate for midwifery practice. Rather than an 'ethic of strangers', mothers and midwives desire and

engage in practices characteristic of the 'ethics of intimates'.

Women in both groups disapprove of power being used to patronise the woman, belittle and silence the critic, or punish those who did not conform to institutional rules and protocols. Disparate relationships for the midwife and a mother-midwife relationship of 'separateness' are more typically identified in narratives concerning hospital midwives.

For these mothers and midwives the concept of 'safety' is broader than the bioethical definition which is based on mortality and morbidity. They want to minimise or eliminate the emphasis on 'fear' and focus positively on the woman's body and ability to birth her baby 'naturally' in most situations. They interpret safety as including more than mortality and morbidity: the woman's comfort and sense of security in a professional-friendship determines how 'well' a woman births. What is 'good' for the woman is considered most frequently to be 'good' for her baby. Feeling 'safe' includes the freedom to birth in an environment that welcomes inclusion of family, and meets spiritual and cultural needs.

'Values-conflict between workplace or service provider ethics and personal/professional ethics' and power 'over' practices are the most commonly intersecting themes. A range of emotions and feelings are manifest when this conflict occurs. Participants said they felt bad, sad, awful, angry and embarrassed. For these participants, beliefs and values are embedded in their social, cultural and historical contexts, and are integral to their ethical deliberation on situations. Personal values and emotions constitute mothers' and midwives' embodied identity, and are a means of evaluating themselves and others as worthy of praise or blame. Several narratives depict the birthing woman in the naughty schoolgirl role, with the midwife or doctor as the harsh schoolteacher. Punishment and 'taking control' of the woman and/or midwife precipitates negative feelings and emotions.

REFERENCES

Anderson T 2000 Feeling safe enough to let go: the relationship between a woman and her midwife during the second stage of labour. In: Kirkham M (ed) The midwife-mother relationship. Macmillan, Basingstoke, pp. 92-119

Beauchamp T L, Childress J F 1994 Principles of biomedical ethics. Oxford University Press, New York

Brown J M, Kitson A L, McKnight T J 1992 Challenges in caring: explorations in nursing and ethics. Chapman & Hall, London

Churchill H, Benbow A 2000 Informed choice in maternity services. British Journal of Midwifery 8 (1): 41-47

Clarke R A 1995 Midwives, their employers and the UKCC: an eternally unethical triangle. Nursing Ethics: An International Journal for Healthcare Professionals 2 (3): pp. 247-253

Fleming V E M 1998 Autonomous or automations? An exploration through history of the concept of autonomy in midwifery in Scotland and New Zealand. Nursing Ethics: An International Journal for healthcare Professionals 5 (1): 43-51

Kirkham M 1986 A feminist perspective in midwifery. In: Webb C (ed) Feminist practice in women's healthcare. John Wiley & Sons, Chichester

Liaschenko J 1999 Can justice coexist with the supremacy of personal values in nursing practice? Western Journal of Nursing Research 21: 35

May R 1972 The meaning of power. In: Power and innocence. Souvenir Press, New York

Rothman B K 1991 In labor: women and power in the birthplace. W W Norton, New York

8

Going to a comfortable place – the ethical voice of mothers and midwives

Whereas both mothers and midwives express dissatisfaction with institutional dominance over childbirth, they speak positively about concepts that constituted 'being with' woman during childbirth. This shared meaning between mothers and midwives, of a woman-centred approach, is constructed from themes identified in their narratives (Thompson 2001).

'BEING WITH' WOMAN

'Being with' woman means that birth practices are woman-centred – not from a gender-only point of view, but from a contextual and 'woman's meaning' sense. Ethical practice with such an orientation ('way of seeing') is relationship-based, expressive of values and virtues rather than normative theory or universal principlism. 'Being with' woman reflects the broader sense of encompassed themes such as 'values-virtues', 'supporting the woman', 'knowing the woman', and 'woman's comfort'. Narratives give almost equal prominence yet distinction to these: that is, all themes are important for ethical midwifery practice but each portrays distinct meaning.

'Values-virtues' occurs when mothers and midwives experience a congruence of values such as respect, trust, valuing individuals, self-pride, confidence, honesty, empathy and character of practitioner. 'Supporting the woman' involves the midwife having her/his prime relationship with woman (including advocacy), 'being with' not 'doing to' the woman, infor-

med choice, communication and time to talk, and power 'for' and 'with' relationships. 'Knowing the woman' requires a relationship based on human engagement where the midwife is an expert-friend, and fulfils a family-social role including follow-up contact. The 'woman's comfort' relates not only to the physical condition of the birthing woman but also to her mental and emotional security: she feels comfortable and secure ('safe' for the woman).

Values-virtues

Virtues and personal character such as those described by Aristotle and more recently, feminist writers (Tong 1993), emerge as a major theme for both mothers and midwives when relating the importance of 'being with' the childbearing woman. Values and virtues refer to both the practitioner's character and his/her approach to practice. For some mothers and midwives, the birthing woman's character is also important for being able to 'connect' with that of the practitioner.

Trust, respect, valuing individuals

Attributes such as trust (and trustworthiness), respect (for persons and ability or expertise, and valuing the individual), confidence, empathy, self-pride and honesty are crucial concepts for both mothers and midwives, in relation to the desired character and approach of the practitioner. Trust comes with a certain kind of relationship, and relationships develop over time and across emotional as well as physical experiences.

Arline, who birthed in a birthing centre, says:

No, no I wouldn't just expect it no. I think that comes from the fact that I had already formed a relationship with her. The fact that I had birthed our first child and she was our midwife and just through all the antenatal care I respected her professionalism, I respected her as a midwife and I'm sure she respected me as a person and as a mother that was able to birth. So yeah I think that's how I come to know that I respect her judgement because I trust her and that's because I had formed a relationship with her which is the key, for me anyway.

Caroline, another mother, views trust from a different perspective. She birthed in a traditional hospital ward setting and although she too refers to the expertise of the practitioner, she implies a more passive role for herself. This is not uncommon for women birthing in mainstream maternity facilities (Kirkham 1986).

Caroline: They've had the medical training to know how a labour, like a text book labour I suppose, would progress; when there should be interference, when there shouldn't be interference and so forth. So I would trust them to know what is right and what is wrong even if I myself think I don't think that's right. I would still, like I said, trust them to know what's the best sort of thing.

Faye: And is respect important?

Caroline: Oh definitely. I mean it's no good going into labour and you've told them how you would like the labour to progress and how it's what you want and what you don't want, and then there's totally the opposite. I would probably feel quite distressed by it actually. I'd be putting my trust in them and they weren't doing as I'd asked. So yeah, respecting my wishes I find, and definitely they're showing they care by doing that.

To this extent, the midwives' respect for the birthing woman is more important for Caroline than mutual respect.

For a midwife to respect a woman who's in labour and what they want, or what they need, is probably the most important thing in the labour. When a woman is in labour she actually doesn't know half of what's going on around her, she's probably not really in control of her emotions, feelings, anything really and to have that respect is probably the only real tangible form of being in control of what's happening.

As a 'new' and first-time mother with very sore nipples and painful breasts, Maree considers respect for, and valuing, the individual are essential values and virtues.

Maree: I think what is important is that they respected that I was in pain and they respected that I would have a view on what was comfortable for me even in terms of positioning the baby. Well the whole thing, they were just very respectful of the fact and [pause] I mean my definition of ethics is if they did something morally wrong or morally right, and 'morally right' to me was that they really considered me and what was the best for me and.

Faye: As an individual?

Maree: As an individual [spoken definitely] and as a new mother, and really appreciated how uncomfortable I was and how new it all was to me and [pause] took charge of the situation in a cooperative fashion which I thought was very good, because I needed their advice but I didn't want them to take over and I thought they were just excellent.

Regardless of whether the midwife is practising in a birth centre, a mainstream hospital ward or an independent community-based midwifery service, as long as the practitioner's orientation is 'being with' woman she considers trust, respect and the valuing of individuals essential ethical features of the mother-midwife relationship.

Katie, an independently practising midwife, recalls a conversation with one of her clients:

I said 'For me this antenatal process is yes, to check the baby, check the blood pressure, those sorts of things. Yeah give you information, but for me the process of antenatal care is to form a relationship with you so that there's trust, there's understanding, there's respect, there's strength in a relationship'.

Diane, a midwife in a birth centre, believes that:

Diane: Women get to trust themselves more when their carer is able to work with them through a process ... we can't always stay for the whole birth if they have a long labour, but the women will trust that – over here we all have the same philosophy of care and they know that.

Faye: Is trust important?

Diane: Oh, I think it's essential. And I think it's a

mutual trust in a way. That the woman knows that you will try and do the best for her and there's a trust there that we know the women are doing the work and they're angling to get as much out the birth as they can, for their sake. It's a huge mutual respect.

Talking with the practitioner occurs when the mother trusts the practitioner and when the mother-midwife relationship enables them to get to know each other. It does not occur when the mother does not trust the practitioner:

Brenda, mother: And this anaesthetist has come in and has gone WELL GIRLIE, and I've gone 'girlie'? Do whatever you like then, but leave me alone. I'm not talking to you, do you know what I mean? Girlie!!

This 'talking with' is related to having 'time to talk', communication, and informed choice, important conceptual components of 'supporting the childbearing woman'.

Kerry-Anne's story from her mainstream hospital practice days, prior to practising in the birth centre, is another example of the expressed importance of trust, 'talking with' and 'time to talk' within the mother-midwife relationship. Trust occurs within relationships and relationships develop over time.

She was in labour and we actually had time before she was in strong labour to talk about her expectations and what she wanted for the birth. So I felt that she trusted me and that we had quite a good relationship after such a short time of getting to know each other.

[and then] I think the 'trust' thing is something that is developed over a period of time rather than right there at the time. So the 'trust' starts early and that's where that if someone is going privately to a doctor and they're seeing him every time, I think that's when the trust builds up. Whereas I think the midwives in the labour ward don't have time to build the trust, but they do 'rely' on the midwife to get the doctor there in time.

Trust and reliance are separate concepts for both the mothers and midwives. Typically, mothers with private obstetricians rely on hospital midwives to notify their doctor in time for her/him to be there for the birth, a point raised earlier by Kerry-Anne in relation to hospital labour ward midwives. Judy, a mother, also thinks that the midwives do not expect or in

some instances want, the doctor to arrive too soon prior to the birth. The doctor's specific role is to arrive at the time of actual birthing. She is not happy that they nearly did not get him there in time:

The nurses all ran in and took me over to the labour ward and I was quite happy with the, from then on, the midwives. The doctor didn't come in, they didn't feel they needed to ring him

[later] Yep, first baby. And oh that's right they hadn't rung the obstetrician by this stage, so they thought oh we better ring him quickly, so they rang and he had left home, he wasn't at home and then just by chance as soon as they hung the phone up he was actually coming in to do a caesarean, so he said 'Oh Judy's actually in here' and poked his head around the corner and it was all action. So it was just lucky that he'd come in, so he was there.

Another example of the importance of trust for the birthing woman comes from Caroline. Her comments indicate a trust in the doctor with a mortality inference; something more like reliance and personal care is expected of midwives.

I would have complete trust in him, my gynaecologist, and what he said went. Don't know why – that's just the way I felt ...Then I was ready to push ... and they said 'Oh yeah, all right you can have a go at it'. One push, the head was crowned and I was thinking where's that doctor, get the doctor here quick. [spoken 'urgently'/anxiously] ...Yeah having my own doctor and one that I knew throughout the pregnancy [and the previous pregnancy] and I had I suppose a good rapport with [doctor's name]. Yes that made a difference. The fact that they did as we told them to do. They probably did know that I had that respect for [doctor's name] by the way I spoke about him. Things like that and I was tickled pink that he was going to be there for the birth. That's probably why they were so panicky when I started pushing and he wasn't there, and they were telling me to stop, wait for [doctor's name]. 'Cause they'd been on the whole shift so they knew. Just talking to the midwife when you're in labour they just know what you need and what you want. They understand how you feel about things, what to say, and what your husband feels and you're totally out of it and your husband's telling them not to do something and things like that.

Mothers build up trust in their obstetricians over a period of time during their antenatal visits. Of equal importance to some of them, however, is the fact that they are paying for the services of that obstetrician and expect that s/he will be there if s/he cares about them. This suggests that contractual ethics (Thompson, Melia & Boyd 1994) is at least a part of the mother-doctor relationship:

But I think it's just because you're in private health and you go in and see this obstetrician the whole time you sort of think, like you still have to pay. I had to pay my doctor for the delivery and no one was there for the delivery and when someone turned up it wasn't even him. So that sort of irked me a bit so I guess I'm always thinking in the back of my mind, I've paid, I'm going to pay this man, he should be there and take an interest. Even though I know they're entitled to their weekends as well. (Judy)

Brenda speaks of her concern that no one had called for the doctor:

Brenda: The midwife said to me afterwards that I probably would have had an episiotomy because I had a small tear, if the doctor had have been there when she was actually delivered, so it was a good thing that he wasn't there, but what if something had've gone wrong. No one said to me, 'We'll get the doctor here'. They waited until she was actually born before they even buzzed him. So I realise that that's a good thing, but who stands where on an issue like that? It's just, I'm not really sure you know?

Faye: How did it make you feel? First of all.

Brenda: Not particularly secure.

When she reviewed the transcript interpretation of 'mother would have preferred that the doctor was present for [mortality-morbidity] safety' Brenda added:

because he was supposed to provide a service!

Self-pride

The value or virtue of 'self-pride', of being proud of one's achievement, is shared by mothers and midwives alike. It is both a value and a virtue that results from 'being with' woman during the childbirth experience. Mothers tend to infer it while midwives more often articulate it. Midwives refer to not only the birthing woman's pride in herself, and the midwife's pride in the woman's achievement, but also to the midwife's pride in her own achievement; that is, pride in her own midwifery expertise and practice. Bev talks about a satisfying experience of birth in one of her later narratives.

I think it was largely about her having a birth plan and being very clear about that. There were no doctors around there, only the night duty midwives. The charge nurse wasn't there, there was no drama, everything was quiet and low key, and it felt really satisfying – for all of us. And they were delighted with their baby and I was delighted with the whole outcome. And it's not often I think that you see a 14-year-old girl feeling empowered in labour but she did ... Well it was 'good' because she had the kind of birth she wanted to have and she was in control of what was happening. And she was supported to allow her to do it the way she wanted to. And that seemed really 'good' to me because so many women want so much less than they hope for. Experiences they try to forget because they've been so awful. Whereas this experience was one that she'll look back on with pride.

Ann says:

And those midwives are just absolutely over the moon because they have been able to have this baby without stitches and things like that, and it's incredible to see the look on their faces 'that we did that without stitches' or 'we did that before he finished scrubbing'. There is that pride there, but not enough have it, not enough midwives have it.

An example of the woman's self-pride in her birthing achievements is seen in Gemma's narrative, derived from a very different environment. Her comments also demonstrate the link between 'birthing well' and the midwife's prime relationship being with the woman.

To me, 'good' in that situation is good for the woman and good for her baby but basically what I believe is that whatever is good for the woman is usually good for her baby. I mean there may be some very rare cases where women don't consider the good of their baby and certainly in those circumstances [the aboriginal women who chose to 'abscond' from the mainland] the women were charged with not taking the good of their baby into account. Whereas I felt that that wasn't so; that in fact these women because they came back home to birth in an environment that they felt supported and safe in – that was the best thing, that was a 'good' thing that they could do for their baby. That was a way that they could birth, as I say, 'birth well' and birthing well is for them to feel satisfied with their experience, to feel that they've done a good job, that they are proud of how they've birthed, their ability to birth, the way they've produced their little baby and all that sort of thing.

And from mothers:

Arline: Oh I felt fantastic [spoken spontaneously and definitely, tone of amazement]. I mean it's yeah, I feel really proud of myself. It's like I feel like I really accomplished something you know, sort of like as well as being a physical and mental thing it's very much a spiritual thing particularly with the birth of [second baby's name] because it was just such a nice birth you know

Brenda: To me it's important because this is me, this isn't pretend, this is real. This is something I'm going to have to, I'm going to live with ... mmm. Yeah [baby's name] was already born and yeah the doctor missed it totally and then I thought, he's going to charge me for this now, and he wasn't even here. I've done it all myself, look, aren't I good?

Caroline: And [second baby's name] she was born, they handed her to me, it wasn't a doctor that got her first, it was me [spoken in a pleased voice] and I was just in tears, I was just bawling. It was just such a lovely feeling, you did it by yourself [last word spoken with emphasis] sort of thing, I didn't have to have suction caps to pull her out and things like that, and I was just so proud of myself [spoken more calmly] and it was great and I breastfed her straight away and she sucked for half an hour on the first side, I was just tickled pink. I was just so euphorious over the whole thing, it was probably, yeah, the fact that there was no outside interference. I didn't have any pain relief whatsoever, although I did use the gas, that's right, I used the gas towards the end and I got it right and [pause] yeah I was just so proud of myself, I thought, this is the way it should be.

Diane, midwife, describes a mother's birthing experience:

Well, third time round, having experienced epidurals and having experienced birth without an epidural and it was once again a long hard one but she did it, and she was proud of herself doing it.

Acknowledging the woman's achievements is an important part of ethical practice. Kerry-Anne compares differing approaches of practitioners.

Even after the birth he didn't comfort her or say to her anything about like 'you did a good job' or anything, that every woman needs to be said to her

after she's given birth.

I've had some other lovely private doctors who have been just absolutely wonderful with the women and then after the birth give them a hug and a kiss and say you did a wonderful job and make that woman feel very powerful about what she's done.

Confidence

Megan describes her first few days of breast-feeding her first baby in a mainstream hospital situation as 'just very difficult'. For her, confidence is a more appropriate concept than 'trust' in the mother-midwife relationship, and in a broader sense the character or personality of the person, the individual practitioner and mother, is very important for ethical practice:

Well, I guess it comes back to that midwife I was talking about. I had confidence in her because of perhaps, maybe it's because of her personality. Maybe it was her, she was the sort of person who I felt I could maybe trust, not so much trust, but her opinion meant more to me than some of the others, and maybe that's just a personal thing.

Katie, an independent midwifery practitioner, also has reservations about using the term 'trust' for the mother-midwife relationship. She discourages the concept:

No, no, it's not trust. It's not trust so much. I respect their rights to make their own decision and that sometimes 'they're' going to think that they made the right decision and sometimes 'they're' going to think that they made the wrong decision. 'Cos we do. We make decisions in life, personal decisions, and sometimes they're right and sometimes they're wrong. So it's not a matter of trust, like I trust the woman to make the right decision. I respect her right to make her own decision.

And, in response to the researcher's question of whether woman-centred practice involved a mutual trust:

Oh absolutely. I expect them to make their own decisions! Do I trust them that they will make the decision? Yes, mostly.

Katie's belief in 'sometimes we make good decisions and sometimes we make bad decisions in life', is shared by Diane, a midwife in a birth centre. Diane discusses this in terms of coming to a Y-junction, a journey metaphor, and making a decision given the information one has at the time.

Kay, whose birth attendant at her second birth was an independent midwifery practitioner, also questions the use of the term trust. Whilst she has trust in a midwife and links the concept of trust with the expertise and character of certain practitioners, she sees trust as an inappropriate concept for the woman to have of herself given that she would never 'distrust' herself. Like Megan, Kay believes that 'confidence' more aptly describes the value-virtue needed in the childbearing woman.

Faye: Is trust important?

Kay: Absolutely [spoken spontaneously and definitely]. You're asking for them to care for you, [pause] to help you towards a safe delivery of your baby, because at that point you become incredibly vulnerable, you've got to trust them. You've got to be able to develop a relationship so you can trust them so when you're in that period of well the total pregnancy but more so in established labour and actual childbirth, you've got to have someone there as a strong advocate that you can trust to probably increase the level of care as you're going through that birth process because it is such a focused event for you. You need to have those people around you that yeah, you can trust, to [pause] just help you achieve that – make any decisions that may be necessary.

So I would not put my trust in all midwives, no I don't blanket them all as experts ... but I don't feel real comfortable I suppose about using that term 'trust' – I don't think I would ever distrust myself. I see it more as a matter of having that trust in a midwife gives me confidence ... that is sort of one area also that [midwife's name] possibly and in some ways, oh I don't know if it's the right word, but maybe nearly discouraged an over amount of trust in her. She was sort of quite clear what her limitations were. She is probably a good example of very ethical behaviour. Do you get what I mean?

Character of person, including honesty and empathy

Character is a major determinant in the midwife's approach and, therefore, the woman's confidence in herself and the midwife. Mothers in particular articulate the importance of the practitioner's character in influencing the mother-midwife relationship because it directly impacts on the woman's confidence, especially the new mother's confidence in her ability to birth, feed and care for her baby. These concepts are identified in Megan's narrative when she discusses her experience of breastfeeding as a new mother.

Faye: Do you think that they sort of unwittingly reinforce your weaknesses rather than nurture your strengths?

Megan: Well, I don't know that they would have reinforced it. I think that if you were a different sort of person it would be easy to have that done. Like 'oh well, maybe I am meant to stay in bed for a few days, or rest more'.

[and]

She was pretty down to earth and no fuss or anything, you know. Just do it in your own time. And so then I guess that then inspires confidence in someone. Rather than some of the others who were not only adamant about the breastfeeding but a bit more gushy and fussy and over the top. But she was the sort of person that, maybe that's where the individual comes into it as well but yeah, I think confidence is very important, particularly for new mothers.

Maree, another mother, explains the importance, for her, of the character of both practitioner and mother, and the reciprocal nature of the concept of confidence.

Maree: You have confidence in some people but you have confidence in them because they've given you confidence. They have showed you [pause] that you, [pause] their whole manner has been what's worked for you and you know that their manner is consistent, it's always the same and it's what you want. So that I think that's why you have confidence in the person and then if somebody else comes in who has a totally different philosophy on how to manage someone or it's just a job or I've just got to do my eight hour shift and leave, and you straight away pick it up.

Faye: Is respect important?

Maree: Oh very [spoken spontaneously and definitely]. I think that's the one thing – respect, compassion and empathy, I think are the three important.

Faye: And you mentioned confidence?

Maree: And confidence, well that's right, yeah.

Faye: Is that the same as relying on someone?

Maree: I think it is, in a sense. Someone can be confident but [pause] not pushy with that confidence. Someone else can be confident and quietly assertive and cooperative, whereas someone else can be very confident, very brash with that confidence and totally non-cooperative because they're 'right', and I think it's that lovely mix of compassion, empathy and respect – confidence in what you're doing, professional ability, competence. All of those things that make up the perfect sort of midwife.

Kay's lasting impression is the difference in relationships between her two births, and the importance of 'knowing' the woman and 'knowing' the midwife. The mother-midwife relationship with the hospital midwives is portrayed as one of separateness whereas the relationship with the independent midwife is one of 'being with' the woman.

I think I got the feeling from the midwives in the hospital setting that they felt as detached from me as I was from them! [spoken slowly and thoughtfully] I mean they were pleasant enough and trying to be helpful but [pause] mmm I don't know that they displayed empathy in a personal way, maybe in a generalised way like 'Oh yes you're pregnant and you're going to go through labour now', but sort of not in a personal sense, no. [The independent midwife's name] probably displayed that with possibly referring to – probably my relationship with [husband's name] or involving him in some way or yeah, and how, 'What can I do to make you happy Kay?' And just having an understanding of my whole family and understanding the things that I'd talked about through the pregnancy, bringing those back 'And you said you liked this, and you don't like that.'

Again, from Maree, the character of the practitioner and 'knowing' the person is very important in determining the approach to practice and the type of relationship that occurs between the mother and midwife. Maree says about one midwife:

she just knew exactly how to, she just had a lovely nature ...

Practice that lacks these concepts of trust, respect, and valuing individuals within rela-

tionship is an inadequate ethical response for midwifery practice.

Supporting the woman

Supporting the birthing woman means providing (i) informed choice (self-determination, not just consent) and communication (time to talk 'with'), (ii) a midwife whose prime relationship is with the woman and who will 'be with' not 'do to' her (including concepts of midwife's presence, and birth journey), and (iii) a power 'with-for' relationship (including advocacy). Examples of such support are given by both mothers and midwives.

Arline explains how the birth centre midwife supported her emotionally, psychologically and practically while at the same time helping her to maintain the central and active role, her self-determination, in the birthing process – a power 'with' mother-midwife relationship:

And I guess the important part of the second stage was that [pause] 'cause I did have a fear, we had discussed my anxiety about tearing, I didn't want to tear, and so [midwife's name] was very good in talking me through, and she had the mirror there so I could see what was happening, she talked me through because my body just wants to expel, like I don't have to push at all. If anything I have to sort of hold it there. So she talked me through that so that I was able to hold his head there for one or I'm not sure how many contractions just to let the perineum stretch a little bit, so that I didn't tear. She was very conscious of the fact that I didn't want to tear and so she did that.

Brenda says:

When I opened my eyes up again after I'd been through this contraction she [first midwife] was there, she was patting my hand, she was just really like your Mum. You know like, 'That was really good dear, you did well'. And it wasn't oh that was three minutes or they're coming every three minutes. When they strapped me up, you know how when they do the epidural and they put the thing around your tummy and the lady [second midwife] said to [husband's name], she's having a contraction now and I was sitting there and going 'SHE'? I'm sitting right here, why can't, and I've just gone oh no whatever, you know, just get on with it, type of thing. So it was totally different. But no I didn't feel like she [first midwife] wasn't caring or she was lax because she was more gentle in her approach. I felt that was more, maybe it was experience too. Maybe because she was older, I don't know, but I just felt really, really comfortable with her. I'd seek her out again.

Ann, a mainstream hospital midwife, says:

I believe that's probably what is good – the person that makes that person feel that they can do it, that gives them the support and energy to get through the labour.

Diane considers that supporting the woman entails a total approach, including the environment:

I think it's much more relaxed here [than traditional birth suites or labour wards]. It's a much more intimate setting and it's probably a lot easier for women to ask the sort of questions that they need to ask and to expose themselves to more of their fears so that they can be more confident by the time they get to birth the baby. It's very important that women are confident in their body's ability to do the task. There's a big mind body connection. A huge one and the more I see women over here the more I see that. So that they have to be able to 'give in' to the process and let it happen or it can go wild ... well certainly I talk to a woman in early labour if I can [pause] and try to give her the confidence to stay at home until I believe that she's at that stage in her labour where she's able to stay home ... I think we're all trying to foster the woman's independence.

Gemma experienced conflict between the 'workplace ethics' and her personal-professional desire to support the woman:

When they [Australian indigenous women of the area] came back on the island of course they would often just 'go to ground' till they were almost ready to have their babies and they'd turn up on the clinic doorstep in the middle of the night and produce their babies – usually quite well without any problems and I guess that to me was a real difficulty because I personally I had a problem with sending these women back all the time over to the mainland when I knew that that's not where they wanted to be and there were really no suitable mechanisms in place to support them over on the mainland ... I mean basically if they came in and had their babies we just supported them and usually they do it very well with no problems and so it was – we didn't say much to them at all. In fact often we were quite delighted with them because they, I guess in a way there was this secret admiration because that they had the fortitude to 'buck the system'.

Utilising a power 'with' approach commonly intersects with 'supporting the woman' and 'midwife's prime relationship is with the woman'. Maree describes the positive nature of the mother-midwife relationship she had with midwives who helped her with breast engorgement and breastfeeding:

But in particular there were two midwives who I just think were the best thing since sliced bread. Both of them were young, neither of them were married or had children and they were just so, their whole approach, their whole manner was just [pause] 'teamwork'. 'OK well', and I'd ask them would you give me a hand, the baby needs a feed will you assist me and just check that I'm doing it right? And [pause] it wasn't 'Yeah that's OK', it was 'That's all right yes but sometimes it helps if you try and sit around that, how do you feel now, would you feel more comfortable or is it an idea if we try a football hold' and you know it was sort of let's work out together. Me and the midwives.

Practical assistance of course is also important.

Maree: These nurses who I thought were particularly good, were on the night that my milk came in and I was very sore and the first one said to me 'All right, well I think what might help is if you hop in the shower and just massage' and she went and got me some vegetable oil and heated it up and she actually got into the shower with me and massaged all around the breast, both breasts and said 'Now lean there, relax against the wall', she really talked me through the whole thing to see if we could get a let-down to relieve some of the engorgement.

Kerry-Anne describes the importance of practical assistance in achieving inclusion of family and thereby supporting the birthing woman:

Oh definitely a midwifery model of care, definitely a woman-centred care or even family-centred care. The whole thing is around the family and I say to the partners 'I really cannot do this birth without you there – you are an essential part of the birth process' ... So you can actually start with the massage of her back or her feet or whatever during labour and then you can say 'Would you like to try and do this now?' and then he takes over ... and then when it comes to the time of the birth the simple things like 'Get her to focus on you now while she's actually pushing, and then see this towel, this warm towel, you're going to hand me that when I say towel. And you're going to look at the clock and tell me the time the baby was born and tell me the sex of the baby' ... All those little things, so it's very family-centred ...

Even when we've had siblings at the birth – one time we had the mother in the bath and I walked into the room and the three-year-old was pouring water out of a jug over her mother, over her tummy, and I said 'Oh aren't you a big help' and she said 'Yes, I always do this when ladies are having babies'. It became her role.

We took a photo of her so that she'll never forget that she did that. And that made all the difference to the mother to look up and see the child doing that for her and feeling that she was in a warm, loving environment while she was giving birth to the next child. So when you ask me what model of care it is, it's very much a midwifery model of care. It's not something you're going to see in the traditional labour ward.

Informed choice (freedom of space and self-determination for the mother)

This is a very strong theme throughout the narratives. Mothers expect it for themselves as individual adults, and midwives expect it for mothers as their right (justice ethics), and out of respect for persons (covenantal and relational ethics) (Thompson, Melia & Boyd 1994). The absence of informed choice conflicts with personal values and is an injustice, as discussed earlier in relation to a lack of self-determination and institutional dominance.

Arline, who birthed her baby in a birth centre, praises the midwives for always consulting the woman or her partner before making a decision:

With the birth centre it's totally what you want and I guess one of the differences there is that at the birth centre they don't routinely offer oxytocin, it's a choice and that's something discussed before you actually, so that it would be part of your birth plan whether or not you want the oxytocin in third stage labour. So that's all pre-arranged, but of course if once you've delivered and there is a large blood loss well of course she'll have to say to you at the time 'Well, I really think it might be advisable, you've had a big blood loss, I think it might be advisable even though you said you didn't want it. You know, these are the risks, maybe we should have it', that sort of thing. Which in effect is what had happened to me. I chose not to have the oxytocin the first time with [first baby's name] they said it might be an idea if this time you do have it and I said that's fine to do

that because I was trusting her judgement and obviously she informed me about the risks about why and the large blood loss or whatever, so yeah. So I did have it. And I will have it again this time for the third one.

Another mother, Judy, who birthed in a hospital ward describes the importance of choice. Her comment does not depict the notion of being 'informed' by midwives. Rather, it emphasises choice for the birthing woman and implies respect for that individual's wishes as well as perceived needs:

Faye: How did they react during that birth to those wishes?

Judy: [pause] Positively – as well as, I think, as fully as they could given that there's so many variables, things could've happened. Like I'd said in the birth plan I didn't want to have an epidural, however if I was in a lot of pain and I asked for it, then of course I was happy, I wanted one. And that I didn't want to have an episiotomy, but if I needed it, yes. So they had those things in the back of their minds.

Megan's narrative discusses how 'difficult' it was for her in hospital when she was learning to breastfeed for the first time, and how she was given so much conflicting advice from midwives. She wanted assistance to learn what to do according to her individual needs and those of her baby, but lactation specialists and devotees of breastfeeding were telling her what to do. Her comments imply an element of paternalism from staff, and she considers respect is important:

Megan: For women in that situation. I mean it's not like they're dealing with people who [pause] are too sick to make up their own minds or too sick to be unaware of what's going on. They're dealing with women who are basically pretty well.

In contrast, Maree's narrative illustrates the congruence of values between her and the midwives attending her, with regard to breastfeeding as a 'new' mother. Women need the freedom to not only make their own decisions but to also implement them, and the following comments demonstrate this within the mother-midwife relationship.

I got to a point where they encouraged me to have her in the room, which I did, but I wasn't getting any sleep, and she was actually quite unsettled, and they said to me 'Look, how are you feeling?' I said 'Look, I feel terrible, I just feel I need a decent sleep' and again they said 'Well, what would you like to do? Would you like us to take the baby to the nursery and you can buzz us and we'll bring her back at any time but we can take her down there, we won't give her anything, it'll just give you some time to sleep and we'll bring her back when the feeds are' and I just appreciated all of that, that these people recognising that, look, I need some sleep or I'm going to fall apart. Just lack of sleep at that stage.

Ann, a mainstream hospital midwife, discusses communication and being informed rather than choice *per se*.

I believe ethically that we need to be aware that people do have rights and they have the right to communication, the right to know what's happening, who's looking after them, why they're being looked after, what the decisions are and why those decisions are being made: not 'this is what will happen'. And they have the right to be able to say to someone 'sit down and talk to me about this'.

Bev, a midwife working in the community and caring for a young woman with mental health problems, is distressed herself as she speaks of how she strived to maintain the woman's 'autonomy', knowing that mother and baby would probably be separated by the health authorities:

Bev: But I did it differently than the way it's traditionally done. I said to her [speaking slowly] I mean I'm not using her real name, I said to her 'Tara, that's very serious what you've just told me and the staff need to know; your baby has to be protected. Because although you feel now that you want to kill him, in a month's time or two months' time when the depression's lifted or it wouldn't lift if you'd killed him, and you'd end up in prison. Can I have your permission to tell?' Now, I would've told even if she'd said no. But she didn't. She said yes. And she was – tears were streaming – and I just felt awful.

Faye: Why?

Bev: Well, I mean I felt dreadful because it was so, I mean talk about being in the middle of this human tragedy, God, on a grand scale.

Diane, a midwife in a birthing centre, examines her interaction with the birthing woman. She reflects on what impact the midwife's own motivation has on that interaction and, in so

doing, has strengthened her initial belief in the importance of self-determination for the birthing woman:

Yeah, and so if you get to this point where a woman is distressed and she wants an epidural and you think oh well she may not, she might give birth soon and she might not need it, you still have to respect that that's where she is at the moment.

Kerry-Anne, another midwife working in a birthing centre, speaks of how the bed has become the focal point of a traditional labour ward or birth suite, and this in itself has reduced women's self-determination:

And when I do actually do a transfer [from birthing centre to birth suite] if this woman doesn't need to be lying down on the bed I make her aware that nothing has changed as far as my midwifery care of her; that she can still make a choice as to where she wants to be if everything is going normally. And it's only if she needs a forceps or a vacuum extraction that she needs to be on the bed. That's only just one little thing.

Ruth's beliefs and practices regarding breastfeeding conflict with those of some of her midwifery colleagues. Therefore, her discussion concentrates on how the midwife's own knowledge, practice and decision-making is a major determinant in providing informed choice for the mother:

Well, I think it comes back to knowledge and I think one of the things about knowledge, knowledge is power and you can't do what you don't know about, and I would say that for us as midwives our imperative is to get out and get educated and to really learn as much as we can and to look, look, and look and look and search and research and check things out and I think that comes with the territory and then we can help women by giving them information so that they can make their choices. Because you can't choose what you don't know.

For Katie, a community-based independent midwifery practitioner, informed choice can quickly become or be perceived as coercion, its antithesis:

I mean it's so difficult then to make sure that you discuss it as much as you can discuss it and you can write it and all the rest of it and, and then [pause] even though you feel like it's all gone over her head, you come to a point where you feel like you can do no more, say no more, explain no more, and continue to be supportive of her decision. And sometimes I'm sure they feel pressured by that process of discussion, why you're trying to get, trying to bang their heads and say 'Will you let this bloody bit of information in and just absorb it for a bit and mull it about and then reflect back to me that you've actually understood what I've been talking to you about'. So it's difficult, it's difficult not to be coercive I suppose, and yet we value informed choice, we value women making their own life choices, including the wrong choices, that's their right to make the choice and make mistakes in their personal decision making just like we all do. It's that notion that, you wanted her to make an informed choice, informed choice equals a risk-benefit analysis from her perspective.

Communication

Time to talk, and spending time with the birthing woman, is very much part of communication and self-determination.

Ann, midwife: But I feel it could have been better if there had been a conference with the parents or there had been a discussion take place with those parents … and took time out to actually speak on a one-to-one and sit on a chair face-to-face and spend time going through what was going to happen.

Bev, midwife: When you're really listening to somebody and following their story all the way to the bottom, you feel something of what they're feeling.

Caroline, mother: In the early stages of labour when you're not sort of full-on all the time, the contractions and you're probably more relaxed and you've got more time in between contractions to talk to a woman and things like that, yeah I suppose that does bring the relationship and trust.

Diane: We work with them to teach them.

Faye: And would that be reciprocal?

Diane: Oh [spoken 'absolutely'] I think every one of us working in the birth centre have noticed much, much more about birth and women by working here and being able to spend the time with them.

Gemma, midwife: We just carte blanc assume that they don't either have the knowledge, that they don't care – one of the things I hear bandied around is that most women attending the public system are low IQ anyway so what would they understand if we explain; 'but we did explain it and she didn't

understand', or she didn't listen. Yes, I think perhaps we should spend more time perhaps on communication skills and actually getting to checking out with people what they have understood and where they're at, and what they want to know too. Some women don't want to know, but that should be their choice, not just because they're kept in ignorance.

Judy, mother: It would have been nice if I'd had the same midwife as when I'd arrived at the hospital until I'd delivered. Just because you've already established the relationship, and I think I was more, well you are more coherent in between the contractions. I could talk normally to them as a normal person without being in agony, but then when it gets into second stage, and transition I just found it was [pause] I wasn't myself, so it would've been nice if I'd had the people that I'd had during the contractions stay with me through the delivery as well. Because they'd sort of seen me as a normal person [smiling] rather than this screaming person.

Kerry-Anne, midwife: We bonded very well. I looked after her right from the time when she came in to hospital for the birth. She was in labour, and we actually had time before she was in strong labour to actually talk about her expectations and what she wanted for the birth. So I felt that she trusted me and that we had quite a good relationship after such a short time of getting to know each other.

Katie, midwife: And I had to butt in and say 'Hang on a minute'. I said to the doctor 'She's indicating to you that she agrees but this is actually just her personality. She hasn't considered all of the options and I'd like to talk about some of the alternatives she has to the things that you're suggesting.' So, and then as soon as I said it she said 'Oh I didn't mean yes, I just meant that I've heard you doctor'. So, so now we say things like, 'Say things to the doctor like yes I hear you, I'll need five minutes to consider that, or, yes I hear you, I just need to get Katie's opinion on the same issue' – so they can buy time. You know? We get them 'buying time' strategies, strategies for getting informed consent.

Megan, mother: The second night I was aware that I really needed to get some sleep. But I didn't want [first baby's name] to have a comp feed, and so that was the only way I could go about it. So, I guess, with their suggestions and [pause] talking it through and having sort of been aware of a few different options, that's how that came about.

Prime relationships

Prime relationship is central to woman-centred midwifery practice. That is, the midwife's prime relationship is with the mother, and the mother's prime relationship is with her baby. The emphasis given by these mothers and midwives to prime relationships surrounding childbirth supports the theory that midwifery practice should be based on a partnership model (Guilliland & Pairman 1995).

Midwife's prime relationship is with mother

Megan: I wasn't there to be looked after. I was there to learn how to look after the baby and make sure everything was right with the baby before we went home.

Mothers, and midwives practising within a 'being with' woman relationship, share a common value of birthing as a physical, emotional and spiritual experience; an achievement, not merely a physiological event. The midwife's prime relationship is with the woman. This contrasts with the approach of midwives who are procedure-oriented and practising as dutiful subordinates or technicians to medical authority and their employer: that is, those with disparate relationships. Maree illustrates this when she discusses her relationship with the midwife who attended her during the earlier part of her labour:

Well she [first midwife] certainly, she was very much a patient advocate. She was there for me and to make sure that the whole experience was right for me, regardless of who the doctor was, and then the second two midwives that were involved, I felt that they were there but they weren't a patient advocate. They were there to do what the doctor said and they were more technicians than midwives in the compassionate sense. That's why I think that first midwife all the way through would have said 'Well hang on, we can't get in that, give her some time to get into this position. How do you feel? Do you want to hop in that position, what would feel more comfortable for you?'

And I remember the time the epidural was put in, the doctor came in to do the epidural and I was in terrible pain, I just could not speak by that time. I could barely breathe. I was gasping for little short gasps of air and I had the second midwife by then, and I always remember he said to me 'OK can you roll over on your side and hop in the fetal position?' and all I could say was 'I can't' and I could just whisper it out because I didn't have enough breath to be, and my husband straight away thought there's no way she can get into that position and I felt that first midwife would have said 'She's in terrible pain, we're not going to get her into that position easily; if we need her in that position so be it, and we'll just try and do it', but the second midwife just didn't say anything. She just stood there and my husband said 'Oh I'll help you do it', and he physically got me over and into the position and but with these terrible contractions the last thing you want to be is curled up ... And I felt that that first midwife would have basically said 'Look she's in terrible pain. You'll just have to hold it here, what position do you want her?': talked to her, saying 'Look I know you're in terrible pain. Let's wait for the contraction to ease and we'll quickly get you over'. You know, again talk me through a contraction into the position instead of trying to bowl me over into this fetal position while I was in the middle of a dreadful contraction.

In addition to the notion of prime relationship, the language of 'bowl me over' reflects a power 'over' approach to the birthing woman with a lack of self-determination for her, and an approach that renders the woman 'invisible'.

In contrast, Maree describes the woman-centred practical assistance she received when learning to breastfeed for the first time. She emphasises the vulnerability of being a 'new' mother and thinks that a second- or third-time mother may have a differing view. Nevertheless, 'prime relationship' is also applicable to multiparous women. The mother as an individual, and her emotional and physical comfort, are the prime focus of two particular midwives attending to Maree and her baby. Unlike Ellie, who also experienced great pain with breastfeeding, Maree is not fearful of her baby's mouth, and her mother-baby relationship is established without disruption. Maree's comments also suggest that continuity of the philosophy of care, that is, 'being with' and supporting the woman, and 'knowing' the person, is ethically important. This is a key contribution of continuity of the particular practitioner.

Then she went off and then the next one came on and the first one had actually handed over to the next one saying 'This lady's milk has come in, she's really very uncomfortable, having difficulties with it' – and the next one was there ready to pick up straight away and

I was very impressed with this lady because it is so uncomfortable and the two times I fed and the time that she was on, because she was feeding three hourly, she actually came, she was with me the whole time, I put the baby on the breast and she actually stood there and massaged both breasts while I fed and it was just the best feeling, it got rid of all the lumpiness in the breasts and the engorgement and then as soon as the feeding was over she took the baby back to the nursery, bought some ice packs, put them on me and she physically tucked me into bed and turned the light out and said 'Now try and get some sleep' and she'd come back and check the ice packs. Same thing when we fed the baby the next time, by morning I felt terrific. I'd had sleep, my breasts felt comfortable, I felt good with feeding and it was just lovely, she just knew exactly how to, she just had a lovely nature and it flowed on from the previous nurse so beautifully, it was without hesitation.

Judy gives another example of how one midwife's prime relationship is with the mother. Her comments also demonstrate that practical attention to the woman's concerns are considered part of the concept of supporting the childbearing woman.

Oh that's right [recalling] he told the nurses not to look because, I don't know why, but he said don't use ice and don't examine her because there's no stitches. But a midwife came on and she said 'Oh I know the doctor said not to, but can I have a look anyway?' I said I don't care, so she had a look and she said 'Look, I think ice would be good', and I said 'Oh well', like the doctor said no ice, she said use ice so I think I had a bit of ice on it for just an hour or two, but looking back I wish I had had ice on it because with my second pregnancy it really numbed everything straight away and it made the swelling go down immediately. Whereas my vulva was really swollen for a long time, quite a few days [with this first birth].

A further example of the midwife's prime relationship being with the childbearing woman comes from Kay. She describes the independent midwife's approach to her during the antenatal period, and the importance of 'informed choice' and 'valuing individuals'.

[midwife's name] came to my home and she wanted to know about 'me'! The obstetrician never wanted to know about 'me' really. No, she didn't [answering herself] and [midwife's name] would focus on just sitting and chatting and having a cup of tea and understanding sort of I suppose what made me tick and what made [husband's name] and I tick as well,

the family. And we discussed everything from the nitty gritty of childbirth as I said she would give me as much information as I wanted, but also would prompt me to think about all sorts of things that wouldn't have maybe come to my mind – and [pause] for a start, she elevates the mother-to-be as an important person, compared to my first experience I suppose.

For Ann, a midwife from a mainstream hospital setting, communication is most important. Rather than having a prime relationship with the woman or having a partnership, she proposes that the midwife should be negotiating 'with' the woman.

Occasionally you get the situation where a midwife is totally involved with that client and the negotiation is quite incredible with: 'We are going to have a baby in 20 minutes but we need to sit down and look at what we are doing to make this more effective. This is where we are at now, this is what we need to do to have this baby.' And I have seen one or two people actually do this with a client now and 'This is what we need to do together. Can you help me by doing this, this and this?' and the client suddenly gets this burst of energy because they are taking control again. But see that's negotiation as well.

Bev's story about a young teenage mother positions the midwife's prime focus on the birthing woman and the mother's prime relationship with her baby rather than placating staff. In addition, the story illustrates the importance of context and relationship, not only for the birthing woman but also for the midwife in terms of portraying the holistic experience of 'good' or 'satisfying' birth.

And [boyfriend's name] starts getting frightened, 'cause he's only 16 himself, seeing her in that much pain and not able to do anything. So he went out and I took her into the shower and put the water on her back and rubbed her and so on ... She moved quickly into second stage, the character of her pain changed again and she stopped being noisy and started pushing; and the staff who had been on there, the two midwives who'd been on all night, they were there in the room and they stayed with her rather than swap over on the day shift, and she just propped herself up on a bean bag in bed and pushed and pushed, and pushed out a beautiful healthy baby, and breastfed straight away, and it was as beautiful a birth as you're ever going to have in a hospital ... and I think it was good because we got a healthy baby sucking at the breast and a healthy happy mother, and a healthy happy father, and there was a lot of love in that room and it felt really good.

Kerry-Anne's narrative, referred to earlier, explains how she endeavours to practise woman-centred midwifery, having her prime relationship with the woman, despite the obstacles of mainstream maternity services.

So I felt that she trusted me and that we had quite a good relationship after such a short time of getting to know each other. She was over the moon when I said to her, 'You don't need any stitches'. This was just wonderful for her, and [pause] he spoilt it. He spoilt the whole thing.

Diane, another midwife working in a birth centre, explains her approach to midwifery practice as woman-centred. She, too, demonstrates that her prime relationship is with the woman, that the woman's self-determination is ethically very important, and that continuity of the philosophy of care throughout childbirth is a feature of ethical midwifery practice.

I think we're all trying to foster the woman's independence and to let her know that no matter who is her attendant in birth she's the one who should be in control of this process. She's the one who should be making decisions.

For Katie, as a community-based independently practising midwife, ethical practice means trying to protect the woman's decision, even if the woman cannot 'own' her own decision. She strongly believes in the woman's right to make or not make a decision. One of Katie's clients wanted a home birth, but her husband did not. This narrative is an example of the midwife using power 'for' the woman in the mother-midwife relationship, despite the fact that Katie does not condone the strategies used by the birthing woman to achieve her birthing aims. The perception of Katie's character is ethically important, too.

She had two hospital births with us, finally we had visiting rights – and this time we cooked up another bloody deal which took forever and a day, even though we haven't got visiting rights we established [doctor's name] as providing back up. The day before she has the baby I'm doing an antenatal visit, she says 'I think I want to have the baby at home … and she didn't want to tell her partner because he would

be very fearful of it and I said I think it'd be a good idea if you did … I got a call at one from him to say she was in labour, come, but is it time for us to go to hospital. And I thought, she hasn't told him … so she has told him that they're going to hospital and he was playing games with me on the phone … they have a very loving relationship but loving relationships are not always honest relationships! … So what she was doing basically is she was making the decision too late into the whole event. I mean I'm not into birth in cars … There's no way we would have got into the labour ward by the time, and she knew that! So, they're manipulative. And she didn't want to own the decision even at the very end she wanted to back out of any of the decisions … So all I was concerned about in my communication was that he didn't feel that I had been part of a cover up and a con job. But at the same time I was going to try and protect her decision to have her baby at home. 'Cos if I transferred her when he wanted me to transfer her – I could have easily said OK let's go, I could've said that easily and she would have gone to hospital, but then I would have been cheating her out of what was her real desire, and that was to have a home birth – even if she couldn't own the decision to have a home birth.

Mother's prime relationship is with baby.
Mothers' narratives demonstrate that during the childbirthing experience, the mother's prime relationship is with her baby:

Arline: So on both occasions, after I had picked the babies up, within minutes of them being born I put them to the breast and they fed straight away, and then he held them and he was able to hold them to his chest which was really nice, and we've got some really nice photos of [partner's name] holding the babies.

Faye: And what about the relationship immediately after the birth with you and the midwife, and with the midwife and your support people?

Arline: [long pause] Immediately after, well once [second baby's name] was born [midwife's name] passed him through my legs and then I sat back down onto the bean bag and obviously [partner's name] was there and my Mum was there and [midwife's name] was there and it was all very, it was really nice, like there was no rush to do anything, they just kind of let me have the time to … so it was all very, it was just a really beautiful atmosphere …

Although I must say there's one thing that was really nice I remember when [second baby's name]'s head was just crowning and [midwife's name] had said, I mean obviously I knew that his head was crowning because I could feel it but she said 'You know if you want to touch his head', and at the time I was in the middle of a contraction and it was like no, no, no! And then once the contraction, it was like, and then I ended up putting my hand down straight away, even just as soon as I said no, no I put my hand straight down and felt the top of his head, and when I look back on that that was something that was really special. It was like just, I dunno it was like, I mean I was connected to him because he had grown inside of me but to kind of like touch him for the first time it was like it gave me, really gave me incentive to just go on, even though it was really quick I felt another contraction but it really encouraged me, like 'he's there', through that last little bit.

Brenda describes a very different environment, one that is procedure-oriented for the hospital staff but which is unique, intense, emotional and overwhelming for her. Being hurried through it denies her the full realisation of the experience, and disrupts the initial establishment of that very special mother-baby relationship.

Brenda: I just felt bombarded with information, like here's my baby and she's looking at me and it really freaked me out – and she just looked up at me and blinked and, and I mean I could cry about it now. It's just like the whole, oh my God, I've had a baby and then I thought I'm not ready for this. All, you know, give her to [husband's name], let me think about this for a minute, you know what I mean? And then what's the time, what's her name, all these things are getting thrown at me and then you've got to – it's too much happening. I think that's what it was more than I didn't 'want' her. But it was more, yeah, it was all a bit of a shock to actually see her, and I just really needed to get used to actually seeing her, and then they want me to make decisions. And so this is a baby, wait a second and I'll deal with what you want me to deal in a minute when I've looked at the baby. And then it was [husband's name], do you want the baby, and I was still kind of like really dizzy.

Faye: Is it just the wrong time to be asking you for decisions?

Brenda: Yeah, totally the wrong time. [spoken spontaneously and definitely] OK, yeah let me, someone write down the time 'cause that's important, but I think the baby, it would have been really nice if someone had have said 'Here's your baby. Isn't she beautiful? Let's have a look' – baby, baby, baby instead of running and doing things and press the button, and don't lift your finger off it and get the doctor and it was just all too much happening

for me to really concentrate on the fact that I had just had a baby. So let's deal with everything else 'cause everyone wants you to be in control and not yell at them and scream at them and be a little bit difficult. So OK I've kind of gone from one mode to another I think – well OK we can deal with this other stuff and then I can be emotional and cry over my baby.

Judy: And then the rest of his body was delivered, that just came out pretty easily and then all the waters just gushed over the top of him, they must have all been trapped behind because my waters hadn't broken at all as far as I knew and he was just lying there like this limp, blimp and I remember saying 'Is he all right? Is he all right?' And the nurse was just, it was probably a split second but the nurse was just there looking at him and the next second the doctor ran in and went 'Oh, the baby's here already' and he quickly picked up the baby 'cause I was saying is he all right? and he needed to be resuscitated and he was very blue and I think he was in a bit of shock from being delivered so quickly so [sighs] he had a low Apgar score initially, he had an Apgar of 2 and then after five minutes it had gone up to 9. So that was all right ... and they took care of the baby and then I had a shower and they brought [second baby's name] back to me and we had a nice feed while I was sitting in the wheelchair, except that he got too smelly because he had also passed a motion inside as well. I said 'What is this odour!?' [spoken with disapproval] and they said 'It's [second baby's name]'. So I said 'I'm not feeding him until you've washed him', oh it was disgusting. So he must have been in a bit of distress inside. Yeah, so I gave him a nice feed and I felt really good.

Faye: So they took the baby and fed the baby?

Megan: Oh no, I'd never let them take the child! [spoken spontaneously and definitely] No. I'd never let them do that. I'd just persevere and say 'Oh, thanks for your advice' and perhaps if they suggested something well I'd take them up on that suggestion simply to [pause] try and shut them up, to be honest. But yeah, I was adamant they never took the child, they never took the baby, and gave her anything but breast milk. Again, I was healthy the whole way through it.

Faye: Yet, most childbearing women are. Childbirth is a 'natural' thing.

Megan: Yes, that's exactly. Yeah, and that's the thing that I guess surprised me, like you know, I'd been pretty determined right from the start I wasn't going to walk around in nighties and pyjamas. I was taking up a couple of tracksuits and that sort of thing. So I was up walking around that night, and I guess my focus and then therefore I expected the nurses to be the same with the baby. So I didn't expect to be looked after, as such, by the nurses, you know. It was more for me looking after, learning to look after the child …

I was sort of surprised by that because I thought, well I'm not, you're not really here to look after me, we're here, aren't we both here to look after the baby and get the baby on track? I guess that probably might have surprised them a little bit, and the fact that I didn't expect to be looked after … I wasn't there to be looked after. I was there to learn how to look after the baby and make sure everything was right with the baby before we went home.

Ellie: When they brought the baby to me I heard 'Feed the baby' but I did not hear – and this is something I wanted to tell you about because I thought about this and thought where, where had the real damage occurred? What I didn't hear, which they tried to stress to me repeatedly, because I was in such a euphoric state from anaesthesia, was 'Feed the baby for five minutes on each breast'. So what in fact happened was they brought me the baby and said 'Feed the baby' which I was, you know, only too willing to do … you'd do anything for the baby, you'd die for the baby at this stage …

'Be with' not 'do to' the woman (includes 'midwife's presence' and 'birth journey')

Integral to the notion of 'be with' not 'do to' is the concept of 'knowing' the person and practising within a 'being with' mother-midwife relationship (partnership).

Arline says the midwife was just 'there':

Well – with [second baby's name]'s birth I was actually in the bathroom and I had the lights off and they were just in the next room, just outside the door, I mean they were only a couple of metres away but they weren't, nobody was 'in my face' or no one was touching me, checking me or whatever. They just sort of allowed me to do my own thing and mainly listened to my breathing and how my breathing was during my contractions and stuff. She kind of gauged where I was kind of thing. So she'd come in and she knew that I was kind of, almost, well she assumed I was almost dilated and I was arguing at the time that I was only 6 cms but no and I was, I was 10 cms and within the short time and I was coming out of the bathroom saying right 'OK I need to push'. And that particular stage, just before I did kneel down at second stage, I felt quite fearful, I was kind of in that transition part where I didn't know where or what I wanted to do and she was really calm and said softly 'Relax and just think about what do you want to do? Do you want to do the same as, do you want to birth the same way as you did for [first baby's name]?' and automatically when she said that it was like 'Yep, that's what I wanted to do' because I knew that that had worked the first time and that I had felt comfortable with that, so straight away I was down on my knees leaning over the edge of the bed. So, yeah that was good.

Brenda discusses the approach of her first midwife in the mainstream hospital ward where she eventually birthed, as 'easy', 'comfortable':

Brenda: [the mother-midwife relationship] was easy, it was comfortable, she was an older lady that didn't worry me at all. And it was all, [sighs] oh she was just so easy to get along with and it was me – 'How are you going dear?' She was around me all the time, she was really 'motherly' and consulting me the entire time. She wasn't saying, 'OK your contractions are three minutes apart' at that stage. She was saying 'That's great dear, that's lovely', encouraging and all that kind of stuff and 'Don't worry, your husband will be here soon, we've called him. He'll be here, don't worry, we'll get you down to the labour ward now'. Reassuring just in everything in her manner was just, she had my best interests at heart, and I really felt comfortable with her. Yeah, that's about all I can say.

Faye: You were saying she [the midwife] was sitting there in the background just feeling the contractions. Did you feel at any stage that she wasn't caring for you?

Brenda: No [spoken definitely] she was most caring. She was always there, she was always 'something'. [This suggests the comparison of being 'nothing']

Faye: Even though she wasn't physically doing things?

Brenda: Yeah, yeah. And she was always, she was right beside me or she was around the room as well, walking around doing whatever she had to do, getting things ready, opening the door when [husband's name] came in and his mother apparently. And she was always around but I didn't feel like I'd been left alone at any stage. I always felt like she was there.

Diane, a birth centre midwife, describes a 'be with' not 'do to' approach to practice based on 'knowing' the birthing woman:

But certainly [pause] it is very much easier for us to assess our women in labour than it is for the staff over there [hospital labour ward]. And we often don't have to do vaginal examinations and things like that here because we know them well enough to know [pause] where they're at in their labour without having to actually do that kind of physical assessment ... I mean I think all of us here can assess where a woman is at in labour without doing intrusive things to her, literally. I would rarely do a vaginal examination on a woman shortly after she arrives. You can usually wait a while and just watch the woman and see how she's behaving and listen to the noises she makes and watch the behaviour and we've all learnt to assess a labour over the phone, so that you can say to a woman, you don't need to be here yet, because you know these women already

Gemma, a midwife, said:

When I say hands-on I don't mean literally. I mean that very much being involved with the birthing woman.

The following comments from Judy echo Arline's initial hesitation to touch the baby's crowning head, and Brenda's disapproval of the notion of physical intrusion into the birth canal during the actual birth:

Judy: No, no, I didn't want to touch him until he came out. [spoken definitely]

Faye: No, no. So they didn't actually work against your wishes at any stage?

Judy: No, no. When I was kneeling up over the bean bag and I said to them, I thought the midwife had her, it felt like she had her fingers sort of against the perineum, going like this, and I said 'Get your fingers out of there' [spoken slowly and deliberately]. I thought she was examining me and she said 'Darling that's not my fingers that's the baby's head'. And I went 'Oh, OK. That's all right.' [laughs] So yeah. I thought they were being mean but they weren't.

Kerry-Anne speaks of her practice:

As though midwives can't observe just by being in the room without actually seeing the woman even. You can listen to her breathing and her body sounds and noises that she's making and you know that she's fine.

Kay describes how the independent midwife attending her for her second birth is 'there' but not 'doing' things to or for her, in contrast to what she describes as a very 'managed' [medicalised, caesarean] first birth:

Yeah and occasionally, well at one stage in particular I suppose, and maybe this is my way of saying, 'Come on get a bit involved here', I was probably starting to [pause] maybe picked up in my dealing of it with the contractions towards the end or during – overly moaning and groaning and she came and whispered in my ear at one stage and she said 'It's all right, you can handle this, it's all right'.

Megan also illustrates the ethical appropriateness of 'physically doing less'. She contrasts the interventionist approaches of the lactation specialists and nursing mothers midwives with the 'hands off' approaches of others, during her first experience of breastfeeding in hospital.

Megan: I was still trying to feed and trying to get used to the whole thing of it ... And this one nurse, the one that I liked, was able to do it, would say 'Look, when she has a break just let me know and we'll change her position then'. Whereas a lot of the others were doing it without waiting for the break. I guess too [sighs and pause] they were just so adamant that their views were right. Quite possibly what she was saying and doing achieves the same results but her attitude was able to get it across ...

Faye: Was she physically doing less than the others?

Megan: Yes.

Faye: And is that good?

Megan: I think so. Mmmm.

Faye: Why?

Megan: Because she was not really crowding in and taking over, but perhaps helping you along the way rather than, rather than taking over.

Faye: It's not hands on stuff, because you said the one who wasn't 'doing'.

Megan: No, that's right. Yeah, it's not a hands-on situation. I just think it's perhaps an understanding.

Power 'with' and 'for' in relationship

Whilst this theme is discussed in detail earlier, it reappears here in brief to indicate that, for these mothers and midwives, it constitutes an important part of what it means to support the woman.

Katie illustrates the use of power 'for' the woman, including advocacy.

Katie: I certainly feel a duty to protect them from the, the coercive behaviour of the hospital. I feel a duty to protect them against harm where it's reasonable and foreseeable, yeah. I don't feel I have any duty to protect them against adverse outcomes that I can't do anything about.

Faye: No, but this one was foreseeable wasn't it?

Katie: I don't have to make their birth perfect for them. That's not my job.

Faye: No, but the harm was foreseeable if she stayed at home?

Katie: Yes, if she continued on the risky behaviour, the harm, the risk of harm is increasing for sure.

Katie also demonstrates how she uses a power 'with' woman approach when she relays the antenatal discussion of roles and responsibilities with her client:

I actually think it's important for me to know the sorts of things that make you vulnerable, I said. 'Not so I can judge you as a character. Not so I can protect you from them. Just so I've got an understanding of the sorts of things that make you vulnerable. Now what are your strengths and weaknesses as a person, and then I as a midwife, my role as a midwife is to capitalise on your strengths and help support you with the things that are weaknesses for you.'

Knowing the woman

'Knowing the woman' is considered by both mothers and midwives to be one of the most important ethical components of woman-centred midwifery practice and, therefore, of 'being with' women. It is important not only for these mothers and midwives, but also for women and midwifery practitioners generally. The mother-midwife relationship ought to be based on the practitioner knowing the individual and the woman knowing her environment. That is, the midwife knows the woman, her ability to birth, and her choices, whilst the woman also knows the midwife, her ability and scope of practice, her expertise. It is a mutual knowing, with responsibility for both parties. Continuity of philosophy of care is also integral to this concept of 'knowing' the woman.

Arline chose to have both her babies at a birth centre:

Arline: That was really important to us to be able to have the same midwife and um [pause] ... so by the time you've gone into labour you've already established a nice relationship with the midwife. She knows – they actually get you to provide a birth plan if that's what you want to do and she's aware of what sorts of things you might like to do and things you wouldn't like to do and so yes, so that's really good in that way, that you know her and she knows you. So you're already relaxed about [pause] labouring or having your baby with her, yeah ...

Faye: Did that make you feel safer because of the friendship, I mean safer at the time of birth?

Arline: Yeah, [spoken spontaneously] yeah it did. The fact that I knew her, like she wasn't a stranger and I knew there was my judgement that she wasn't going to, and she knew what my expectations were, she was well aware of what my needs were and so she was able to fulfil them and I think that made me feel safe knowing that she wasn't going to be some crazy mad woman coming in and telling me to lie up on my back on the bed, you know, like – so yeah just the fact that I knew she was going to let me do ... Of course if something untoward happened then she wasn't going to let me just keep going obviously, she was going to say 'Well, hey, look'.

In her narrative, Brenda indicates that when mother and midwife do not 'know' each other the relationship is one of 'separateness'. Her story also reflects that the procedure-oriented hospital midwife is more likely than woman-centred, partnership-oriented birth centre midwife or independently practising midwife, to have disparate relationships and therefore, inadequate ethical responses.

Brenda: Because I wasn't making eye contact with them, maybe that's why they were talking to him, rather than me. [pause] Yeah, I think I was making a little bit too much noise as well.

Faye: How did you get that impression?

Brenda: Well being told to shh for a start, I remember, and then crying, I was crying the whole time and just crying and screaming into the mask, yeah.

Faye: Why were you crying?

Brenda: Oh it hurt. That's how I, I release a lot of my tension through my tears and, and I'll cry just like that. The Kosovo refugees arrived, I cried, that's just me, kind of like a thing that I do and yeah I cry a lot ...

Faye: Some people talk about the continuity of care.

Brenda: I believe that that's going to be particularly important in this birth. [spoken spontaneously and confidently] If I had have had that lovely little midwife the whole time, I reckon I would have behaved beautifully because she was so encouraging. Whereas I felt like I really had to cooperate with the second one and I knew I had to 'behave' myself and quieten down and everything for the second one.

Judy describes how she needed the stern voice of the midwife during the actual birth, providing an interesting contrast to other narratives. However, she follows that comment with one of wishing she had had continuity of practitioner, and implies that a closer relationship might have helped her.

Well there wasn't really time, it just all happened so quickly, but I mean apart from that they were excellent. I remember the nurse saying at transition stage I find that really it's a horrible feeling of being totally out of control, and I must have been screaming because it just seemed to help to scream [spoken quietly and thoughtfully] and the midwife said 'Just stop it. Just push into your bottom this screaming isn't doing anything', [spoken quietly and 'kindly' but definitely] and I said 'I can't' [spoken in a mock 'scream'] and she just said in a very sort of stern voice,'Stop it'. And I needed that otherwise I would have just kept screaming I think. So even though it sounds harsh, people have said, oh that's not very nice, I did need that; yes ...

It would have been nice if I'd had the same midwife as when I'd arrived at the hospital until I'd delivered because you've already established the relationship, and I think, well you are more coherent in between the contractions. I could talk normally to them as a

normal person without being in agony, but then when it gets into second stage, and transition, I just found it was [pause] I wasn't myself, so it would've been nice if I'd had the people that I'd had during the contractions stay with me through the delivery as well. Because they'd sort of seen me as a normal person [smiling] rather than this screaming person ... I'd sent in a birth plan – and they already knew about me before I turned up which I thought was really nice ... I think that would be a good idea to meet the midwives throughout the pregnancy as well.

Kay: When I was in labour with my first baby we went to 'the private hospital' and I had a midwife caring for me there who probably gave reasonable care, but didn't seem really skilled or very empowered to develop a good relationship with me. I mean I didn't know her prior, so I walked in there and [pause] it's very difficult to suddenly develop a rapport.

[comparing the relationship she had with the independent midwives for her second birth]

That they did the right thing by me and I guess what enabled them to do the right thing by me was that we had many lengthy discussions beforehand to understand each other's philosophy I suppose, and to understand my [sighs] wants, hopes, desires [pause] and we checked that we 'agreed' I suppose, so their ethical behaviour was in getting a good understanding of what each other's [pause] role is, and responsibilities and she checked with me, yes she did check with me [confirming her own thoughts], if – do you want to have this done, or do you want to have that done, blah, blah, blah. Yes, so she checked with me ...

Faye: Hm mm. Would it be accurate to say you got to know them?

Kay: Absolutely.

Faye: Yes. So you got to know them. Is continuity of care important?

Kay: Absolutely, yes. It's the whole crux of it I think, empowering women in taking some control and giving them that view and that confidence that they're able to do it because in establishing rapport and a relationship with a midwife gives you an opportunity to what, [pause] to probably explore and understand your real desires in how you want to be cared for. By being, by having a continuity of care in the type of midwives that I had in the second birth, I was able to dictate the terms of the environment that

I eventually gave birth in, and that affected my attitude towards it.

Faye: Why don't you remember much about the midwives in the first birth, do you think?

Kay: Because of, I would say their – what's the word I'm looking for, their 'presence' and their – I guess they weren't very assertive women. I could see that they probably deferred to the obstetrician to be making decisions.

The concept of 'knowing' the woman and the woman 'knowing' the midwife appears to be one that Madonna, a mainstream hospital midwife, has not really considered before. When she does, it appears to raise administrative issues rather than ethical concerns for her at first, but on reflection she re-focuses on the individual and relationships. Madonna occupies an administrative position within the midwifery staff, which could account for her approach, to some extent.

Faye: Do they [pregnant women] see a midwife antenatally?

Madonna: No. Only for the 'booking-in' procedure and introduction to the hospital, that's the only time. Parenting classes.

Faye: Do you think they would benefit from that?

Madonna: From seeing a midwife? [pause] Yes I do, but once again it would be sort of setting up, you would have to set up a practice whereby you had, they would see the same midwife once they came in because you sort of feel sorry for these ladies, they come in, the only person they know or are familiar with is the obstetrician or the doctor, and if he doesn't make it, it's his weekend off or something, then we're all total strangers to them. Unless they have been through the parenting programmes, in which case, yes, they do form a very strong alliance with the girl, the midwife who has taken them through those programmes.

Faye: Does that make a difference to the birth?

Madonna: I think so.

Faye: How?

Madonna: Because they've had a familiar person, somebody that they [pause] trust, with them.

Somebody they have confidence in, somebody they know and they feel they can relate to.

Woman-centred midwives explain why 'knowing' the 'person' is so important for their practice.

Bev: What we should be doing as midwives, is trying to understand how our partner [the childbearing woman] sees their own best interest. Sharing knowledge with them so that they've got a good understanding of their own best interests and then working to promote their best interests – instead of trying to impose our views of what's good for them.

Diane: Women get to trust themselves more when their carer is able to work with them through a process, and working in the birth centre now I know just how different women birth when they have learnt more about themselves and when the midwife caring for them, she knows more about them. By the time we get to birth the woman here we've got a pretty good idea of how she's going to behave in labour – and of course we know a lot about a social history – and that comes out if we ever care for a woman who isn't one that we've cared for all the way through the antenatal period ... if you have somebody that you don't know, it's very difficult to assess where she's at when she arrives, or it's even more difficult, and that's what labour wards have to work with all the time.

Kerry-Anne discusses the importance of the mother and midwife knowing each other in order to develop a partnership. Her comments also refer to self-pride in her expertise as a midwife.

Faye: How do they 'know' that you 'know' [the midwife's expertise]?

Kerry-Anne: I think that's right from the beginning when you first meet the woman. My practice is that when I first meet a woman we talk about her, first of all, [pause] about what she wants for the birth and maybe if she doesn't even know anything about it she just presumes that she wants a natural birth. So we'll talk about her expectations and what she needs to learn, what she needs to read, the classes that she needs to go to, to achieve what her expectations are. And then, at the end of the interview I give them the option of knowing a little bit about me. So I usually say to them 'Well we've been talking about you and your family, now do you want to know anything about me?' And some of them will say no, and be a bit embarrassed, and others will say 'Yeah, what about you?' So then I tell them a bit about my professional experience, where I've worked, how long I've been a midwife, and then I tell them that I am extremely good at looking after women in pregnancy and labour, and I'm very proud of the fact that I'm very good at doing that. So that I think I'm giving them – I'm not trying to show off to them – I'm trying to give them confidence. And I say to them 'Now midwifery is my specialty, but anything to do with other things I don't know a lot about and so there may be times during the pregnancy that I will suggest to you that you go and see your GP [general medical practitioner], OK? – especially if you've got a cough or a cold, or you've got something other than to do with the pregnancy. I will advise you to see your GP because he is the expert in that'.

Kerry-Anne further contrasts her current birth centre practice with that of her earlier practice in mainstream hospital labour wards, and the inadequacy of the latter in facilitating a mother-midwife relationship built on partnership or 'being with' the woman:

Kerry-Anne: What can you do when she's actually gone to the private doctor and the contract is between her and him? She's seeing him antenatally and she feels that she knows him and he's her doctor and he's going to do everything right for her.

Faye: And you're just a fly-by?

Kerry-Anne: And I'm just a fly-by – she's only just met me. She doesn't really know what my role is because I haven't really had a lot of time to spend with her in the labour ward, even though I've had a little bit of time before to talk about how I can help her with her pain relief and all that sort of stuff and that when she's ready for delivery I will let the doctor know and that sort of thing. And then when I ring him he can't come and then I go in and say to her 'Doctor can't come and I'll just go ahead and birth your baby, and I'm an experienced midwife and I will be able to do that quite safely for you'. But she doesn't really know. She's paid a doctor. She's gone privately to a doctor and she expected him to be there.

Katie, an independently practising midwife, relates the importance of knowing the birthing woman and her family, for her role as a midwife, so that she can support the woman in achieving the kind of birth she wants. In addition, she identifies the resistance encountered sometimes for making explicit the 'knowing' of self – perhaps because of the way in which people interpret the questioning and perhaps because of the chal-lenge of 'owning' decisions that such a 'getting to know you' process poses for the individual.

I said, OK at our next visit one of the things I want to focus on is roles and responsibilities, ours and yours ... So, I get there and he [the husband] wasn't home yet. So I was feeling her whole tummy and I look at her little face, and there's a few tears in her eyes, and I said 'What's going on for you?' She said 'I'm just feeling very, very vulnerable' and I said, 'What is it that makes you vulnerable?' [these last questions spoken in a 'soft' voice] and then he walked in the door ... and she said to him something like 'It's started'. And he said, 'What, 20 questions?' And so I looked up and smiled at him, and then I looked back and smiled at her and I said, 'We need to talk roles and responsibilities. I actually think it's important for me to know the sorts of things that make you vulnerable'. I said 'Not so I can judge you as a character. Not so I can protect you from them. Just so I've got an understanding of the sorts of things that make you vulnerable. Now what are your strengths and weaknesses as a person, and then I as a midwife, my role as a midwife is to capitalise on your strengths and help support you with the things that are weaknesses for you' ...

Continuity is everything. Is everything. Continuity of care changes the essence of you as a midwife. Because you get to see the humanness of the person you are looking after in much greater, in much, much more intensified and detailed way. So even the people that would never be friends, 'cause they're just different sort of people, different politics, different personalities, different whatever, you get a real appreciation of them, where they've come from, who they are, and what their strengths and weaknesses are.

Expert-friend

Mothers and midwives with a 'being with' woman orientation liken the mother-midwife relationship to a 'friendship' but include the concept of expertise, not 'expert'. Arline's comments about the professional friendship she had with her midwife and the midwife's character are quoted in Chapter 3, when discussing what is considered 'fair treatment' in differing relationships, and the acceptability and expectation of partiality amongst close friends and relatives.

Diane, a birth centre midwife, discussed the concept of expertise.

Faye: Do they see you as an expert?

Diane: I hope not ... They are independent learners and they come to us seeking resource material so that they can. A lot of them have got plans by the time they come here, as to how they want things to go and they're just trying to get all the information together that they need to be able to achieve that. And I think over in the other class [mainstream hospital] it's often not seen by the women in the same way; they're not as motivated to achieve something. They're there to get the information that the hospital is going to give them.

'Getting to know' and trust the patient/client has been defined by healthcare professions as 'familiarity', and discouraged by both hospital institutions and the 'objective' scientific method. More recently, midwives have disagreed with this teaching:

Above all else the women we care for will also care for us if we trust them. This goes against our training, which implies that the patient is not trustworthy, but only if we trust the women we care for will they feel able to trust themselves (Kirkham 1986 p.37).

Faye: The word friendship. Does that mean anything to you?

Diane: Very much so. Oh yes, we form wonderful friendships at the clinic and that's interesting because this was something that when we started nursing we were told it was a very poor thing to do, it was unprofessional. But who do you care more about than a friend? You know, family and friends you care more about so I think it's important if you do have a friendship and I don't feel guilty about calling some of them my friends at all. I thoroughly enjoy the relationship.

Again Judy, a mother who birthed within a mainstream hospital ward, appears to provide a contrast to some of the other narratives. She describes similar features of character for the midwife during earlier stages of labour, but during the actual birth the midwife's approach alters – as do the personnel themselves. At that stage, Judy portrays more of a detached approach by hospital midwives, and the 'expert' schoolteacher-to-be-obeyed image. Her distinction between what professionals and friends would and would not do also illustrates Toulmin's (1986) argument that we expect

markedly different conduct from people depending on what the relationship is between the parties. A degree of partiality between close relatives and friends is acceptable and expected.

Faye: When you said they were 'friendly', was that both for [first baby's name] and [second baby's name] – the midwives?

Judy: Yes they were. I think for [first baby's name] they were friendlier, more sort of jolly because we had a bit more time, and then the first two with [second baby's name] were very friendly and the next two that came on sort of 'at the business end of things' ... I knew that like, as I said, the midwife telling me to stop screaming and to start pushing, a friend probably wouldn't say do that, she would just say 'Oh, if it helps just keep screaming' or something. So, that was sort of the business-like and professional part of it.

Faye: And a friend you need to get to know, don't you?

Judy: Yes, yes, so they were friendly, but not.

Faye: Do you look on them as being the experts? Is that a word that comes to your mind?

Judy: Mm. Yeah, I think they're experts, yes. When [second baby's name] was born and the doctor came in and said 'Ooh the baby's here', and there's the baby lying on the bed and he went 'Ooh sorry I didn't make it'. I really was very, very happy at that stage with everything and I still am very happy. I was really happy, and I said 'Oh that's fine I've had terrific care from the midwives, I didn't need you', and he went 'Oh thanks a lot' and he was really taken aback by that.

Katie, an independently practising midwife, als considered the concept of 'the expert'.

Katie: They don't look at it in terms of that traditional notion of distant expert. We definitely are a resource to them. We've definitely been blamed. I've been to over a thousand births. They've been to two or three. You know, their own. [sighs]

Faye: Is that on a friendship basis more than an expert basis?

Katie: Oh absolutely. But that doesn't diminish, I don't think that diminishes your obligations in terms of your clinical expertise. And professional background and experience. Yeah, you're definitely a friend, you're definitely a trusted family friend, and sometimes you get quite a lot of tears at those six weeks [postnatal] visits, and it's not a dependence or anything else, it's a friendship, it's a weird sort of friendship that comes for pregnancy and finishes at six weeks after the pregnancy.

Pairman also found that women and midwives describe their relationship in terms of partnership and friendship. In her research, Pairman concludes that terminology used by mothers and midwives varied because of their different contexts. Midwives worked within a professional context, but

the women were not constrained by professional dictates and describe the relationship as they experience it [as friendship] ... [both] recognised its time-limited nature (Pairman 2000 p.211).

Kay, a mother, described her own experiences:

Kay: Well, see, because I've talked about two different experiences with midwives, I see my second experience with those midwives as possibly rare, because [midwife's name] and [second midwife's name] probably have unique experiences and have developed a particular view of the process of childbirth. So to call them [midwives] 'experts', no I would not – I mean in general, midwives experts – because I can see that there's at least, probably two main schools of thought. A midwife can sometimes be as pro-intervention as some obstetricians and I am aware that not all obstetricians are pro-intervention, but so I would not put my trust in all midwives, no I don't blanket them all as experts.

Faye: Kay, some people talk about friends and friendship and the midwife being a friend or friendships being developed. Can you comment on that in those two experiences?

Kay: Well I certainly regarded [independent midwife's name] as a friend and [second independent midwife's name], [pause] different kinds of friends I suppose. [long pause] Mind you [independent midwife's name] probably became a little more professional in her manner once we were in hospital as well so there wasn't so much a relaxed matey attitude, there was sort of let's help you the best we can and I understand what you want and that sort of approach. Certainly in the hospital birth, the first birth, no I just stepped into a strange environment, I didn't feel that anybody was there particularly as my friend. I felt as though I had gone into an environment where I would get the best 'medical' care but in the back of my mind I had

hoped that that equalled helping me to achieve a natural childbirth. I was under the assumption that was the goal of everybody!

Kay's comments suggest that the midwife's approach is altered by different settings, a finding of van der Hulst (1999) in The Netherlands and a claim made by Thompson, Melia and Boyd (1994).

Madonna, a mainstream hospital midwife, seems more hesitant about defining the mother-midwife relationship beyond the hospital stay duration and her description of friendship sounds more like 'acquaintance':

Faye: Maybe that's part of why we do acknowledge people in the supermarket and so on, because there's that relationship still. Does it go on for longer than just the birth, do you think? Or is more like a friendship?

Madonna: I think it's more like a friendship. Mm [pause] I mean many of them I don't recognise them at all, I don't remember them, but the fact if they look at me and smile and they've got a baby I think, oh, OK they remember me from hospital, I've no idea who they are.

Kerry-Anne, a birth centre midwife, to some extent confirms that not only do others view the mainstream hospital midwife differently to birth centre midwives, they also view themselves differently – based on the primacy of relationship:

I really feel that some women that are going to the general labour ward do not even understand what the role of the midwife is. Even in the labour ward, I think, especially private patients see the midwife maybe as the doctor's helper – not as a professional in her own right, who can make decisions and be accountable for her actions. Whereas in the birth suite it's a different relationship with the women altogether because you know them antenatally. You've educated them through your classes on one-to-one and so they see you very much as the professional, and also as a friend.

Midwife's family-social role

The 'midwife's family-social role' is described as the midwife's role towards the new family and towards society generally, as a professional practitioner. The midwife is part of the social construction of family, part of introducing and receiving the new baby into the family and the 'new' family into their social network or society. Knowing the woman and her family, respect for individuals and difference, involves a personal interaction with mother, baby and family. This aspect of practice is another central concept of a woman-centred, 'being with' woman orientation.

Arline birthed in a birth centre:

Arline: I think they sat down and had a cup of tea, I don't know. I'm not actually sure but no it was very yeah very social again. Sounds like a bit of a garden party, but no they did just kind of sit around and I think they did have a cup of tea – while I was in labour, which was fine. I couldn't care what they were doing as long as they were leaving me alone. And my Mum was there for the birth of [second baby's name], and that was another fantastic thing about the birth centre that you can take your children, I mean your other children. So we were able to take [first baby's name] up and that was, because I'd never been apart from her overnight anyway, so that was important that she was able to stay with us, so it wasn't like all of a sudden we'd gone and where had we gone kind of thing, so she was there too, so that was really nice and my Mum was there and that was really nice too.

Faye: And was your mother actually present for the birth of [second baby's name]?

Arline: Yes [spoken enthusiastically] she was. I remember once I'd knelt down and I turned around and had a quick look to see who was there and I said 'Oh you better grab Mum if she wants to come' sort of thing. And so they asked her and she said great, so she came and she was present which was nice because it was actually her birthday, he was born on her birthday. So that was part of kind of like a nice birthday present for her, so yeah so that was good and that was nice.

Faye: So it was very much a family thing?

Arline: Oh totally [spoken spontaneously and definitely] yeah and I hope the next one will be the same, and have them all there again, hopefully.

Diane, a birth centre midwife, speaks of one particular mother-midwife relationship and also refers to her practice generally.

Our relationship was very good and I saw her afterwards at a picnic, 'cause I used to run a picnic for these women after work -

Katie, an independent midwife, said:

I went into the six week (which was really a nine week) postnatal visit with a client who'd just had her third baby with us, and we put out everything, and then I trot across the road and round the corner and have lunch with one current client and two previous clients. I mean, I didn't need to see any of them, but I like to see them, and they like to see me ... And then we catch up with each other at picnics. Four times a year we have picnics in the park, anywhere between 30 and 80 people turn up for them, and you catch five minutes or only two, if you're lucky; you go home exhausted. And they come just to see you, to see how you're getting on and they send you lovely things like this lovely – they found it, they were just snooping around in some sort of shop and they found this really, really, really old midwifery book! So you know, they bought, they bought it for me. They went 'Oh look at that really old midwifery book. Katie'd love that'. Or you get something through the post, or something dropped on the step. Like recently, one of my ex-clients dropped a book. She found a book in the shop called *The Midwife's Daughter*. The child's book. So she just dropped it in, just wrapped it up pretty and dropped it on the steps for [Katie's daughter's name]. So you know they keep in touch with you in irregular [pause] lovely ways. So in that respect we're not expert at all. But, they do rely on expertise.

In addition to the 'silencing' affect of power 'over' relationships, as discussed earlier, Kerry-Anne expresses a sense of sorrow at the disruption that occurred to the mother-midwife relationship when an obstetrician stitched an intact perineum:

Faye: How did the relationship between you and the woman proceed after that?

Kerry-Anne: It sort of ended, I'd say. I didn't follow through. I didn't visit her in the wards and maybe I should've but I just felt so bad about it that I couldn't bring myself to even go and see her again. And I've never heard from her since. I can't even remember her name. I just remember very much the incident, and the disappointment.

Those hospital-based midwives whose practice does demonstrate a power 'with' and a 'being with' woman approach, also indicate that they value relationship highly. That is, they make follow-up contact with the mother after the birth and are interested in her. Ann explained:

They are the people who are willing to step, that have a respect for themselves and for the people they work with, but they also have an interest in people and that's their motivation their interest and perhaps that caring aspect too. And so it's not always done in the work time. Sometimes it's in the meal break, sometimes it's after work that they will go and see the client and ask them how they're going ... And I thought it is quite incredible, we have quite an extended family. I believe [pause], you always believe that you walk out and leave the work behind but I don't think you can in that situation. [pause] Because you go to the supermarkets and I go to a church, you might go to a function, your work is there, people know you [long pause]. So I guess we have a very high profile. We don't realise this but I believe midwives have a very high profile in the community. We're the first people that they identify with and we're the first ones that they rush up to in a supermarket with their children to show us what their children look like, but we don't use that. I think it's because we don't maybe realise the potential that we have or the importance that we have.

Caroline birthed in a mainstream hospital ward, and says this of the midwives:

Even though they said 'Oh we'll see you tomorrow and make sure we find out what happened', they did show a lot of concern and I felt that they did really care [pause] and I thought this was wonderful, they did show that care.

Judy also birthed in a mainstream hospital ward, and she comments on the midwives who made contact with her postnatally.

Yes I felt they were very caring. And they came and saw me up in the ward later and just popped their head in one day and said hello, which I thought was nice of them to contact me afterwards and just to see how I was getting on there and they said 'Oh, it was really quick, wasn't it', yeah that was good. We sort of had a brief rundown of it. But there wasn't a long time to establish any sort of relationship.

Follow-up contact by midwives is not only evidence of caring but is also an important part of the midwife's family-social role. It occurs either at the midwife's instigation within the healthcare facility or at the family home within independent midwifery practice. Sometimes it occurs by chance in the wider societal environment, in which case the contact is initiated mutually or by either the mother or midwife. This latter encounter can occur early, during the postnatal period, or even years later as Ann's narrative illustrates. Ann assisted a young couple antenatally when they arrived at the hospital seeking induction, and later in the neonatal intensive care nursery, she cared for their baby who subsequently developed cerebral palsy.

Ann: They really blamed the hospital, blamed the staff for not listening and for not taking on board what they had said and really were quite angry that their baby was affected in this way ... occasionally I see them in the supermarket. This little girl – now she's five years of age – can't walk, can't talk, just no control ...

Faye: What was your feeling there?

Ann: It brought back a lot of the – because they mentioned the nursery and they mentioned how everyone was so good to them there ... and I looked at them and thought to myself ... they know what the outcome is for their baby, they know that the situation is going to be long term but [pause] they tell me they didn't have the courage yet to try for a second child and to me I felt that was very sad [Ann sounded sad herself as she recalled] because obviously they haven't got the trust yet [pause] to even have another child, if that child is going to be OK. So ethically I thought they don't really trust us: that's the feeling I got – the trust – that if there was a concern or worry they couldn't bring that to us.

Megan experienced difficulty with breastfeeding and conflict with the approaches of some midwives in the postnatal ward. The midwife with whom she did have a 'connection' occasionally has social contact with her.

Megan: I just see her like at the shops, and that sort of thing.

Faye: Yeah, and what sort of a relationship do you have?

Megan: Oh it's lovely. She always fusses over [first baby's name]. She actually was there for [second baby's name] but I didn't have as much to do with her when I had [second baby's name]. And I think it's lovely that she remembers both the kids. She remembers both the children's names. Now, how many other babies would she have done that? She remembers pretty much when their birthdays are and I had a hard time breastfeeding [second baby's name], as I mentioned earlier, and she always jokes about 'Oh well', you know she had some comment about 'Oh this is the one that's sort of thrown the nursing mothers into turmoil'. Or some comment like that. Because of what you'd gone through and the frustration that I'd obviously expressed to her at different times in the hospital. So yeah, certainly not friendship but somebody that it's always nice to run into.

Faye: Do you think that's part of the role of the midwife, or part of the continuity of care?

Megan: Oh, well it's a lot to expect of them. Really, to be able to remember every woman that they've ever looked after. But I think that maybe that is rare. Like with any profession, there's the ones that enjoy it and it becomes their lives, and then there's the ones that do it as a job. And she's obviously one of the ones that, you know.

Woman's comfort: security, 'safe' for the woman

As opposed to the notion of 'safety' from an objective, scientific, mortality perspective, a woman-centred relationship helps the child-bearing woman to feel comfortable, 'safe', supported and secure in her environment. It involves not only physical but also psychological, emotional and spiritual support.

Whilst physical comfort of the woman is important for both mothers and midwives, the other interpretation of 'comfortable' is related to 'freedom of space', and psychological and emotional 'security' for the woman. She needs both external and internal autonomy: the physical ability and opportunity, as well as the mental capacity and opportunity, for self-determination.

Faye: Is 'doing good for you' going to be 'doing good for this unborn baby' anyway?

Arline: [pause] Yeah, yeah, yeah I think yes doing good for me is yeah, because then it allows me to feel comfortable and positive about what's the process that's happening where I think, because I think birthing is largely psychological, I mean obviously it's a physical thing but a lot of the management of the pain, well I don't like to call it 'pain' but yeah I think a lot of that has to do with how you work your own mind with it [and] um, feeling safe. Well I guess [pause] I mean that's the most vulnerable time I think in a woman's life is [spoken slowly and thoughtfully] while she's birthing so you want to be able to feel [choosing words] safe in that you know there's no judgement or there's no kind of criticism like she

should be doing this or she shouldn't be doing this, so just like I guess it's coming back to that, just allowing me the freedom to do what I want.

Both mothers and midwives express sentiments regarding women's 'comfort' and security. Gemma particularly portrays the lessons she learnt as a midwife practising within an aboriginal culture in a remote area of Australia.

Gemma: But in rattling my cage it also helped me to realise that the most important dimension to childbirth is the woman and her comfort and her trust in her body's ability to birth and all those sorts of issues, and that's very much related to the environment in which she births. If she feels the environment's safe even if we as health professionals think it's the most unsafe, grotty horrible environment that could be, that doesn't matter – that's safe for her.

Judy: Well it did happen with the second pregnancy but only because my doctor went on holidays and only with one of the doctors not with the other one. So I didn't feel there was that same level of concern from them but at least you were comfortable with the midwives.

Brenda: If I think I can do it, I think I should be allowed to try. If there's nothing wrong with the baby and there's like no chance that I'm going to die or something like that, I think that I should be given – I have the right to have my own baby. I, you know, what gives the doctor or a midwife for example, the right to make these decisions for me? If I'm not in any danger why can't I continue to labour by myself?

Faye: And for safe and comfort I'm thinking things like support, an environment they can relax in.

Diane: Yeah and when you say safety and comfort I think they need to know that they can tell you anything and know that it will be in confidence and that you will respect that. And it might be telling some of these parts of their life that might have an influence on their birth, something that makes a difference to way they birth.

Kay: And then honesty and assertiveness needs to come from the mother too, to say, to be able to feel comfortable enough too I suppose to feel free to express her wants and desires and her hopes.

Valuing individuals, acknowledging difference, and having a commitment to a woman-centred mother-midwife relationship is not depicted in narratives of midwives employed in procedure-oriented birthing practices.

WAYS OF SEEING

Metaphors used by mothers and midwives

Metaphors convey new insights by using comparisons, and a truth that is sometimes not previously acknowledged by the particular profession. Moral metaphors are culturally determined, highlighting and suppressing certain features of experience.

Caroline describes what it was like for her when her newborn baby was taken away for oro-pharyngeal suction by the paediatrician. Her metaphor of 'football pass' suggests efficiency and product outcome – even that the baby was an inanimate object – the baby is transferred from one location to another in the fastest possible way. Her description however, suggests that it is not right for her to be separated from her baby, that the baby is handled with indecent haste and carelessness, and that she is anxious and powerless to prevent it happening.

But I'd never seen anything like this. As soon as he was born, no sooner had the cord been cut then Dr P walked in, it was like a football pass, Dr M passing straight to Dr P and off they went. Wow, where's my baby going? I mean I had no idea what was going on ...

By far the most commonly recurring theme in metaphors is that of 'journey'. Both mothers and midwives refer to the concept of journey. It suggests that their way of seeing birth, their meaning of birth, is that of process, uncertainty, experience and learning, and achievement. It is transformative. Birthing is not merely about the efficient outcome, of being 'given a healthy baby' – a 'product'. Birthing is part of the broader process of becoming a mother, of conceptually and physically developing the mother-baby relationship.

Arline, a mother who birthed both of her babies in a birth centre, says the following in relation to the birth process:

And I saw the top of his head. Then once I reached that point well you know I just love it from then on 'cause that's like you're almost home kind of thing.

And in relation to knowing what to do for the second birth, Arline says:

I guess being the second you're more, the way had been paved.

Kay compares her first birth, a caesarean operation in hospital under the care of a private obstetrician, with her second birth, a vaginal birth in hospital under the care of an independently practising midwife:

I then did – from [obstetrician's first name]'s recommendation, I did have an epidural because I had no other path to follow I suppose ... [about the second birth experience] but it's just a natural course, it has to take its own course ... I had to take full responsibility for choosing to go that way ... so it's a bit of a mountain to climb but I was determined enough to try it.

Megan suggests the journey metaphor when discussing establishing breastfeeding in hospital.

Because she was not really crowding in and taking over, but perhaps helping you along the way rather than, rather than taking over.

Brenda uses the metaphor of journey when she articulates aspirations for her second impending birth:

So, yeah, I think that all those things are important and that's what I'm looking for in this birth is to build a relationship, hopefully previously while I'm pregnant with maybe meeting some of the midwives and feel comfortable with going to the place I'm going to go to.

Diane rejects the idea of mothers thinking of midwives in the birth centre as 'experts', and explains the difference in the mother-midwife relationship in a birth centre compared with her previous practice in mainstream hospital ward:

I hope not – I think they see us as somebody who can help them steer a clear path through that [not 'experts']. I think they see us as a guide through a journey and it's a very important journey in their lives and I think they see us as somebody who can help them steer a clear path through that ... what I say to women is when you reach a decision point in your labour for instance, you need the information to make a decision. And what you have to do is make that decision based on the information that you have at the time and if you take the right side, if you're at a Y-junction and you take the left arm

Gemma defines what she considers is a 'good' midwife in terms of journey:

I'd describe a good midwife as being someone who has a sound knowledge base but a midwife who is able to just be with a woman, to journey with her on her birth journey whatever that be for that woman. But when I say a sound knowledge base I mean she is actually responsible for, to protect the woman and she's responsible for the woman's safety – and the baby of course.

Katie uses a 'journey' metaphor when she talks about her main ethical concern as a midwife practising independently in the community:

I worry that I honour and respect her ability to decide or not to decide, to plot her own course.

Wurzbach (1999) argues that language, discourse and metaphors reflect social organisation, and construct our identity and subjectivity. The metaphor of 'journey' used by both mothers and midwives confirms their common meaning of identity for the childbearing woman. This contrasts with the military style, control language of power 'over' relationships. Those mothers and midwives whose orientation is 'being with' woman, identify the childbearing woman as a central and active figure in what is her personal and unique experience. To a great extent the childbirthing woman is self-determining, interacting with her body, her baby and changing circumstances, and making the best decision with the information available at the time. The experience requires endurance, motivation and confidence in one's ability. It is centred on the woman herself, her baby, and the temporal nature of the process of birthing. The desired 'destination' is to birth a healthy baby with the woman's physical and psycho-emotional integrity intact. The woman's birthing achievement has a lasting impact on her. Those women whose first childbirth experience deprives them of this journey, often aspire to it with subsequent pregnancies. Brenda is such an example. A personally satisfying experience transforms the 'pregnant woman' into a woman who has grown and birthed a baby, into a mother who is utterly desirous of establishing one of the strongest relationships of her life – the mother-baby relationship.

Personal transformation

Mothers and midwives relay stories of personal transformation as the result of ethical responses within childbirth practices.

Altered way of seeing

The following are examples from mothers and midwives, of their altered 'way of seeing'. Reference is also made to 'opening my mind'.

She [obstetrician] really played down the actual event of childbirth, and I can see that more clearly a number of years now down the track and having experienced something very different. (Kay)

Gemma, a midwife, portrays the positive effect on her practice of experience in a different cultural context. It opened her mind and altered her way of seeing, her orientation:

Yes, it did open my mind to thoughts that there is another way. I had to think hard about what I'd been taught – about safety, about the issues involved, the very hospital training that I had and where it fitted into all of that and it sort of is a conflict when you first start challenging those beliefs or learning that you had ...

For me personally [pause] it had a really positive effect on me because up until then I'd been fairly much a hospital-oriented midwife believing that the only place to have a baby was the safety of a hospital and all that sort of nonsense, and those women [Australian aboriginal women in a remote area] taught me that that's not so; that in fact if a woman births where she feels comfortable then she births well usually, and that for each woman that may be some place different and that it should be that as health workers we should support women's choice and support their comfort, and if they feel comfortable in a level 3 whizbang hospital then that's where they should be and we should support them there. But if they feel comfortable at home or where ever then that's where they should be supported ...

Changed practice

Personal transformation affects not only ways of seeing but also ways of acting, of practising.

Caroline's transformation occurs through her own life experiences, and her experience of birthing her babies:

Oh well, I was, I suppose by the time I had fallen pregnant with three of them I wanted things to be, I'd really changed my outlook on life. I'd changed my diet, I'd realised what a healthy, balanced diet can do for a person, and I was determined that I wanted it all natural. I didn't, I don't like drugs in any way, shape or form, and [pause] the fact that I actually wasn't offered any drugs in any of those labours is probably – I found [pauses and sighs] I suppose it's not really an ethical issue, but to me it is important that I wasn't pushed to have an epidural or Pethidine or anything like that.

Kay contrasts her first, operative, birth to her second, vaginal, birth and suggests her changed outlook or 'practice' of birthing:

Well I kept probably convincing myself that because of the previous talks [with the 'independent' midwife] that it can be that way if I view it that way; take control as much as I can with my own thinking and how I'm going to respond to this and deal with this ... I never even thought of having drugs while I was in labour [second birth]. It didn't occur to me which I was sort of surprised at in a way later. It didn't occur to me to even have them.

Diane, a midwife, attributes some of her transformation to her birth centre workplace philosophy and environment:

Diane: Well there's a big mind-body connection. A huge one and the more I see women over here the more I see that. [and later] I would rarely do a vaginal examination on a woman shortly after she arrives ...

Faye: And it's important to know them, to get to know them, and them to get to know you?

Diane: Oh very. Yeah and they really want you there but I think most of them now, and they probably were dependent on us initially, and we were probably all a little bit guilty of making them dependent on us because it made us feel good, but we're much less likely to do that now and I think we're all trying to foster the woman's independence and to let her know that no matter who is her attendant in birth she's the one who should be in control of this process. She's the one who should be making decisions. And so, they're not – it's a different relationship [to mainstream hospital labour ward].

Brenda: Whereas now, this time, bugger everyone else, I'm gonna cry over my baby if I want to, that's the type of thing that I'm feeling now ...

Faye: Some people talk about the continuity of care.

Brenda: I believe that that's going to be particularly important in this birth. [Brenda did not have this orientation/value for her first birth.]

Kerry-Anne says that the incident when the obstetrician stitched what she believed to be an intact perineum affected her practice in that she now always explains to women that she does not cut an episiotomy unless they give her their permission and unless she judges it necessary.

It affected my practice in as much as I always talk to women that I'm going to be helping birth, about their wishes for episiotomy or tears, or whatever they want. So that is a big part of my practice. Even if I meet a woman who I've never met before antenatally and I'm going to be birthing her baby, at some stage I will mention I do not do episiotomies unnecessarily ... If you are going to tear with this epis, from the scarring with this one, what do you want me to do? So they're more or less giving me permission to do whatever I think at the time.

SUMMARY

The unprompted language of these mothers and woman-oriented midwives is that of relationship, context and virtues-values. They overwhelmingly propose that ethical midwifery practice involves 'being with' woman during childbearing. For the mother and midwife to 'know' each other and for the midwife to support the birthing woman in ways that empower her, is central to the concept of 'being with' the woman in partnership. Acknowledging the woman's achievements and working 'with' her induces positive feelings and emotions for both of them.

Human engagement is the site of ethics for these mothers and midwives. An ethically adequate mother-midwife relationship is open and honest; trusting and respectful of persons, and of the woman's ability to birth. It is consultative and woman-centred, and features continuity of carer and philosophy of care. In such relationships, the midwife shares her knowledge and power 'with' the woman, in an equitable and mutually respectful partnership. These women also value friendship, and consider one has a prime responsibility to particular others. Context and character of moral agents are important features of ethical childbirth practices and this supports the claim that ethical practice occurs prior to, during, and after any dilemma or problem resolution.

The metaphor of journey recurs across mothers' and midwives' narratives. Birth is not only a social construction and an experience unique to the woman, it is also a journey with an uncertain but natural course. Language, discourse and metaphors reflect social organisation, and the mother/midwife identity and orientation. In the vast majority of instances birth is not a life-threatening dilemma. 'Safety' for the woman and baby also means the freedom for the woman to express herself, to 'let go' and 'do what is right for me', with the physical and emotional support of the midwife. These birthing women see themselves as self-determining, interacting with their body, baby and changing circumstances, and making the best decision with the information available at the time. The woman needs to subordinate herself to her body and mind, not to the birth attendant. The practitioner is sought for her/his expertise, not as the distant and powerful 'expert'.

Some mothers aspire to a woman-centred environment prior to any experience of it. Many mothers and midwives, however, undergo a personal transformation when they experience a woman-centred birth environment after that of the institutionally dominant, mainstream Western-culture maternity services. Their way of seeing or orientation is altered, as is their practice or way of acting. Midwives speak of 'opening my mind to other ways', needing to rethink issues of 'safety', and having previously-taught-beliefs challenged. Mothers' comments resonate with the concept of empowerment – a belief and confidence in themselves and their ability to birth their babies. They indicate that, for their next birth, they would actively seek an environment that is supportive of them as individuals, and in which midwives 'know' them.

REFERENCES

Guilliland K, Pairman S 1995 The midwifery partnership: a model for practice. Victoria University of Wellington, Wellington, NZ

Kirkham M 1986 A feminist perspective in midwifery. In: Webb C (ed) Feminist practice in women's healthcare. John Wiley & Sons, Chichester

Pairman S 2000 Women-centred midwifery: partnerships or professional friendships?. In: Kirkman M (ed) The midwife-mother relationship. Macmillan, Basingstoke, pp. 207-226

Thompson F E 2001 The ethical nature of the mother-midwife relationship: a feminist perspective [unpublished Ph D dissertation]. University of Southern Queensland, Toowoomba, Queensland, Australia

Thompson I K, Melia K M, Boyd K M 1994 Nursing ethics. Churchill Livingstone, Melbourne

Tong R 1993 Feminine and feminist ethics. Wadsworth Publishing Co, Belmont CA

Toulmin S 1986 How medicine saved the life of ethics. In: DeMarco J P, Fox R M (eds) New directions in ethics. Routledge and Kegan Paul, New York

van der Hulst L A M 1999 Dutch midwives: relational care and birth location. Health & Social Care in the Community 7 (4): 242-247

Wurzbach M E 1999 The moral metaphors of nursing. Journal of Advanced Nursing 30 (1): 94-99

Checking our course – values and philosophical foundations of the midwifery profession

Mothers and midwives reject intrusiveness and institutional dominance over childbirth practices (Thompson 2001). They overwhelmingly describe ethically adequate practices as those that reflect 'being with' the woman. Birth is a unique, intense, intimate, physical and spiritual experience for the woman, not merely a physiological event with a 'product' outcome. The use of power in relationships is the central theme of their narratives. Whilst they may seek to take advantage of the benefits of medical science, technology and expertise, they consider it important that practice acknowledge and be guided by the authenticity of knowledge gained from personal experience – how they feel and how it is for them. Practices and language that 'take over' from the woman and render the individual invisible are considered unethical and unacceptable. Practices and approaches based on generalisations and normative theory are also interpreted as ethically inadequate for these mothers and midwives.

What, then, are the values and philosophical foundations of the profession? To construct an ethic that truly reflects values of midwifery practice, it is necessary to deconstruct existing frames of ethical response and reconstruct an ethic for midwives based on the lived reality of mothers and midwives. The following discussion examines conceptual theoretical frameworks implicit in midwifery research, literature and organisational structures. In so doing, it is hoped to identify taken-for-granted assumptions. Mothers' and midwives' real life experience is compared and contrasted with the profession's conceptual frameworks.

THE PHILOSOPHY AND THEORY BEHIND MIDWIFERY PRACTICE

Ways of knowing: midwifery's epistemology

Knowledge gained from personal experience, and practice that is guided by the particular rather than reductionist, normative theory, are important for mothers and midwives. The midwife who is praised and sought after is the one who helps the birthing woman do 'what is right for me'. Mothers and midwives alike use the metaphor of journey, including concepts of uncertainty, having a natural course, the way has been paved, the woman 'doing' it herself, and respecting her ability to 'plot her own course'.

What is the epistemology of midwifery? How do we conceptualise our reality and our images of the world?

Unlike the objective, single-truth of positivism and the scientific method, midwifery practice is based on multiple sources of knowledge including knowledge gained from personal experience. While the midwifery profession endorses the benefits of scientifically acquired knowledge it also acknowledges the legitimacy of personal experience and lay knowledge (Flint, Poulengeris & Grant 1989; Sleep 1992; Mander 1992; Hall 1994; Davis 1995; Cioffi & Markham 1997; Kelly 1997).

What does it mean to be 'with woman'? Jane Hall offers the metaphor of walking with the woman on part of her life journey, as she travels through the deep and profound experience of birthing:

to sense a woman's needs as she travels and to assist her to meet them in a way which not only promotes the safe delivery of a healthy baby, but which is enhancing and empowering for herself and her family (Hall 1994 p.65).

Significant life experiences such as birthing can be a time for new knowledge, understanding and strength. For the woman this transformation occurs within the context of her family, community and culture.

For the midwife who accompanies the traveller, it demands a 'knowing', a 'being', a 'relating' and a 'doing'. The science of midwifery, the 'knowing', involves both the conventional means (such as drugs) and a range of strategies such as massage, therapeutic touch, relaxation, visualisation, music, aromatherapy, movement, hydrotherapy, heat and cold – strategies which are determined in partnership by the woman according to her experience and by the midwife according to her knowledge and skill. The analytical and objective aspects of the domain of knowing do not speak to the experience of the journey itself or to the deep connection inherent in 'being with woman'. Andrea Robertson suggests that women may have been hoodwinked into trusting the wrong people during birth; that rather than placing faith in medical men we should have believed in ourselves more. She also claims that

if birth was not so sexual perhaps it may be easier for women to express their needs (Robertson 2000 p.2).

It is essential that midwives be able to accept difference (a stance the postmodern feminists adopt), that they believe and trust in the woman's ability, and that midwives be willing to let go of their need to control – themes which have emerged in the present narratives. The goals and mode of care should be determined largely by the woman and her family.

To operate from [an analytical and objective] knowing alone is to stand on the side of the road,

only stepping onto the road to perform specific tasks and providing care according to a predetermined set of outcomes (Hall 1994 p.66).

This induces the image of the marathon runner clutching at refreshments as s/he runs past the 'drinks stop'. Those handing out the refreshments do not 'know' what the athlete's journey has been like; although they have watched many runners pass by they have seen only glimpses of each runner. Other runners and those accompanying the runners on their journey develop an understanding of the experience of the marathon, the process of achievement.

Doctors are expensive and in a hurry, but pregnancy and labour are long, as is the real work of the midwife (Kirkham 1986 p.37).

Mothers and midwives see the need to 'know' the woman in order to identify individual needs and responses to the birthing process (Thompson 2001). To seek a balance in the art and science of midwifery is to respect the 'humanness' of our work, something that is missing with reductionism and objectivism. For example, the influence of Socrates and Plato can still be seen today in the way that abstract theoretical knowledge is seen as superior to skilled activity; a socially constructed view of knowledge. The duality of mind and body endures in the notion that personal meanings are subjective and reality objective; the body is merely a vehicle through which the mind can experience the external environment. All of this has been further criticised by feminists. Not only have woman's ways of knowing not been acknowledged in such a male-oriented social construction but attributes ascribed to women such as 'emotional', 'intuitive' and 'personalised' are

devalued by a Western, technologically oriented culture where rationalism and objectivism are more highly valued (Davis 1995 p.152).

When the childbearing woman and midwife know each other's strengths, limits, desires and ways of responding, it leads to decisions that are particular to the individual rather than based on generalisations (Flint, Poulengeris & Grant 1989; Davis 1995). A woman is more than a psychological, physiological and social being, molecular and atomic components. Like Hall (1994), Davis criticises references to 'the breech in room one' as objectifying human beings and contrasts that approach with the holistic perspective of the independent midwife, one of whom explained that she needed to spend time with [the birthing woman], to get to know her, watch her, learn her likes and dislikes over a whole range of things, not just birth. Mothers and midwives in the present analysis also explain how important it is for the midwife to spend time with the birthing woman, to get to know and respect her and her identity as an individual. In particular, Katie's narrative details how she likes to learn what makes the woman vulnerable, what makes her and her partner and family 'tick', not only with respect to pregnancy and birth but in other areas too, so that she can support her in those aspects during birth:

'We need to talk roles and responsibilities. I actually think it's important for me to know the sorts of things that make you vulnerable', I said. 'Not so I can judge you as a character. Not so I can protect you from them. Just so I've got an understanding of the sorts of things that make you vulnerable ... then I as a midwife, my role as a midwife is to capitalise on your strengths and help support you with the things that are weaknesses for you...'

Mothers, in particular, emphasise the authenticity of experiential knowledge and a 'knowing'. They express the need to 'go with your body', to 'have space to do what is right for me'. Describing her second birth, in a birth centre, Arline says:

I was actually in the bathroom and I had the lights off and they were just in the next room, just outside the door. I mean they were only a couple of metres away but they weren't 'in my face', no one was touching me, checking me or whatever. They just sort of allowed me to do my own thing and mainly listened to my breathing and how my breathing was during my contractions and stuff. She kind of gauged where I was kind of thing. So she'd come in and she knew that I was kind of, well she assumed I was almost dilated and I was arguing at the time that I was only 6 cms but no I was 10 cms and within the short time I was coming out of the bathroom saying right 'OK I need to push'.

This type of knowledge seems different from both the 'application of theory' type and the type of knowledge one gains from habituated and experiential learning that results from repeated situations. Often, the woman birthing for the first time will also 'know' what she wants to do, albeit that the multiparous woman will 'know' better the alternative strategies for 'how' she wishes to birth. For example, Arline continues:

And that particular stage, just before I did kneel down at second stage, I felt quite fearful, I was kind of in that transition part where I didn't know where or what I wanted to do and she was really calm and said softly 'Relax and just think about what do you want to do? Do you want to birth the same way as you did for [first baby's name]? And automatically when she said that it was like 'Yep, that's what I wanted to do' because I knew that that had worked the first time and that I had felt comfortable with that, so straight away I was down on my knees leaning over the edge of the bed. So yeah that was good.

While the notion of 'instinct' for human beings is not embraced, it does seem likely that when the woman knows her own body well, she synthesises knowledge from other related but different experiences, much like what might be referred to as 'intuition'. Davis (1995) raises the idea of the pregnant body as a 'knower' in contrast to the Cartesian view, and whether the embodied knowledge that a pregnant woman holds is different to instincts. A birthing woman uses embodied knowledge such as being able to 'get in tune' with her body; her body dictates what she needs to do to birth her baby such as rocking, walking or moaning, and she experiences a mind-body unity rather than split.

Mothers and midwives emphasise the importance of treating the childbirthing woman as an individual; of informed choice, continuity of carer and philosophy of care, respect for people as human beings, and of valuing the individual. Kay, a second-time mother, whose care was given by an independently practising midwife, says:

[midwife's name] came to my home and she wanted to know about 'me'! The obstetrician never wanted to know about 'me' really. No, she didn't [answering herself] and [midwife's name] would focus on just sitting and chatting and having a cup of tea and understanding sort of I suppose what made me tick and what made [husband's name] and I tick as well, the family. And we discussed everything from the nitty gritty of childbirth, as I said, she would give me as much information as I wanted, but also would prompt me to think about all sorts of things that wouldn't have maybe come to my mind – and for a start, she elevates the mother-to-be as an important person, compared to my first experience.

The values of choice, control and continuity are integral to midwifery practice. Personal knowledge is important because it reflects what is unique to the individual. Women want to be treated as individuals, each pregnancy is unique and special, and to be 'with woman' implies giving of oneself in an authentic and empathic way. Personal knowledge is gained through the experience of working with women and by reflecting on one's personal and professional practice. It allows for the humanness of both the woman and the midwife, and deepens their relationship.

Midwives who have grown accustomed to fragmented, task-oriented practice, or those midwives who have not experienced any other system of care but the one described, may find it difficult to form the committed personal relationship necessary for individualised care (Kelly 1997 p.197).

This concept of commitment to personal relationship is expressed in the present analysis as the 'family-social role of midwife' and is characterised by the midwife's perceived importance of 'follow-up' contact with the mother postnatally. Midwives who adopt a woman-centred partnership approach seem to develop this commitment, whereas those who are more procedure-oriented, such as practitioners in science/technology-oriented workplaces, do not.

Diane, a midwife at a birth centre attached to major hospital: Our relationship was very good and I saw her afterwards at a picnic, 'cause I used to run a picnic for these women after work.

Katie, a community-based midwife: I went into the six week (which was really a nine week) postnatal visit with a client who'd just had her third baby with us, and we put out everything, and then I trot across the road and round the corner and have lunch with one current client and two previous clients. I mean, I didn't need to see any of them, but I like to see them, and they like to see me ... And then we catch up with each other at picnics. Four times a year we have picnics in the park.

Faye: Do you think the mother-midwife relationship goes on for longer than just the birth, or is it more like a friendship?

Madonna, a midwife at a major hospital: I think it's more like a friendship. I mean many of them I don't recognise them at all, I don't remember them, but the fact if they look at me and smile and they've got a baby I think oh, OK they remember me from hospital. I've no idea who they are.

Unfortunately, Kelly (1997) reverts – albeit as a small part of her discussion – to the abstraction of moral philosophy and principles-based decision making to guide midwifery ethical and moral knowledge. As argued earlier, this is an inadequate ethical response for midwifery practice given that Western (male) moral philosophical theories and universal principlism are based on generalised norms, the rightness or wrongness of 'actions', focus on dilemmas and 'issues', and deliberately exclude context, relationship and the particular in their quest for objectivity. The former are more appropriately the ethics of strangers. Midwifery requires an ethic of intimates – an ethic of engagement.

Like nursing, midwifery has rapidly increased 'research awareness' amongst students and practising midwives, and has formalised research skills into curricula (Sleep 1992). Whether or not it is realistic to expect that practitioners will introduce research into the workplace is debatable, when service and management are not always receptive to change. Innovation is not always valued by clinicians or employers, especially if it threatens their beliefs, values, attitudes and behaviour. Proceduralisation, delegated responsibility, the operation of a double standard, medical dominance, and the hierarchical structure of midwifery mitigate against such advancement. They necessitate counter measures such as challenging authority, playing power politics and gaining peer support, developing intellectual curiosity and the power of reflective thinking, facilitating critical reading skills, promoting, evaluating and valuing innovation, and fostering skill acquisition and clinical judgement. Several of these reactionary forces and counter measures have indeed emerged in the present midwives' narratives.

Experience is a significant basis of learning because it is the interaction of the individual with the environment and all aspects of that person's life including formal learning experiences (Mander 1992). Experience can challenge traditional thinking and broaden the vision and understanding of a discussion. A phrase that appears in the present narratives is 'open my mind' to ways of seeing.

This belief in personal experience produces conflict for practitioners in a workplace setting which deliberately excludes context and the so-called subjective from its objective empirical knowledge, problem-solving and decision-making.

Ethical theories and principles 'incorporated'

Next, midwifery literature is examined to identify those ethical theories that form the basis of childbirth practices, within a Western Anglo-Celtic cultural framework. One focus is whether ethical principles are incorporated into healthcare practices at both the individual practitioner level and at the institution and government level. For example, do healthcare facilities and governmental departments promote duty or obligation, and principles-based ethical decision making for maternity services? Do the profession and practitioner endorse that orientation? Is there cohesion between the institution's approach and the individual practitioner's values or are other ethical orientations influencing practice?

Governmental reports on childbirth services and practices

Again, Australia is used as an example and a prompt to consider such influences in other communities. Frith (1996), for instance, considers the issues of choice and autonomy as a central theme for ethics and midwifery, referring to the UK Department of Health 1993 report, *Changing Childbirth*, which stipulated that maternity care should be woman-centred.

Having a Baby in Victoria, the final report of the ministerial review of birthing services in Victoria (Victorian State Government 1990) is one of the most comprehensive examinations of its kind in Australia for that time. The review demonstrates dialogue across differences and alternative forms of knowledge, and shows how administrative and professional interests maintain a technocratic model of maternity care despite the efforts of others to replace it with a 'woman-centred' approach (Reiger 1999).

Nine years later, the Australian Federal Government published the report on the Senate inquiry into childbirth practices, *Who's Rocking the Cradle?* (Australian Federal Government 1999). According to this report Australian women value the safety of their babies and themselves during birth above all other considerations, giving this as their prime reason for choosing to give birth in a hospital. However, they were generally concerned about the extent to which childbirth has been medicalised and the resultant increase in obstetric intervention. The committee considered that (i) there was no medical justification for the high rate of caesarean section birth (at over 20% it is one of the highest in the world – also discussed in Chapter 2, in the medicalisation of healthcare) and (ii) the variation between publicly and privately insured women was unacceptable. Hospital birth centres were the favoured settings because practices within them enhance women's birthing experience and the climate was conducive to cooperation between midwives and obstetric specialists. The committee also recommended that the government continue to fund midwives to assist at home births for women at low risk, and noted that many women in the current mainstream system were being denied continuity of care. Women were particularly neglected in the postnatal period following the move to early discharge from hospital after birth because reduced community services have resulted in women being at home without help. The first week after birth was critical for women because it was then that they were establishing successful breastfeeding, learning how to care for the baby and adjusting to the psychological changes of motherhood.

These inquiries (UK Department of Health 1993; Victorian State Government 1990; Australian Federal Government 1999) report on service satisfaction, not the ethics of childbirth practices *per se*. However, evidence from them and the present narratives indicates that mothers and midwives want to be valued as individuals, and need 'human engagement' from maternity services and childbirth practices. A relationship approach to mothers and childbirth rather than a procedural-'product' orientation offers this 'engagement' in an adequate ethical response for midwifery practice.

The high incidence of obstetric intervention and the neglect of women's needs are criticised by mothers and midwives alike. The mortality-morbidity emphasis, and priority of the principle of beneficence over that of autonomy within technology-dominant, medicalised childbirth labels the woman as defective and renders her invisible during the process and experience of childbirth. The analogy of a 'machine' requiring fuel and repair, rather than an interactive person with needs, has long been applied to the human body in a scientific, mind-body split approach to healthcare – a 'product' philosophy rather than an 'experiential' engagement philosophy. Such abstraction is an ethically inadequate response to the embodied experience of birth. As argued earlier, in Chapter 5, the words of women are often used to further the work of a medicalised system rather than to demonstrate the value of women's work in childbirth. Medically owned and operated technologies enabling scans and plans for date of birth, elective surgical birth that is 'effortless' for the woman, and early discharge from hospital to reunite family quicker, are presented as giving women more control – but they have not transformed women's work in childbirth to being valued for itself. Rather than supporting women towards achievement in birth, women are viewed as defective, as 'requiring' techno-medical control for birth. Using the Australian example again, a caesarean section rate among privately insured women aged 35 years or more having their first baby under the care of an obstetrician is over 40 per cent (Australian Federal Government 1999). If this rate is based on physiological necessity only, it suggests that nearly half of the primigravida women in that group cannot birth their babies vaginally, and this is hard to believe. Early discharge from hospital has meant that not only are women not receiving the help that they previously did in hospital, but they are also being left with less help at home at an earlier stage in the postnatal period, because funding cuts have reduced community services (Australian Federal Government 1999). These changes to childbirth practices have furthered the work of the economically-oriented healthcare industry and the medicalisation of childbirth, reinforcing existing power relations. Recent reports clearly show that mothers and midwives are not satisfied with that current situation.

Theory of caring – midwifery

Generally, midwifery encompasses the concept of caring. The profession officially endorses 'caring' through its philosophy, code of ethics, standards for practice and various position statements. These are produced and ratified by midwives for the International College of Midwives and the specific national organisations.

Dickson (1996) draws on nursing theorists, for example Watson and Benner, to develop a theory of caring for midwifery, stating that caring prevents the person from being reduced to the moral status of an object. Although this redresses the problem of reductionism and objectivism, it does not offer an adequate ethical response for midwifery practice. It does not address the imbalance of power in relationships, of dominance and subordination, for example.

To use 'caring [for]' as the central value of the practice is to perpetuate the dominant role of stronger and superior protector-provider – it reduces rather than maintains the well and capable birthing woman's independence and self-determination.

[A]lthough providers may be well-meaning and nurturing in their care of childbearing women, their approach is most often nurturing to weakness, rather than strength ... Birth is not only about making babies.

Birth also is about making mothers – strong, competent, capable mothers, who trust themselves and know their inner strength (Rothman 1996 p.253-4).

If a power 'with' relationship, a woman-centred partnership, is the guiding value for midwifery practice then the well, capable birthing woman is the active decision-maker, determining what kind of assistance, if any, she needs and when that assistance is required. The midwife or other birth attendant, such as the doctor, is a resource person rather than the dominant provider and controller.

Babies, who have been turned into medical products, the products of the procedures of delivery, get presented to their mothers. In the bad old days, there might be a 72 hour wait. In newer times, the baby gets turned over quickly, cleaned up and wrapped like a package, instantly recreated from part of the mother's body to product of the hospital. It is the staff who presents the baby to the mother, in obvious contradiction to what has just happened: the mother presented the baby to the world (Rothman 1996 p.255).

As mothers and midwives indicate (Thompson 2001), adequate ethical responses in midwifery are contextual and temporal. They are based on relationship, not the duty-based rules of being responsible for the wellbeing of the patient, the abstract generalisations of right and wrong 'actions', or the dichotomies of mother's versus baby's rights, and quantity versus quality of life. It is sometimes forgotten that the ratio of birth to death is 1:1, and since medical science and technology have prolonged life and prevented many illnesses and diseases, we begin to think that all problems are solvable, an implication of modern bioethics. Problems that the woman herself cannot deal with alone will arise from time to time. Likewise, there will be circumstances previously agreed to, implicitly or explicitly, by both the woman and the midwife, when the midwife appropriately uses her power 'for' the woman in the role of her advocate. In that case, and according to the present mothers' and midwives' narratives, the power balance moves away from the woman temporarily and only indirectly since it remains the woman's informed choice, not mere consent, that guides practice. The balance of power returns towards

the woman relatively quickly. So that although there is a shifting of power within the partnership, the balance of power rests predominantly with the woman and endures over time. On the other hand, the 'caring [for]' emphasis implies that the midwife will 'do' for the birthing woman because she cannot 'do' for herself during childbirth. Yet, 'not doing' is often the true quiet art of midwifery (Kirkham 1986). 'Being with' woman, empowering the mother to have confidence in her own ability to birth her baby, is a 'hands off' approach.

Furthermore, the midwifery-specific concepts of 'presencing', 'knowing' and understanding, ensuring client control, and interacting are endorsed; linguistically, illness-oriented explanations drawn from nursing theorists are not. The latter conflict with feminist-oriented midwifery concepts. Such explanations refer to the patient, healing, cared for, recovery and 'promoting' independence, as if it were 'restoring' independence. The language at times changes to client, equality and self-responsibility, choice of services, control of the experience and continuity of care (the three Cs) when authors specifically use the term midwifery. This latter 'shift' indicates the different nature of the two practices, nursing and midwifery. Midwifery formally incorporates 'caring' into acknowledging women as persons based on mutual relationships of respect, trust and the dignity of all members of society (for example, Australian College of Midwives Incorporated (ACMI 1995) Code of Ethics and others such as NMC Code of Professional Conduct). However, adopting a theory of caring for midwifery places the concept of 'caring [for]', rather than one of a power 'with' partnership, central to midwifery and, therefore, central to any ethical response within midwifery practice. For similar reasons, applying the term 'therapeutic' to the mother-midwife relationship is inappropriate in most instances. The linguistic nature of such a label implies a 'defect' or illness in the child-bearing woman, ascribes more power to the midwife/practitioner than the mother, positions the professional in the elite expert role (in keeping with the medicalisation of childbirth), and reinforces the static power imbalance of the status quo; that is, in favour of the institution, not shared 'with' and between individuals.

Ethical principles and the midwifery discourse

Critiques of the scientific method have focused on its purported objectivity, universalism and lack of context – deficits when addressing ethical concerns. The application of ethical principles for decision making in the clinical area, however, enjoys enduring support from some healthcare professionals, especially when these principles are complementary to or accompanied by context and relationship.

The ethical principles most commonly discussed in midwifery literature are beneficence and autonomy, mainly because of the emphasis placed on individualism by ethical theories such as deontology and utilitarianism.

Proponents of consequential utilitarian ethics and principlism for midwifery discuss respect for persons, the exercise of individual rights and 'rational' autonomy, as needing to be limited or circumscribed for the common good, for universal fairness and justice. Beneficence and non-maleficence dominate ethical decision-making for the practitioner, and consistent with normative bioethics, rationale is based on the obligations and good acts of the professional, usually in life-threatening situations. Whilst midwives do have a responsibility to keep up-to-date with current research and knowledge, the present discussion adopts a different way of seeing regarding the rest of their argument. For example, Jacqueline Richards claims that

our professional reputation is undermined when we offer such conflicting advice [between beneficently passing on benefits of 'advance' to clients and justifying her actions to colleagues] (Richards 1997 p.165).

Such a view focuses on the professionals and describes a mother-midwife relationship of separateness rather than a prime relationship with the childbearing woman – of disparate relationships for the midwife. Relational feminist ethics places principles such as individual rights of justice secondary to the relationship and shared goal of the mother and midwife. Furthermore,

Ballou believes that in nursing – and the present discussion suggests therefore, by default in some approaches to midwifery – autonomy

is confused with concepts of professionalism, power, image, control, authority, accountability and independence ... [but concept analysis showed recurring themes of] self-governance within a system of principles, competence or capacity, decision making, critical reflection, freedom, and self-control (Ballou 1998 p.102).

Whilst autonomy is political in nature, the truest form comes from the person's own action and evolves internally. It is important to note that the present discussion does not critique the particularity of any author's definition of autonomy. It focuses on the philosophical method central to bioethics and the independent assessment of acts according to moral principles (McGrath 1998).

Woodward (1998) investigated nurses' and midwives' individual understandings of what it is to care. Findings suggested that principle-based ethical theory lacked the particularity and relationship necessary to guide ethical decisions about individuals, and there was tension between autonomy and beneficence. Rather than rejecting beneficence however, Woodward proposes that patient autonomy and practitioner-guided beneficence should be balanced to protect the moral integrity of both patient and practitioner. Paternalism is justified when rationality is impaired, significant harm is likely without intervention, and the person will agree retrospectively. This part of the argument is still immersed in principles-based ethics and normative theory. On the other hand, Breeze (1998) writing about nursing ethics and the intellectually disabled person, puts forward the deontological and utilitarian assessment of autonomy – that in order to exercise autonomy one has to be rational. She argues that such an assessment has the potential to be subjective and value laden. Again, the present discussion is critical of assessing individual 'acts' according to abstract principles, void of context and relationship.

Woodward (1998) raises the importance of dialogue between practitioner and patient, and draws on the feminist and Aristotelian perspective of moral agency being constituted from and motivated by good reasons, not merely doing good acts. However, the argument oscillates back towards principlism by concluding that beneficence, or 'doing good', which is derived through caring

should not be uncritically superseded by contemporary emphasis on autonomy [because] This disregards the intrinsic morality in a caring relationship, deprives the patient of the qualitative component of care and personalized application of knowledge and skills, threatens to diminish the source of practitioner motivation and may result in self-reproach and retribution through frustrated moral agency (Woodward 1998 p.1051).

Debates which focus on 'patient' and 'dependency' retain a normative bioethics gaze. When they refer to midwifery, they more typically reflect midwifery practice in a medicalised hospital setting or environment and as mentioned earlier, settings directly influence variations in the exercise of power in practices (Thompson, Melia & Boyd 1994). The term 'patient' is used frequently and the ethical argument remains guided by principlism rather than relational or virtue ethics. For example, the argument suggests that 'doing good', beneficent acts, will create a nurse-patient relationship and thus practice will be ethical, but one needs to ask if the practitioner is deciding what is 'good' for the 'patient' and again question the distribution of power in such a relationship. Neither is the influence of the mother's and midwife's character adequately addressed. Nevertheless, despite these differing interpretations, the influence of feminist ethics is beginning to emerge in the more recent midwifery discourse.

When autonomy is taken to mean independence based on rational decision-making and self-governance, debate on the collective autonomy of midwifery practice is fundamentally flawed (Clarke 1995a; Fleming 1998) needing corrective action by midwives (McKay 1998; Wagner 1998). For Stella McKay autonomy of midwifery practice depends on the midwife acting as an advocate instead of 'giving' autonomy to the woman because the latter implies midwife-control. That is,

lack of autonomy may have less to do with professional issues and more to do with the feminine role. In general women are still not identified with positions of authority and control ... [midwives] need to assume greater responsibility and acknowledge the accountability that comes with power (McKay 1998 p.18).

There is some interdisciplinary support for 'autonomous' midwifery practice too:

widespread, irrational, non-scientific statements made by obstetricians against independent midwifery have nothing to do with safety, but everything to do with fear of competition (Wagner 1998 p.20).

This echoes the earlier statement that autonomy is political in nature.

Given that language portrays our philosophical and social orientation, the use of the principle-based term 'autonomy' rather than 'informed choice' illustrates how our way of seeing determines our way of practice, and vice versa. Examining discourses can reveal underlying assumptions and make explicit the values of the practice. A practitioner focused practice is guided by principles and duty or obligation ethics; what can and ought the midwife 'do' as a professional practitioner? Language such as 'informed choice' and 'active role' for the childbearing woman describes a practice with a mutual and shared goal, a practice that is woman-centred in a mother-midwife partnership.

The British survey by Churchill and Benbow (2000) reports on 'informed choice' in maternity services and an 'active role' in decision making. In that survey, women indicated that (i) there was more active decision making in midwife-led antenatal clinics than maternity units, (ii) environmental and/or structural factors affected women's perceptions of participation in decision-making more than the personnel involved, and (iii) midwives were the primary source of information to women in most antenatal care settings. A longitudinal survey of women attending mainstream maternity services in Australia compared women's knowledge of pregnancy, fears for self and baby, and locus of control, in single-baby pregnancy and twin pregnancy (Thompson 1992). Findings demonstrated that magazines, books and pamphlets were the most helpful sources in both early and late pregnancy, and midwives were the second most helpful source of information in early pregnancy for both groups of women. By the 32nd week of pregnancy other pregnant women were the second most helpful source of information for women with a single-baby pregnancy, and midwives and doctors remained the most helpful source for those with a twin pregnancy. All women, regardless of the type of pregnancy, believed less in the third trimester that events in pregnancy and childbirth were determined mostly by their own behaviour.

Midwives experience conflict when beneficence dominates the childbearing woman's autonomy, resulting in paternalism towards the woman and sometimes the midwife (Toohill 1997). Knowledge and technological advances offer more options for reproductive health which means that respecting autonomy in the presence of competing principles becomes more difficult. According to Sharp (1998) there is an institutional and policy 'macro' level of practice and an individual 'micro' level of practice. The latter achieves 'good' through interaction with the individual woman. Midwives have an instrumental role (cure, diagnosis and treatment) and an expressive role (caring, helping, comforting and guiding). Advocacy at the macro level is recommended to reverse the devaluation of normal processes and promote practices that value accomplishment and empowerment for the childbearing woman. Sharp talks of self-determination rather than 'rational' autonomy as discussed in Chapter 3, and persuasion after confirming the woman's goals and assumptions rather than beneficence, regarding the wellbeing of herself and her baby.

This review of the midwifery profession's literature reveals that contemporary practice emanates from two generally differing belief and value systems. One consists of the medicalised childbirth practices based on scientific rationalism, universal ethical theories and abstract principlism. The other, more recent, espouses the values and orientation of relational and feminist-virtue ethics, for example caring as the essence of moral agency, the centrality of context and particularity, and the ethical imperative of redressing power imbalances in relationships. Sentiments expressed in mothers' and midwives' narratives (Thompson 2001) and the literature are similar: midwives experience more conflict when the former approach is imposed on their practice, and more congruence when practice is based on relational or feminist values – engagement ethics. A relational and feminist orientation to ethical midwifery practice, therefore, presents as more appropriate than the currently dominant normative bioethics.

WAYS OF SEEING AND CONSTRUCTION: ORIENTATION

Practitioner definitions of midwifery practice

The way members of an occupation or profession define themselves influences both their interaction with other occupations in the workplace and the future direction of their profession (Scoggin 1996). Philosophical agreement with midwifery ideologies and increased years of practice are the most predictive variables of a positive midwifery occupational identity, and the primary identification of nurse-midwives is not with nursing (as it is at the beginning of the occupation), but with midwifery. This supports the argument that the way we see determines the way we practice, and settings impact on the practice and the practitioner's orientation. Furthermore, practitioner orientation reflects that the practices of nursing and midwifery are different in nature.

Another argument of the present analysis is that tradition does not deny creativity or change – rather, traditions such as those of the midwifery community endure because critical and internal examination verifies those values and beliefs which best guide their practice. It is the old values that provide legitimacy or authenticity which are passed on and

This process provides continuity within a culture because a form, even though changing, embodies some of the norms and values that served it well in the past (Scoggin 1996 p.41).

Consumers and midwives alike are questioning the appropriateness of medicalised childbirth for the majority of women, and are indicating their desire for informed choice and a return of emphasis on self-determination for the birthing woman. Safety is important, but it is not the only thing that matters. The woman's experience of childbirth as part of the human condition, and her engagement within relationship, are central to an adequate ethical response in practice.

Smythe and Kerins define independent midwifery practice according to employment status and one's accountability position in the decision-making process:

The [independent] midwife provides continuity of care from pregnancy, through labour, and in the postnatal period. Hospital practice is described as referring to midwives who are employed by an institution and are directly accountable to other midwives or managers, and who do not provide continuity of care. While independent midwives may practice 'in' hospitals, they are not employed by the hospital, and therefore are not hospital midwives. Decision making is described as the process of making judgements about the actions or non-actions of practice (Smythe & Kerrins 1994 p.3).

Parratt (1996) argues, on a philosophical basis, that all midwives can practise independently regardless of their place of practice or employment status, if they adopt the partnership midwifery theory. Based on the work of Leap (1991 cited in Parratt 1996), Parratt distinguishes between the self-employed midwife who is able to choose her/his working hours and workload, and the midwife who practises independently because s/he has

experience, diverse reasons for entering midwifery practice, sees birth as a social event, believes birth is usually a normal event, that is, a trust in women's bodies that they can give birth without intervention, provides continuity of care, provides real choice in options for place of birth, promotes the woman and the midwife having equal but complementary responsibilities, promotes a relationship of trust and mutual respect with the woman, and adopts her own style and way of practice (Parratt 1996 p.24).

These attributes certainly do characterise a midwife working in partnership with the childbearing woman. However, regardless of how desirable they are according to one's personal philosophy and private capacity, as Parratt suggests, midwives practice in relationship with other healthcare practitioners and facilities, with government departments and professional registration bodies. It is the imbalance of power in those relationships that constrain the midwife's independence and the adequacy of the ethical response within midwifery practice.

Practitioner-identified philosophy of midwifery practice: values and beliefs

Midwives consider that open communication, adequate life skills, a nurturing and caring environment, and a democratic management structure are prerequisites for empowerment of childbearing women – and midwives; paternalism and advocacy, when it legitimises a paternalistic approach, are constraining factors (Too 1996). Narratives in the present analysis, especially Diane's, concur with Too's (1996) findings.

Katie, the independently practising midwife, discussed the primacy of women being 'informed' and 'owning' their decisions, of the midwife 'knowing' the woman and her family, and of her sincere aim to support women's wishes while providing safe professional care for community-based childbirth. Informed choice could quickly become or be perceived as coercion, its antithesis:

I mean, it's so difficult then to make sure that you discuss it as much as you can discuss it and you can write it and all the rest of it and, then even though you feel like it's all gone over her head, you come to a point where you feel like you can do no more, say no more, explain no more, and continue to be supportive of her decision. And sometimes I'm sure they feel pressured by that process of discussion, why you're trying to bang their heads and say 'Will you let this bloody bit of information in and just absorb it for a bit and mull it about and then reflect back to me that you've actually understood what I've been talking to you about'. So it's difficult, it's difficult not to be coercive I suppose, and yet we value informed choice, we value women making their own life choices including the wrong choices, that's their right to make the choice and make mistakes in their personal decision making just like we all do. It's that notion that, you wanted her to make an informed choice, informed choice equals a risk-benefit analysis from her perspective.

Smythe and Kerins (1994) surveyed practising independent midwives in Auckland, New Zealand with regard to decision making. The beliefs and values that guide clinical decision making for those participants were safety, close partnership with the woman and her family, and anticipation of problems. Other important beliefs and values, however, concerned supporting the woman's personal/cultural views on birth, the woman feeling as though she's done a good job with her birthing, providing informed choice on all available options, that the woman often has an inner knowledge of herself and her baby, and that being positive can change the energy and enhance the process whereas negative energy, looking for problems, inhibits the process. This latter belief is also integral to the narratives of Katie, Diane and Kerry-Anne. Other narrative evidence in the New Zealand research demonstrated that making the decision was not necessarily a problem; the problem was overcoming barriers such as conflict between midwife and doctor. Those findings concur with the present narratives. Midwife-doctor cooperation and conflict is an example of the use of power 'alongside' or abuse of power 'over' colleagues, respectively.

Again, the philosophical orientation of midwives in the present narratives is not unique to them. It is echoed by some who recently entered the profession, and perhaps that reflects a revised approach to the 'way of seeing', the orientation in practitioner preparation programmes. Student nurse-midwives who sculpted in clay their individual and personal philosophy of midwifery practice, and then described the sculpture to others, depicted the centrality of women within the context of their communities (Vande Vusse 1997 p.47). Common images were the availability of the nurse-midwives' supporting hands, vulvas with crowning fetal heads, and people sitting in

groups as small diverse communities. In their descriptions, students frequently commented that the nurse-midwife was assisting quietly without taking the main focal position, that the focus of practice was on the self-determining women and families, and that a reverence for life was important.

Relationship

Policy initiatives make midwifery practice

more daunting, challenging and complex, and some midwives have stated that they do not get the support they require within the current model of statutory supervision ... skills to take innovative and truly woman-centred care forward must become a priority (Deery 1999 p.251).

Ruth Deery promotes the therapeutic relationship between midwives and their clients, because of its success in social work, mental health nursing, counselling and psychotherapy. She asks supervisors of midwives and midwifery managers to consider such an approach, plus clinical supervision, as enhancing the way midwives learn to relate to one another. Furthermore, she notes that the midwife-client relationship is changing and although she does not identify the change she highlights

the amount of energy used when midwives use themselves as a therapeutic resource for women (Deery 1999 p.251).

Clinical supervision would help here.

Jeanne Siddiqui (1999) suggests that key elements of the relationship between the woman and midwife are authenticity of being, conscience (embracing engagement and the feminist notion of 'virtue' in caring), commitment (again, part of caring, and including advocacy), presence, compassion, empathy and empowerment. She is critical that midwifery philosophy (in Britain) is based on utilitarian principles, claiming that codes and charters only provide guidelines and do not necessarily empower the professional to act with authority. Her proposals resonate well within the present discussion. Disappointingly, she also refers to the mother-midwife relationship as a 'therapeutic' relationship and thus the reader reverts again to thoughts of medicalisation and the need to 'fix' or treat. The linguistic nature of the term 'therapeutic' teaches us to again view childbirth from within the expert-patient, illness-disease model. This latter approach conflicts with Siddiqui's strong feminist theme of developing a shared philosophy and shared values – the midwife as a personal source not 'elite expert', the application of intuitive skills and ways of knowing, and the empowerment of women. Referring to midwifery education, Siddiqui states

however thoroughly students are taught fundamental skills such as temperature taking, aseptic technique, etc., if they are not overtly taught the elements of caring within midwifery, they may have difficulty in responding appropriately when faced with clients in all or any situations. Midwives who have entered midwifery with a nursing background may need to 'unlearn' many of the approaches and models used in caring for the sick (Siddiqui 1999 p.113).

This has also been my experience during ten years as a midwifery educator, and forms part of the basis of the claim that nursing and midwifery are different practices. They are different by their nature; not merely because of different ways of 'doing' or 'not doing' in the midwifery example, but because of different ways of 'seeing', of orientation. Although skills and techniques are important

Of the two elements in a tradition ... skills and techniques, and ways of seeing – Gombrich emphasises the latter (Langford 1985 p.9).

Attitudes

There is a general consensus amongst midwives that ethical sensitivity and responsiveness to women during childbearing, and in relation to their reproductive health, is not only complex but also oriented to the empowerment of women and uniqueness of the particular woman (Cullen 1995; Too 1996; Sharp 1998; Siddiqui 1999; Hall 1999; Churchill & Benbow 2000). This runs counter to the universalism of deontology and utilitarianism, and the abstraction of principlism.

In the 1960s the emphasis was on the woman:

If the woman can be encouraged to be upright and mobile, labour is likely to progress more quickly and the woman will feel more in control, especially if she is encouraged to change position from time to time in order to become as comfortable as possible (Myles 1964 p.181).

As discussed in Chapter 2, medicalisation followed. By the late 1980s literature began (re)focusing on the birthing woman more and on medical technology and intervention less. However, the emphasis was still on the hospital environment and the wisdom of medicalisation for childbirth.

The discrepancy between the desired and the achieved levels of home birth, however, and the prevailing attitudes towards it, suggest that it is health service staff who are hindering women from having home birth, rather than women being 'unfit' for it ... the daily practice of midwives demonstrates behaviour, decision-making and attitudes which still lean towards fulfilling the utilitarian goals of the NHS rather than the individual needs of women (Clarke 1995b p.270).

Common responses of hospital midwives towards home birth consistently deny the woman autonomy and respect (Clarke 1995b). They do not respect the woman as an end in herself. Rather the woman is manipulated for the ends of obstetric or hospital management policy. Jennifer Hall (1999) reports on how her friend described the contrast in attitude and behaviour of midwives who attended her first and second home births. The first midwife was unobtrusive; she was present but calm and relaxed, trusted that women (and thus she) could give birth on their own without medical assistance, and the equipment was in the corner of the room unopened until required. The midwife at the second birth, apparently an experienced home birth attendant, transformed the couple's bedroom into a mini-hospital room – a place that is normally one of intimacy, and often a place where personal, private possessions are kept. She was on the other side of the room involved with the equipment when the baby was being born, indicating that she did not 'believe' the mother's warning about the speed of the first birth. The midwife returned to the equipment soon after the birth, taking longer to discard unused items than she had to open them. The second midwife's panic would have 'terrified' the father had he not experienced the first home birth.

Fear among midwives is generated by the experiences gained within hospital settings ... the assumption is also made that the hospital is the safest place, despite the evidence [to the contrary, for example, Guilliland 1999] ... medical care is seen to help, so it becomes expected for labour, and midwives then feel pressured to 'produce' a perfect child and become terrified in case they do something wrong (Hall 1999 p.226).

These embedded and embodied views indicate the integral role of relationship and context, the personal and the particular, for an adequate ethical response in midwifery practice.

SUMMARY

This chapter compared mothers' and midwives' narratives, in particular the midwife's perspective, with current literature, under three themes: (i) ways of knowing, (ii) ethical theories and principles 'incorporated', and (iii) ways of seeing (practitioner orientation).

Explicit and implicit ethical values within the midwifery profession resemble those of the midwife's real life experience (Thompson 2001), when their focus is woman-centred rather than theory-driven and problem-oriented. Their personal narratives and recent midwifery literature do not parallel the dilemmic, problem-solving approach of bioethics. Practitioners' ethical orientation and responses vary between practice settings in both the lived reality and literature. Non-institutional settings are more conducive to 'being with' the woman in an intimate, relaxed mother-midwife relationship.

Ways of knowing (epistemology)

Authentic or legitimate information and knowledge come from multiple sources including the woman's personal experience. The embedded and embodied nature of 'birthing' knowledge is emphasised by the present mothers and mid-

wives and acknowledged in current literature. Birth is a journey. For the midwife who accompanies the traveller, it demands a 'knowing', a 'being', a 'relating' and a 'doing'. The science and 'knowing' of midwifery involves both conventional means such as drugs and a range of strategies that are determined in partnership by the woman according to her experience and by the midwife according to her knowledge and skill. This holistic and consultative approach contrasts with the reductionist mind-body duality of problem-solving bioethics. A birthing woman uses embodied knowledge such as being able to 'get in tune' with her body. Her body dictates what she needs to do to birth her baby such as rocking, walking or moaning, and she experiences a mind-body unity rather than split.

Personal narratives show that the domain of knowledge also means the woman and midwife 'knowing' each other. It is important for the midwife to spend time with the birthing woman and to learn her likes and dislikes over a whole range of things, not just birth. When the woman and midwife know each other's strengths, limits, desires and ways of responding, it leads to decisions that are particular to the individual. Personal knowledge gained through working with women and reflecting on practice focuses on the humanness of both mother and midwife, and deepens their relationship.

Ethical theories and principles 'incorporated' (including governmental reports)

Findings from governmental reports resemble some of the values and philosophical beliefs identified by participants in the present research as appropriate for childbirth practices, but the lack of attention these reports receive from powerful public authorities indicates their different 'gaze' and ethical perspective.

When narratives from these mothers and midwives are compared with the literature, ethical principles are incorporated into healthcare practices at both the individual practitioner level and the institutional and governmental level, where the practice setting is a mainstream hospital ward. Relational and feminist virtue ethics guide practice in birth centres and independent midwifery services.

Healthcare facilities and governmental departments promote duty and obligation, and principles-based ethical decision making for maternity services. In that setting, the profession and practitioner endorse a normative, 'ends' or 'consequences' orientation. Administrative and professional interests maintain a technocratic model of maternity care despite the efforts of others to replace it with a 'woman-centred' approach. While statistics paint a favourable picture, many facets of modern obstetric practice work against the empowerment of women and erode the role of the midwife. Individual mothers and midwifery practitioners experience conflict between institutional workplace/service provider ethics and personal/professional ethics when the individual's values align with woman-centred practices. In this sense, therefore, analysis suggests a lack of cohesion between the institution's approach and the individual's values.

Ways of seeing (practitioner orientation)

Midwives' primary identification shifts from nursing at the beginning of their occupation, and medicalisation of birth in mainstream settings, to midwifery, with increased exposure to midwifery traditions and woman-centred birth practices (Scoggin 1996; and see narratives from Bev and Diane).

Midwives in the present analysis emphasise the importance of ethical midwifery practice being guided by their experiential knowledge and 'what was right for the woman'. Their narratives reflect the feminist criticism that the powerful and public sphere relegates women's concerns to the disempowered and private sphere, and demonstrate the inadequacy of normative, values-and-context-free, problem-solving bioethics for midwifery practice – criticisms shared by Siddiqui (1999). These midwives speak of open communication, trust, respect, confidence, pride, and continuity of carer and philosophy of care. Birth plans can empower women by increasing their active involvement in decision making, in and outside mainstream settings (see also Too 1996), but as Diane's narrative demonstrates, birth plans can also precipitate threat and punishment. Woman-centred midwives use language of relationship, context, virtues-values, and character of moral agents: they are critical of institutional and 'expert' dominance over childbirth practices, and speak of quietly assisting the birthing woman (Thompson 2001; Deery 1999). These midwives express negative feelings and emotions when workplace or service provider ethics conflict with personal/professional ethics' and when power 'over' practices disempower the mother or midwife. Contrary to birth centre or independently practising midwives, who are portrayed as working 'with' the birthing woman, hospital midwives are depicted as being hostile towards difference (Clarke 1995b; Hall 1999), and having disparate relationships (Thompson 2001). The mother-midwife relationship with them is one of separateness – 'no proper relationship', as Katie says. A practitioner-focused practice is guided by duty or obligation ethics, what the midwife can and ought 'do' as a professional practitioner. Language such as 'informed choice' and 'active role' for the childbearing woman describes a practice with mutual and shared goals, a woman-centred mother-midwife partnership.

REFERENCES

ACMI 1995 Code of ethics. Australian College of Midwives Incorporated, Melbourne

Australian Federal Government 1999 Who's rocking the cradle: Senate inquiry into childbirth practices. Australian Federal Government, Canberra

Ballou K A 1998 A concept analysis of autonomy. Journal of Professional Nursing 14 (2): 102-110

Breeze J 1998 Can paternalism be justified in mental healthcare? Journal of Advanced Nursing 28 (2): 260-265

Churchill H, Benbow A 2000 Informed choice in maternity services. British Journal of Midwifery 8 (1): 41-47

Clarke R A 1995a Midwives, their employers and the UKCC: an eternally unethical triangle. Nursing Ethics: An International Journal for Healthcare Professionals 2 (3): 247-253

Clarke R A 1995b Ethics and midwifery practice: the links between moral responsibilities, midwives and homebirth. Midwives 108 (1292): 270-271

Coiffi J, Markham R 1997 Clinical decision-making by midwives: managing case complexity. Journal of Advanced Nursing 25: 265-272

Cullen M C 1995 Australian midwives' practice domain. Knowledge and wisdom: the keys to safe motherhood. 9th Biennial Conference, Australian College of Midwives Incorporated, Sydney

Davis D 1995 Ways of knowing in midwifery. Knowledge and wisdom: the keys to safe motherhood. 9th Biennial Conference, Australian College of Midwives Inc, Sydney

Deery R 1999 Improving relationships through clinical supervision: 2. British Journal of Midwifery 7 (4): 251-254

Denzin N K, Lincoln Y S (eds) 1994 Handbook of qualitative research. Sage, Thousand Oaks, California

Department of Health 1993 Changing childbirth. HMSO, London

Dickson N 1996 A theory of caring for midwifery. Australian College of Midwives Incorporated Journal, June: 20-24

Fleming V E M 1998 Autonomous or automations? An exploration through history of the concept of autonomy in midwifery in Scotland and New Zealand. Nursing Ethics: An International Journal for Healthcare Professionals 5 (1): 43-51

Flint C, Poulengeris P, Grant A 1989 The 'know your midwife' scheme: a randomised trial of continuity of care by a team of midwives. Midwifery 5 (1): 11-16

Frith L (ed) 1996 Ethics and midwifery: issues in contemporary practice. Butterworth-Heinemann, Oxford

Guilliland K 1999 Managing change in midwifery practice: the New Zealand experience. Future birth: the place to be born conference, Birth International, Camperdown

Hall J 1994 Directions for midwifery education – learning to be 'with women'. Midwifery and the Community: 3rd National Research Forum, School of Nursing, Faculty of Health Sciences, La Trobe University, Melbourne

Hall J 1999 Home birth: the midwife effect. British Journal of Midwifery 7 (4): 225-227

Kelly M E 1997 Exploring midwifery knowledge. British Journal of Midwifery 5 (4): 195-198

Kirkham M 1986 A feminist perspective in midwifery. In Webb C (ed) Feminist practice in women's healthcare. John Wiley & Sons, Chichester

Langford G 1985 Education, persons and society: a philosophical inquiry. Macmillan, London

Mander R 1992 See how they learn: experience as the basis of practice. Nurse Education Today 12: 11-18

McGrath P 1998 Autonomy, discourse, and power: a postmodern reflection on principlism and bioethics. Journal of Medicine and Philosophy 23 (5): 516-532

McKay S 1998 The route to true autonomous practice for midwives. MIDIRS Midwifery Digest 8 (1): 17-18

Myles M F 1964 A textbook for midwives. Livingstone Ltd, Edinburgh

Parratt J 1996 Practising midwifery independently: for the majority of midwives? Australian College of Midwives Incorporated Journal, September: 23-28

Reiger K 1999 Birthing in the postmodern moment: struggles over defining maternity care needs. Australian Feminist Studies 14 (30): 387

Richards J 1997 Too choosy about choice: the responsibility of the midwife. British Journal of Midwifery 5 (3): 163-168

Robertson A 2000 The pain of labour – a feminist issue. ACE Graphics, Camperdown

Rothman B K 1996 Women, providers, and control. Journal of obstetrics, gynaecology and neonatal nursing 25 (3): 253-6

Scoggin J 1996 How nurse-midwives define themselves in relation to nursing, medicine, and midwifery. Journal of Nurse-Midwifery 41 (1): 36-42

Sharp E S 1998 Ethics in reproductive healthcare: a midwifery perspective. Journal of Nurse-Midwifery 43 (3): 235-245

Siddiqui J 1999 The therapeutic relationship in midwifery. British Journal of Midwifery 7 (2): 111-114

Sleep J 1992 Research and the practice of midwifery. Journal of Advanced Nursing 17: 1465-1471

Smythe L, Kerins R 1994 Decision making in independent midwifery practice. Midwifery Research Forum, La Trobe University, Melbourne

Thompson F E 1992 Women's knowledge and experiences in twin and singleton pregnancies [unpublished Master of Nursing Studies dissertation]. Department of Nursing, La Trobe University, Melbourne

Thompson F E 2001 The ethical nature of the mother-midwife relationship: a feminist perspective [unpublished PhD dissertation]. University of Southern Queensland, Toowoomba, Queensland

Thompson I K, Melia K M, Boyd K M 1994 Nursing ethics. Churchill Livingstone, Melbourne

Too S-K 1996 Do birth plans empower women? A study of midwives' views. Nursing Standard 10 (32): 44-48

Toohill J 1997 Paternalism and the parent with an intellectual disability. Birth Issues 6 (4): 11-14

Vande Vusse L 1997 Sculpting a nurse-midwifery philosophy. Journal of Nurse-Midwifery 42 (1): 43-48

Victorian State Government 1990 Having a baby in Victoria: final report of the ministerial review of birthing services in Victoria. Victorian State Government, Melbourne

Wagner M 1998 Autonomy: the central issue of midwifery. MIDIRS Midwifery Digest 8 (1): 19-21

Woodward V M 1998 Caring, patient autonomy and the stigma of paternalism. Journal of Advanced Nursing 28 (5): 1046-1052

Plotting our practice – values and philosophical foundations of the birthing environment

The values and philosophical foundations of the birthing environment are reflected in the discourse of practitioners as well as the more official discourse of the profession. Continuing on from the profession's discourse, therefore, and in order to identify taken-for-granted assumptions in the practice environment, this part of the discussion compares and contrasts mothers' and midwives' narratives with values that are specific to workplace ethics, as expressed by midwives. Firstly, the power of language and conceptual theoretical frameworks implicit in organisational structures of practice and decision making are examined, and lastly, comment is made on the notion of a midwifery partnership.

THE POWER OF LANGUAGE

Not only does our way of seeing determine how we conceptualise experience, but language, too, structures our experience. Ways of seeing our world and ways of describing our world are closely connected, and like ways of seeing, language habits are acquired from and shared with others who belong to the same linguistic community (Langford 1985). Maree, a first-time mother, speaks of hospital midwives and doctors trying to 'bowl her over' into a fetal position while she was in the middle of a contraction, to insert an epidural cannula. Another mother, Brenda, describes how incensed she was at being called 'girlie' when she was noisy during her birthing. On the other hand, the metaphor of 'journey' is used in several narratives to portray the positive experience and achievement of birthing.

Birth language

The impact of language used by midwives and other healthcarers in relation to childbearing women has received increased attention in recent years. Firstly, language presents a certain image of the profession. Secondly, language is not neutral: it is symbolic of conceptual meaning – of our way of 'seeing'. Given that midwives in most Western societies enter their practice via nursing, and generally practice in a hospital setting, medical terminology is accepted and internalised. Thirdly, language generates and maintains power, and the techno-scientific language used in hospital reinforces the professional's control and the woman's powerlessness as a passive recipient of the type of care that professionals deem necessary (Carboon 1999). Machin and Scamell found that, in England, the medical metaphor continues to dominate the ethos of intrapartum care: women, vulnerable in labour,

are reassured by the safe boundaries set by medicalisation and are more susceptible to the symbolic messages of that environment (Machin & Scamell 1997 p.84).

Midwives describe their experiences of decision making in independent practice as consultative, well-documented, a balancing act, demanding, professional, worrying, and satisfying: the least typical descriptions are logical, caught in the middle/can't win either way, tense, sleepless nights, no problem, disappointing, OK (Smythe & Kerins 1994). Their chosen additional words were inspiring, great, self searching, good communication, clear, learning from mistakes, safety, woman/family oriented, partnership, fruitful, mind expanding, educative, questioning practice, building self-esteem, constant evaluation, lovely, reflective, challenging, and appreciated.

The language used by midwives and other birth attendants reflects their attitudes and, regardless of how correct their individual philosophy is, can objectify the woman who is giving birth. For example, to identify the unborn baby as an 'R.O.A.' and the mother as a 'multip', or to speak of the midwife as having 'done the delivery' dehumanises the woman, places her in a passive role, and reaffirms the midwife's need to be in control.

Truthful language that puts the mother and woman at the centre is a humble language where the midwife is not the star of the performance [for example, 'I attended that birth' rather than 'I delivered that patient'] (Zeidenstein 1988 p.75).

Far from being minor, to use objective obstetric and medical language for birth is to influence the ingrained beliefs and actions of the midwifery profession, and words that diminish the woman's uniqueness and humanity reduce the sense of mutual respect. Zeidenstein urges us in particular, to replace 'normal spontaneous vaginal delivery' with 'spontaneous vaginal birth':

Are not all births normal anyway? The use of normal in the case of birth predisposes the possibility of an abnormal vaginal birth (Zeidenstein 1988 p.76).

A concept analysis of normal labour

Midwives view the concepts of natural and normal labour as not mutually inclusive (Gould 2000). Although language is flawed, it is through language that further understanding and professional knowledge is developed and shared. Because midwifery knowledge is enmeshed within the medical model, many midwives believe that natural childbirth is normal, but that normal childbirth can include common interventions and thus does not have to be natural. Furthermore, there is vast interprofessional dissonance in understanding the term 'normal labour'. The obstetrician, epidemiologist, psychologist, anthropologist, sociologist and midwife all define the term differently: according to Wagner (1994 cited in Gould 2000), the midwifery belief is that normal labour is defined by the woman and not others. This is consistent with the woman-centred, woman-governed midwifery model of care but not with the more medically-defined model found in obstetric and midwifery texts. The latter define labour according to the 'normal in retrospect medical model', a definition also criticised by Kirkham (1986) and later, Page (1995). Definitions that are individual to each woman make the midwife's normal practice parameters difficult to quantify. Gould argues, firstly, that midwives have consequently been coerced by the medical profession's measurable parameters of normal labour ('normal in retrospect') at the expense of other crucial but equally difficult to define elements of the labour process. For example, the mother's persona, the sensations the woman actually experiences, and the fact that aspects follow each other sequentially at their own pace to have the optimum effect, are ignored in the quantifiable-measurement model. Secondly,

if labour was perceived as necessary work leading to achievement, as described in many of the original uses of the word 'labour', women might be able to move away from the passive role in labour which the medicalisation of childbirth has introduced ... [and as] The Winterton Report (Department of Health, UK 1992) points out our society needs other measures of success in the maternity services as well as safety, including elements of the social side of midwifery practice (Gould 2000 p. 425).

In order to work truly with women, midwives need to understand the social and political forces which shape the reality of women's lives.

If we want to support the normal we will need to understand epidemiological trends, to hold advanced clinical skills, and be able to challenge what is meant by normal (Page 1995 p.356).

This requires that midwives practice outside the confines of institutions, that they practice in the communities where women live and work.

PRACTICE DECISIONS AND CONFLICT BETWEEN WORKPLACE AND PERSONAL/PROFESSIONAL ETHICS

The conflict of values between workplace ethics and personal/professional midwifery ethics is a major theme in the present mothers' and midwives' narratives. It intersects with the theme of power 'over' and is identified in both mothers' and midwives' narratives. Midwives and mothers are often 'silenced' by medical dominance and authority in such conflicts. Typically, the midwives placate the 'system worker' to protect the mother and deliberately avoid future contact with the individual practitioner to avoid recurrence of such conflict. Kerry-Anne's narrative tells how she did not carry out written routine orders for all primigravida women under a particular obstetrician's care, to have an episiotomy – 'I couldn't bring myself to actually cut this woman unnecessarily' – how she 'calmed down and calmly walked back into the room and gave him the catgut and stood by him while he sutured her', but that she

never confronted him [obstetrician] ... And from then on I made it my business not to be around when he had a primigravid patient in case I was asked to do the delivery. Because I still felt that in the same circumstances I would not be able to do an episiotomy just because it's written on someone's card – that that is his procedure for primigravids.

Mothers' stories tell of how their support person formed an alliance with the staff through fear for the woman's and baby's safety, negating previously discussed agreements between them and the birthing woman.

Brenda: I couldn't have any more gas, I'd had too much gas. Would you like to have an epidural? And [husband's name] was going Yes! And just stop the

pain, and I don't know what I said about it, but [husband's name] said yes and that was fine by me, whatever he said went. I was too busy rocking and I had my eyes shut .. And I've gone 'Oh well, I'll have it then'. And I was strong, like I wasn't going to have it, I was going to do it just on gas, and he's gone 'Give her the epidural'. He's my support partner and he's going 'Just stop the pain, give her an epidural', so I've curled up, and they've done it.

Her husband also coached her during the actual birth, in accord with staff wishes and 'rules':

I'm thinking everyone can see me and I'm over this bar and I want my clothes on and I don't really like this ... so I wrapped my leg around it so that they couldn't make me stand up, and [husband's name] untangled my legs for me and made me stand up [spoken in exasperation]. So as a support person he was doing all the right things for the staff but not for me sort of thing.

Conflict between workplace and personal/professional ethics is not peculiar to midwifery. Nursing literature also reports on the congruency between nurses' values and job requirements, calling for integrity (Koerner 1996), the ethical wellbeing of the environment nurses work in (Olson 1998), and the role conflicts and ethical challenges as seen from a feminist and critical-theory perspective (Padgett 1998).

The tendency to focus first on the moral quandaries in clinical situations is probably sound, both because of their immediate appeal, and also because they focus directly on the nurse-patient relationship. They also illustrate the tensions experienced by nurses in accepting responsibility for the well-being of patients, between their personal feelings and moral beliefs on the one hand and their professional responsibilities on the other (Thompson, Melia & Boyd 1994 p.67).

Historically, 20th century midwifery in the Western world has been under the control of medicine, administratively, philosophically and clinically (Clarke 1995a; Fleming 1998). Generally this remains so at the beginning of the 21st century, and because medicine and midwifery endorse different epistemologies and philosophies, individual midwifery practitioners experience conflict between workplace and personal/professional ethics.

Western medical practice, as discussed in earlier chapters, is based on universal ethical theory, primarily utilitarianism, and the epistemology of science and technology. It is guided by the Hippocratic oath which emphasises cure rather than care, an interventionist philosophy. Western medicine does not accept as legitimate, alternative ethical approaches or the empowerment of women 'alongside' the professional, most of whom are male.

Clarke (1995a) claims that, in Britain, midwives are the 'professional piggy in the middle'; that is, between the employer (the National Health Service) and the professional/registering nursing body (the NMC). Neither the professional independence and autonomy of midwifery, nor the underlying philosophical differences between the code of professional conduct and the workplace are acknowledged. With regard to professional independence, the (British) Midwives Act of 1902 promised better education and registration but surrendered professional and clinical autonomy to medical control. The Royal College of Midwives cooperated with doctors, agreeing that midwives would attend normal births only and offer relatively unskilled nursing assistance. From 1920 until the 1980s when it was abolished, the Central Midwives Board admitted midwives as members, but statutory law forbade midwives to comprise the majority of membership. The majority of members had to be medical practitioners and therefore, rules for midwives were medically controlled and the scope of midwifery practice strictly limited (Clarke 1995a; Fleming 1998).

Cecilia Benoit delineates three competing approaches in the postfunctionalist debate on service professions – professional dominance, professional decline and patriarchal control:

Fusion of service ethic and technical expertise grants service professions monopoly over possession and transmission of knowledge, autonomy to organize working conditions to their own choosing, and authority over clients and allied occupational groups ... professionals located inside the medical-industrial complex are under constraint to follow protocols of their private employer – increased productivity and decreased costs. The result is a reduction of patient services that are not profit-making (e.g. preventive and primary care) and shorter lengths of hospital stays (Benoit 1994 pp.303,309).

In the clinical area, the obstetrician has 'ownership' of patients yet the (British) code instructs midwives to 'safeguard and protect the interests of individual patients and clients'. Similar contradiction between code and workplace exists in Australia:

midwives are responsible for their decisions and actions and are accountable for the related outcomes in their care of women

and

midwives use their professional knowledge in an endeavour to ensure that women are not harmed by conception, childbearing or birthing practices in all environments and cultures (Code of Ethics, ACMI, Sections IC & IIC).

Mainstream midwives rarely have an opportunity to use their own skills and clinical judgement in areas fundamental to their role (Clarke 1995a; Fleming 1998; Thompson 2001). Kerry-Anne, a midwife in the present narratives, did not want to cut the woman unnecessarily and despite 'standing orders' to the contrary from the consultant obstetrician, assisted the woman to birth with an intact perineum. Kerry-Anne feels she and the woman were later 'punished' for her disobedience. Furthermore, control over natural childbirth processes by obstetricians has reduced the midwife's ability to practice outside the medical framework; that is, the deskilling of midwives.

The UK Code of Professional Conduct instructs midwives to 'justify public trust and confidence' but in the example given by Clarke

if [the midwife] tells the women the truth, in order to safeguard and protect their interests, the public view of the integrity of the consultant is damaged, as well as the reputation of hospital standards [risking initiation of disciplinary action by the employer against the midwife] (Clarke 1995a p.250).

Again, the Australian Code of Ethics for midwives (ACMI 1995) presents a similar conflict, as typified by Kerry-Anne's experience of the obstetrician who claimed that suturing of the woman's perineum was necessary even though the midwife's judgement was that of an intact perineum. If the midwife tells the woman the truth, in order to (i) 'maintain standards of personal conduct which reflect credit upon the profession' (Section IC), (ii) 'provide care ... while also working to eliminate harmful practices within those same cultures' (Section IIA), and (iii) 'ensure the woman is not harmed by ... birthing practices' (Section IIC) (ACMI 1995), the public view of the integrity of the consultant is damaged, as well as the reputation of hospital standards, and the midwife risks disciplinary action against her by the employer. Kerry-Anne was 'silenced'. In Australia and the United Kingdom, midwives have to

provide midwifery care within a wall of silence because midwifery care is defined by the employer (and probably, in consultation with obstetricians), and not by the midwifery (semi)profession itself (Clarke 1995a p.250).

Finally, whilst there is nothing wrong with adopting a deontological philosophy for midwifery ('individuals are ends in their own rights'), there is a major problem when midwives are expected to practice that philosophy within a utilitarian system (Clarke 1995a). The latter is concerned with large numbers of people, not individuals; a system wherein the individual is a means of helping other individuals achieve their own ends. The utilitarian philosophy requires that midwives conform to the policy of hospital birth, for the greatest good of the greatest number (Clarke 1995b). Thus, not only is there a philosophical conflict, but there is also a conflict between the assumed and the real status of the midwife as an employee.

If doctors, not midwives, are the gatekeepers to maternity care on the macro level (Fleming 1998) some midwives become protective gatekeepers on the individual level when informed choices and decisions are to be made (Levy 1999a). 'Protective steering' meant that midwives wanted to meet the wishes of women, provide unbiased advice, but acknowledge their own strong feelings regarding certain issues, and establish a balance between supplying enough information for the woman to make a choice whilst not frightening her with too much information. Interestingly, Levy (1999a) takes terms from the 'journey' metaphor to describe the processes by which midwives facilitate informed

choices during pregnancy: 'orienting' and 'exploring', 'territory mapping', and 'protective steering'. Protective steering involved consideration of the pregnant woman, and not professionally compromising herself or upsetting her colleagues. The individual and relationship appeared to be central to all of these aspects. The conflict those midwives experienced, however, was again the constraint of their powerless position in the organisation's hierarchy. They felt powerless to impose the consequences of their advice upon other professionals.

This patriarchal-related disregard and powerlessness of midwifery is characteristic of the paradigm conflict in service professions:

Even midwives holding nursing degrees and formal certificates fall short of recognition as legitimate service professionals because they lack 'esoteric knowledge' imperative to successfully dealing with inevitable 'uncertainty' (Benoit 1994 p.313).

The culture of midwifery in the National Health Service in England specifically is imbued in service and sacrifice, and highlights the conflict for individual practitioners:

midwives lacked the rights as women which they were required to offer to their clients (Kirkham 1999 p.732).

Resembling the broader, oppressed position of women, the specific cultural characteristics of the practice were identified as internalised self-sacrifice, guilt and self-blame. There was a lack of adequate support or protection within the workplace for midwives, and the fact that they referred to their own needs as 'selfish' reflected poorly on a supposedly caring practice. Given that maternity services are (male) medically controlled, and language and institutions are (male) gendered (Kirkham 1999), the utilitarian approach of maternity service institutions supports Rosemarie Tong's (1993) claim that ethics, too, are gendered. It also supports the claim that the existing gendered orientation of institutional maternity services is ethically inappropriate for the female-oriented practice of midwifery. As proposed earlier, the conflict evidenced in research (Levy 1999b; Kirkham 1999; Thompson 2001) depicts a lack of cohesion. This is not only social or practical cohesion, but a lack of ethical cohesion for midwives working in a utilitarian system when their practice values are embedded in a different philosophy, for example, deontological, relational or feminist-virtue ethics.

THE MIDWIFERY RELATIONSHIP

The present analysis shows that an ethically adequate mother-midwife relationship is a partnership wherein the midwife's power is exercised 'with' the woman. Guilliland and Pairman (1995) propose that midwifery ought be seen as a partnership between the childbearing woman and the midwife. They claim that the childbearing woman's primary relationship is with her baby and that she is responsible for decision-making in relation to herself and her baby. On the other hand, the midwife's prime relationship is with the childbearing woman. The organisation's needs ought not dominate the needs of the individual woman.

Guilliland and Pairman (1995) distinguish the concept of a midwifery partnership from those developed by the nursing theorists, Parse, Newman and Christiansen. Parse's elements of 'true presence' and 'going with the person wherever the person is rather than attempting to judge, change or control the person' are applicable to midwifery. On the other hand, the theories of Newman and Christiansen are not. Newman's partnership refers to the relationship between professionals rather than between nurse and patient. Christiansen's theory of partnership focuses on the profession rather than the individual practitioner or patient-client. Neither of the latter interpretations of partnership suit midwifery practice.

The midwifery partnership works with the woman [during pregnancy and childbirth] to achieve and define her own environment and experience, and seeks to place power and control with the woman regardless of setting ... The midwife facilitates the woman's expanded consciousness or specific lived experience (Guilliland & Pairman 1995 p.32).

Feminist beliefs are integral to a philosophy of midwifery partnership; for example, childbirth is socially and culturally constructed, 'nor-mal' is medically constructed, and working with women in their own environments, valuing each woman's life experience and their ways of knowing reveals that there is a range of 'normal'. A knowledge of the particular woman and the need to do relatively little [intervention] but to observe and experience ['with' the woman] the sense of the rhythm of the labour are essential skills for the midwife. Continuity of caregiver is fundamental because a trusting relationship develops over time and with this trust the woman develops confidence and increases her ability to make informed choices, another central concept identified in mothers' and midwives' narratives (Thompson 2001). The interrelated theoretical concepts of Guilliland and Pairman's (1995) midwifery partnership are individual negotiation, equality, shared responsibility and empowerment, and informed choice and consent. The woman and midwife both use these concepts within the partnership. This co-authorship further illustrates the feminist nature of the proposed mother-midwife relationship.

Finally, the implementation of such a partnership is enhanced at the macro level by governmental policy. For example, increasing people's control over their lives, increasing their autonomy and integrity, promoting trust and partnership between the healthcare user and the healthcare provider, and encouraging individuals to accept responsibility for their health are guidelines for informed choice and consent, published by the New Zealand Department of Health, and provide an important mechanism for empowerment.

SUMMARY

This second part of the discussion on values within the midwifery profession reviewed the debate over decision making in the practice setting, and conflict between workplace and personal/professional ethics. Maternity services are medically controlled, and language and institutions are gendered. Ethics, too, are gendered. In mainstream maternity services midwifery practice is not 'self-determining'; midwives are controlled by the medical profession, employer and registering bodies. Underlying philosophical differences between a code of professional conduct and the workplace are not acknowledged. In the clinical area, the obstetrician has 'ownership' of clients, yet midwives are expected to be accountable for related outcomes in their care of women. Mainstream hospital midwives rarely have an opportunity to use their own skills and clinical judgement, and when they do they can be punished.

Finally, the most recent trend of thought is that partnership forms the basis of midwifery philosophy and practice, with the concept of a primary relationship being central to that ideology – another major theme in mothers' and midwives' lived reality. The midwife's prime relationship is with the woman while the mother's prime relationship is with her baby.

REFERENCES

ACMI 1995 Code of ethics. Australian College of Midwives Incorporated, Melbourne

Benoit C 1994 Paradigm conflict in the sociology of service professions: midwifery as a case study. Canadian Journal of Sociology 19 (3): 303-329

Carboon F 1999 Language power and change. ACMI Journal 12 (4): 19-22

Clarke R A 1995a Midwives, their employers and the UKCC: an eternally unethical triangle. Nursing Ethics: An International Journal for Healthcare Professionals 2 (3): 247-253

Clarke R A 1995b Ethics and midwifery practice: the links between moral responsibilities, midwives and homebirth. Midwives 108 (1292): 270-271

Fleming V E M 1998 Autonomous or automatons? An exploration through history of the concept of autonomy in midwifery in Scotland and New Zealand. Nursing Ethics: An International Journal for Healthcare Professionals 5 (1): 43-51

Gould D 2000 Normal labour: a concept analysis. Journal of Advanced Nursing 31 (2): 418-427

Guilliland K, Pairman S 1995 The midwifery partnership: a model for practice. Victoria University of Wellington, Wellington NZ

Kirkham M 1986 A feminist perspective in midwifery. In: Webb C (ed) Feminist practice in women's health care. John Wiley & Sons, Chichester

Kirkham M 1999 The culture of midwifery in the National Health Service in England. Journal of Advanced Nursing 30 (3): 732-739

Koerner J G 1996 Congruency between nurses' values and job requirements: a call for integrity. Holistic Nursing Practice 10 (2): 69

Langford G 1985 Education, persons and society: a philosophical inquiry. Macmillan, London

Levy V 1999a Midwives, informed choice and power: part 1. British Journal of Midwifery 7 (9): 583-586

Levy V 1999b Protective steering: a grounded theory study of the processes by which midwives facilitate informed choices during pregnancy. Journal of Advanced Nursing 29 (1): 104-112

Machin D, Scamell M 1997 The experience of labour: using ethnography to explore the irresistible nature of the biomedical metaphor during labour. Midwifery 13: 78-84

Olson L L 1998 Hospital nurses' perceptions of the ethical climate of their work setting. Image: Journal of Nursing Scholarship 30 (4): 345

Padgett S 1998 Dilemmas of caring in a corporate context: a critique of nursing case management. Advances in Nursing Science 20 (4): 1-12

Page L 1995 Renewing midwifery: science and sensitivity in working with women. Knowledge and wisdom: the keys to safe motherhood. 9th Biennial Conference, Australian College of Midwives Inc, Sydney

Smythe L, Kerins R 1994 Decision making in independent midwifery practice. Midwifery Research Forum, La Trobe University, Melbourne

Thompson F E 2001 The ethical nature of the mother-midwife relationship: a feminist perspective [unpublished PhD dissertation] University of Southern Queensland

Thompson I K, Melia K M, Boyd K M 1994 Nursing ethics. Churchill Livingstone, Melbourne

Tong R 1993 Feminine and feminist Ethics. Wadsworth Publishing Co, Belmont CA

Zeidenstein L 1988 Birth language: a renewed consciousness. MIDIRS Midwifery Digest 8 (4): 418-419

11

The discourse of other travellers – literature on women's experiences

Chapter 10 discussed the actual life experiences of mothers and midwives (Thompson 2001) from the midwives' perspective, and compared them with the midwifery profession's values as reported in current literature. In this chapter those narratives are discussed from the mothers' perspective, comparing them with contemporary literature on women's experiences of birth and the midwife's approach.

Mothers in the present narratives are very homogenous in their values and beliefs of 'being with' the woman in the mother-midwife relationship. The ethical aspects of 'being with' woman during childbirth that matter most to them are the virtues of trust, respect, informed choice and self-determination which involves open communication, power 'with' and sometimes 'for' the woman, a prime relationship with the woman, supporting and 'knowing' the woman, 'being with' not 'doing to', character of practitioner, woman's comfort including feeling safe and secure, and the midwife's family-social role, for example in follow-up contact after birth. This suggests that ethical deliberation which is appropriate during birthing focuses on particularity and a personalised ethical response – an ethic of engagement.

Self-determination recurs across the mothers' narratives as 'freedom' – freedom to do what is right for the woman as an individual. This is so regardless of whether she births in a birth centre with midwives, with an independently practising midwife in attendance, or within a mainstream hospital ward.

THE BIRTH: WOMEN'S EXPERIENCES

These mothers overwhelmingly want to be able to safely 'do what is right for me' at birth, to have freedom of space and self-determination, and to be valued as individuals. Arline explains what for her, are the advantages of a birth centre:

Arline: ... there's lots more options in terms of what you can do and they encourage you to move around. Stay upright if that's what you want to do. You don't have to hop on the bed to birth, you can do it wherever you want to birth, in the shower, on the floor, on the toilet, on the birthing stool, over a bean bag, over the bed, or I mean if you want to lie down then lie down. There's no one there saying 'Right, OK, up on the bed now'. So you just kind of just do your own thing and they support you to do that.

Faye: What is it about a midwife that is supportive?

Arline: I guess for me allowing me the space to do what I wanted to do. That was it. She supported me in this and even though she was 'there' she wasn't really there and so that was important for me because I didn't want anyone, I didn't even want my partner around me while I – in second stage everyone, come in! you know, no problem, but while I'm just in the first stage I very much go within myself and just do my own thing and so yeah, I think just allowing me the space to do what I needed to do.

'Safety' during birthing for these women means more than a consideration of physiological mortality/morbidity. It includes the woman's 'feeling' safe; feeling emotionally, socially, culturally and physically comfortable and secure – and at ease.

Brenda birthed in a mainstream hospital ward.

Well the first midwife that I had put me at ease, she was quite happy with whatever I wanted to do like I wanted to crouch up in the chair, I wanted to sit in the chair backwards and she'd let me do that and she didn't get in the way, she kind of went around me to get to my tummy to feel the contractions and then I wanted to have a shower, I just wanted just [husband's name] and I in the shower, and so she went out and she was fine about that, 'Let me know if you need me'.

This expression of being 'at ease' indicates two important ethical themes. One is the woman's comfort and feeling of 'security'. The other is that of ethical values congruence, a theme which is generally absent in current literature.

Being 'at ease' is reported by Walsh (1999) in relation to the professional-friend role of community-based midwives who work in partnership with each other and provide continuity of care, and by Shields et al (1998) regarding women's relationships with staff in midwife-managed care. The latter research examined satisfaction with midwife-managed care and 'shared-care', and showed that women receiving midwife-managed care recorded more comments about what they liked while women having 'shared care' had more comments about what they disliked.

Lack of self-determination in the present narratives came from the women who birthed in mainstream hospital settings, and referred to decision making. The woman not only wants to be informed and have the opportunity to make and participate in decisions about herself and her baby (external 'autonomy'); she also wants to be psychologically able to do so (internal or mental freedom). These mothers acknowledge the need for expertise and professional knowledge but disapprove of the way that many women are coerced, frightened, 'over' powered and disempowered in the birthing situation. They seem to be saying that it is ethically wrong, firstly, to use paternalism and fear-for-safety to subordinate the childbearing woman, and secondly, to employ strategies such as 'haste' which often implies emergency and safety, and 'dismissal' to exclude the 'other' and deny her the right to self-determination. Tew is also critical of the obstetricians' misuse of science to mystify mothers and the public in their unsuccessful attempt to uncover the physiological mysteries of safe childbirth:

They appeal to ethics to sanction practising orthodox, untested therapies and to abstain from trials to test the effectiveness of alternatives (Tew 1990 p.294).

She doubts the ethics and appropriateness of obstetric care decision making being left to those whose perspective, although highly advanced scientifically, is restricted in terms of the human experience of childbirth. Subsequently, the 1992 Winterton Report and the 1993 *Changing Childbirth* report, in England, said that encouraging all women to give birth in hospitals cannot be justified on the grounds of safety (Clarke 1995; Ogden, Shaw & Zander 1998).

Although mothers in the present narratives express a need for the mother-midwife relationship to be primarily one of power 'with', they also rely on the midwife's advocacy from time to time – for the midwife to exercise her power 'for' the woman, but still from the individual's perspective. Differences in cultural beliefs and expectations contribute to such an individual perspective (Rice 1999). Megan's narrative illustrates her strong protective feelings towards her baby and her desire to keep her baby near to her. Kerry-Anne, a midwife, expressed her conflict with the impersonal care in mainstream hospital postnatal wards. Protocol discouraged women from interacting with other women's babies because it was seen as 'not right'. Again, Rice (1999) reports similar difficulties with protocols, experienced by Hmong women in Australia. The women wished to protect their newborn by keeping the baby near, on the bed with them, but were not allowed to do this because their caregivers saw the practice as dangerous. Research indicates that (i) there is a lack of information and choice for women, (ii) health professionals, particularly doctors, act as the experts on childbirth and their decisions are considered more important than those of the women, and (iii) women feel that they have no control of their own bodies, resenting hospital policy and practices (Thompson 2001; Rice

1999). An English study revealed distinct cultural differences between women with a relatively low socio-economic status and those with a relatively high socio-economic status, and recommends an element of caution when advocating 'informed choice' across the board (Machin & Scamell 1997). To universally enact an 'informed choice' policy may alienate the women most in need of support, advice and information because of its cultural inappropriateness. One clear message may not be effective in a diverse society. Empowerment and informed choice may not always be relevant, and for advocacy to be appropriate it needs to be sensitive to cultural difference.

We must give all women the opportunity to perceive childbirth outside the current dominant hegemony ... (Machin & Scamell 1997 p.83).

Machin and Scamell found, too, that women in the higher socio-economic group had not expected to be so overwhelmed by the change in setting for labour, to one of crisis. Their usual ideological 'props' of control and autonomy gave way to those of the dominant culture, the medical model, because that was the cultural tool offered to them at the time by their attendants.

Because birth is a ritualistic practice even the most determined anti-interventionist women may be easily swayed by the assuredness of obstetricians and midwives who may have the powerful metaphor of the safety of science on their side (Machin & Scamell 1997 p.84).

Dominance and submission are strongly reflected in the present narratives. For example, Brenda and Caroline, and their husbands as support persons, are transformed into passive, cooperative recipients of epidural pain relief and medical induction of labour respectively, and if it had not been for the midwives Caroline's medical induction would have gone ahead. Kay relinquishes her wish for a natural birth to that of emergency caesarean section under general anaesthesia. Other research claims that fear, and in particular fear for the baby, is the dominating negative feeling during emergency caesarean section delivery (Ryding, Wijma & Wijma 1998). This is understandable,

but the question needs asking whether fear 'induced' into women through the status quo, through the medicalised control of birth in the Western world, leads to so-called emergency caesarean operations. Women in the present narratives report that positive attitudes help women to birth 'well' while negative attitudes inhibit them, and their narratives illustrate the effect of such fear on the woman and her family. After the birth of her first baby, Kay felt as though she had just survived a life-threatening event: she was grateful to the obstetrician for saving her and her baby's lives but she remains doubtful whether that surgery was really necessary. She still believes that she was not allowed to try for herself and that she was not provided with accurate or adequate information during the pregnancy or intrapartum period. Antenatally, the obstetrician spoke of where the baby might go to school and did not discuss Kay's wish for natural birth. Kay said that during labour the obstetrician made quick visits and gave no explanations. Finally, she was rushed to the operating room. Similarly, Handler and colleagues found women's satisfaction with prenatal care settings included

respect, treatment as individuals, and understanding of their personal experiences. They emphasized that they want procedures explained, their questions answered and to be asked questions about both their medical and emotional status ... the amount of time spent waiting was often juxtaposed in the women's minds with the amount of time spent with the caregiver (Handler et al 1996 pp.33-34).

It was ethically important to Kay that she be enabled and empowered to try to birth her second baby naturally, an experience she felt was denied her for her first birth. It was outside mainstream, medicalised maternity services therefore, that she was given the confidence and professional support to attempt a natural birth (VBAC) and avoid the inevitable 'once a caesar always a caesar', long-term sequelae of the 'cascade of intervention'.

In their narratives, these mothers convey the concept of privacy in terms of the midwife's 'presence' and 'being with' not 'doing to', sub themes of 'supporting the woman'. Arline speaks of the midwife being there for her but not there – 'nobody was 'in my face' or no one was touching me, checking me or whatever.' Similarly, Brenda says her first midwife did not get in the way, she went around her, whilst the second midwife, the harsh schoolteacher, arranged epidural pain relief in response to Brenda's crying. Kerry-Anne, one of the mid-wives, tells of how a woman who screamed during her birthing was told to shut up and her husband sent from the room because she was not 'behaving' herself. Ogden, Shaw and Zan-der (1998) also report that women birthing in hospitals have problems with privacy when they want to make a noise in childbirth.

Closely linked to the theme of supporting the woman and the concept of privacy is the con-cern about damage to the perineum: the fear of tearing and not wishing to have an episiotomy. Judy recorded in her birth plan that 'I didn't want to have an episiotomy, but if I needed it, yes'. Megan's comments are the same, but Arline actually feared tearing. Diane, a midwife, describes how an obstetrician cut an excessively large episiotomy on a woman who subsequent-ly required intensive physiotherapy and surgical repair of vaginal-bowel damage. According to her narrative, the doctor's power and gender were the issues at stake. Debra Salmon's (1999) feminist analysis of women's experiences of per-ineal trauma in the immediate post-delivery period found that the doctor-'patient' relation-ship, particularly in relation to gender, not feel-ing heard, and a lack of information and advice were the most significant influences. She also found the use of terms such as 'torture' and 'punish' alarming, with some women even feel-ing brutalised during their experience of sutur-ing. Findings indicated that women's health is marginalised and the competence of the practi-tioner in suturing after childbirth needs more recognition. Inadequate pain relief was a com-mon comment, and being 'patched up' was a persistent theme – not a highly technical process where muscle layers have to be carefully identi-fied and sutured appropriately.

There was a clear indication from the data that the women experienced doctors' maleness as a significant element in their experiences ... [one of several examples was a woman and her female GP several weeks later] believed that the male doctor 'did not know what a vagina looked like'. This could indeed have resulted in him failing to sew correctly (Salmon 1999 p.252).

A midwife had that particular woman look in a mirror and it was then she saw that part of the labia was stitched back on itself.

Invasion of the birth canal is another vital part of women's concept of 'being with' not 'doing to', and is vehemently disapproved of by several of the mothers in the present analysis. Brenda says: 'Before that, everyone wanted to stick their fingers there and now no one wants to even tell me I'm OK!' Judy says: 'When I was kneeling up over the bean bag I said to them, I thought the midwife had her, it felt like she had her fingers sort of against the perineum, going like this, and I said 'Get your fingers out of there''. She thought they were 'being mean' but they were not. Again, the impact of setting on practice is identified in these narratives as well as in current literature. Narratives involving birth centre and independently practising midwives lack these odious expressions and portray a practice of respect and affection for persons, of minimal or no invasive techniques, as compared with main-stream practices. Ogden, Shaw and Zander report that women who birthed in hospital

expressed their experiences using powerful and evocative language and can vividly recall how they felt at the time. In particular, the results provide insights into the effect of the place of birth on the actual birth experience (Ogden, Shaw and Zander 1998 p.345).

This fierce protection of the birth canal and ethical disapproval of its invasion, could be related to the mother's protection of her baby, her prime relationship with the baby, as well as the integrity of her own body. If so, it requires further exploration in future research. The effect of setting on the ethical response in practice has also been discussed in Chapters 3 and 4.

Hall and Holloway (1998), amongst others, categorise women's experiences of labour and birth in terms of 'control'. Narratives in the present analysis, however, rarely use the term 'control', rather they speak of 'doing what is right for me', 'encouraging and supportive', 'not getting in the way', power and empowerment. These are terms of human engagement and are more positive expressions than 'control'. Furthermore, such positive terms suggest human engagement 'with' another, and therefore may more accurately depict the nature of ethically adequate childbirth practices and mother-midwife relationships.

Although none of these participating mothers describes the experience of home birth, those who birthed in a birth centre and Kay, who employed a home birth midwife, discuss their experience of birthing in very similar ways to those who have birthed at home (Morison et al 1999). Arline explains how in the birth centre you can birth wherever you want to; the literature reports the importance of mobility and 'control' over birthing positions for women birthing at home. Brenda birthed in a mainstream hospital ward and is critical of not being able to spend time with her newborn baby as soon as she was born, time to realise that yes this is a baby, her baby. Conversely, Arline details how she and her partner had skin contact with their baby at the time of birth, in the unrushed environment of a birth centre. Literature reports how couples at a home birth spend time alone with their baby, undisturbed by their carers, and have their privacy protected by others present in the house. Being more relaxed at home, and more 'tensed up' in hospital, is another distinguishing feature of non-institutionalised, non-medicalised birthing. Gemma, a midwife in the present narratives, strongly believes that when and where the woman feels comfortable and secure she will birth well, and that may mean different things and places for each woman. Again, this is a belief echoed by women in the literature (Morison et al 1999).

Actual life experiences of mothers and midwives show that procedure-oriented medicalised care undermines the woman's confidence in her ability to birth her baby, and the birth becomes the attendants' not the mother's birth. Brenda tells of how it was time now for pain relief and how she had to birth over the bar. No one was taking any notice of Maree's vigorous shaking during birth because they were busily getting ready for the delivery and they had to arrange a paediatrician – a similar story to that told by the midwife Ann, about anxious parents not being heard. Ellie describes how she wept from the pain every time her baby was presented to her for breastfeeding yet the midwives were not allowed to recommend anything except a nappy to bite into and to advise viewing the instructional video.

When the birth is taken out of the woman's hands by obstetric and technological intervention, and policies, she and the midwife are disempowered and the mother-midwife relationship is one of separateness, of disparate relationships. Communication and individualised care are integral to an ethically adequate response in childbirth; a response more typical of the ethics of intimates and a focus on the particular than normative theory, standardised protocols and objective problem solving. Current research confirms that other mothers who birth in hospitals also feel they are not listened to and are not told information they want to know (Ogden, Shaw & Zander 1998). Antenatal classes and individual hospital midwives fail to impart coping strategies for labour to women (Spiby et al 2000). Diane, a midwife from the present analysis, raises the question of empowerment via antenatal education and whether it places women at risk of being punished during a birth in mainstream services. Kay, a mother, praises the independent midwife she employed for her second birth, for providing her with 'ways of dealing with labour', and condemns the private obstetrician from mainstream services, for not addressing during any of their antenatal meetings, her desire for a natural birth.

I would just dearly love to see, that at that point a general practitioner is obliged by health policy, to give women impartial, unbiased information on what is possible with childbirth and what options there are. I mean the full medical model, I'm sure will always suit some women but it's not easy to find any other choices at the moment.

Mainstream hospital settings and procedure-oriented practices render the birthing woman invisible and disempower her support person. Brenda and Caroline tell of how their husbands were doing all the right things for the staff, but not for them. Maree's husband was the only person who took any notice of, and offered any explanation for, her violent shaking. Yet despite his own medical training he seemed powerless as her advocate. On the other hand, and with the exception of Madonna, these participating midwives (Thompson 2001) present as woman-centred and portray the labouring woman as the focus of the birth. They see the father/partner's support as integral, as does literature on home birth (for example, Bondas-Salonen 1998).

The fathers described themselves as both supporters and observers at the birth. As supporters they were involved in such actions as massaging, holding and encouraging their partner. As observers, the fathers examined how the environment affected the birth and took actions to maintain harmony (Morison et al 1999 p.35).

Interviews with independently practising Dutch midwives concur with the present discussion, that the setting or 'location' of birth has consequences for the professional functioning of midwives (van der Hulst 1999). The Dutch midwives say that home births are more time-consuming, their visits with the woman are more and their presence longer, their approach is more informal and the interaction with the birthing woman is easier than in the hospital. Again, the present analysis sees that the notion of being at ease demonstrates a congruence of values as opposed to values conflict evident in narratives of institutional dominance. Expectant parents are more active at home than in hospital, often doing small domestic jobs. The midwives' relational care is more intense and woman-centred (van der Hulst 1999). This leads the discussion on to the character and approach of the midwife/birth attendant.

THE MIDWIFE'S APPROACH: WOMEN'S EXPERIENCES

'Knowing' the midwife is a very strong theme. Arline, Kay, Megan and Maree in particular consider it important that the midwife share similar beliefs to the woman because of the continuity of philosophy of care. This group of mothers (and midwives) consider continuity of carer important for ethically adequate practice that meets individual needs. Arline actively sought the midwife whom she knew and who knew her. The mothers and midwives from birth centres or 'independent' midwifery practice usually refer to each other as friends or professional-friends, and current literature reports similar findings (Morison et al 1999; Walsh 1999). Hospital midwives are more frequently referred to as 'friendly' and 'professional', not 'friends'.

No it wasn't like a friend. They were friendly and business-like and professional. Because a friend may not do what's best for the situation because they're too wrapped in you feeling pain or something like that, so I think they were friendly to me. (Judy, mother who birthed in a mainstream hospital)

This varied, though, between individuals and with the impact of the setting on their orientation towards early labour and actual birth.

I think that my first midwife treated me like a friend, yeah. It's the trusting and the making you feel comfortable, and she's not making herself a stranger. She's trying to get into your circle of comfort and I felt like she was trying to protect me, and friends do that for you as well ... just so open in her manners and everything. (Brenda, mother who also birthed in a mainstream hospital)

Well I certainly regarded [independent midwife's name] as a friend ... [independent midwife's name] probably became a little more professional in her manner once we were in hospital as well so there wasn't so much a relaxed matey attitude. (Kay, mother attended by independent midwife, in hospital)

Katie, an independently practising midwife, defines the professional-friendship between her clients and herself as:

You're definitely a friend, you're definitely a trusted family friend ... and it's not a dependence or anything else, it's a friendship. It's a weird sort of friendship that comes from pregnancy and finishes at six weeks after the pregnancy.

In Chapter 5 it is argued, as have others (Gilligan 1982; Tong 1993; Noddings 1984; Norberg & Uden 1995), that gendered morality does not acknowledge care, personal relationships, and attentiveness to contextual detail. Virtue theorists, too, have discussed the value and richness that friendship affords (Friedman 1993). Our commitment to and partiality for particular persons differs from commitment to abstract moral values, principles and rules (Toulmin 1986), rules that dictate right and wrong action. Indeed, moral growth and transformation of abstract moral guidelines may be possible through our commitment to particular persons such as friends (Friedman 1993). Because equality, respect and affection are central to Friedman's argument, it is relevant to the present analysis which identifies self-determination, trust, respect and character as major themes in most narratives, and 'love' in some. Equality between friends is not formal or quantifiable. It exists through personality, attitudes, emotions and overall character.

One friend's superiority in one area, for example, in breadth of life experience, need not give that friend a privileged place in the relationship ... (Friedman 1993 p.189).

Hierarchical relationships lack this balance and mutuality, fostering master-apprentice positions. With friends, her/his interests and 'best' interests are central to one's actions, goals and aspirations, and their success is cause for our own joy. Whilst respect for persons as moral equals and respect for a person's specific worth are different, both types of respect are committed to certain abstract moral guidelines or standards. To that extent, our commitment to the person is subordinate to our commitment to the relevant moral standards – it is not intrinsically a commitment to that person. Commitment to a particular person involves some readiness to be attentive to her, to take her seriously, and to act on her behalf. It counterbalances our commitments to abstract moral guidelines. According to Friedman, affection does not necessarily involve assumptions about the inherent moral worth of the person; it attends to someone's unique particularity. Friendship is

a close relationship in which trust, intimacy, and disclosure open up for us whole standpoints other than our own (Friedman 1993 p.198).

Again, they are concepts identified by the present mothers and midwives as ethically important in the mother-midwife relationship.

In the narratives presented here, women tell of previous negative experiences, and contrast them with the positive experience of having a midwife who knew them, focused on them as individuals, and genuinely involved the woman's partner and existing children. Walsh (1999) identified similar themes and found that all other themes filtered through the 'professional as friend' relationship that women had with their community-based midwives. Like the language used in some of the present narratives, Walsh reports depersonalised terms such as she/he/they statements about hospital caregivers during negative experiences. In her narrative Kay, a mother, describes vividly her negative experience and feelings towards her obstetrician whose first name she uses, but says that she does not really remember anything about the hospital midwives at her first birth.

According to this group of mothers, essential features of an ethically adequate mother-midwife relationship – of 'being with' the woman during childbirth – are open consultation, exercising power 'with' the woman, trust, respect (especially with regard to valuing the individual), confidence, character of person, and an environment in which the woman feels comfortable and secure. These ethical values are echoed by a group of Swedish women who describe the midwife's 'presence' during childbirth as

to be seen as an individual, to have a trusting relationship and to be supported and guided on one's own terms (Berg et al 1996 p.11).

Affirmation and familiarity with the midwife and surroundings indicates a valuing of individuals, identified in the present analysis as 'knowing' the woman. A trusting relationship between mother and midwife develops from good communication, skill and expertise, and includes the midwife's character, professional knowledge and proficiency as well as the women's feeling of security:

Keywords were friendliness, openness, safety, interpersonal congruity, intuition and availability (Berg et al 1996 p.13).

In the present analysis this is interpreted as a congruence of 'values-virtues' such as respect, trust, confidence, moral character and 'self'-pride (mutually felt; for mother's achievement, and for midwife's skill and expertise). The relationship is empowering and exercises power 'with' not 'over' the woman because the midwife's prime focus is 'being with' the woman during childbirth. Again, these sentiments identified in the present analysis relating to the distinctive nature of midwifery practice are also expressed by Berg et al when they claim that

knowledge about the relationship between the birthing woman and midwife is acquired over the years. It is a tacit knowledge embedded in practice (Berg et al 1996 p.14).

Having the knowledge, skills and communication to coach a woman through the journey of childbirth, being encouraging, supporting, and respectful, and having a positive mental attitude were also identified by Icelandic women as the elements of empowerment necessary for 'caring encounters' during childbirth (Halldorsdottir & Karlsdottir 1996).

Fleming (1998) examined the interdependent nature of the midwife-client relationship in New Zealand and Scotland, and developed a conceptual model of attending and presencing, supplementing and complementing, reflection and reflexivity. Reciprocity is the basic social process of the model and context is integral to the concepts midwives and clients discuss. She too identifies the difficulty for midwives wishing to practise within a women-with-midwife partnership, of 'knowing' and 'thinking' outside Western philosophy parameters, and of escaping the powerful dominant discourse. Her recommendation for further research into intimacy, knowing, sensing and intuiting the other to reduce the feeling of unease is addressed to some extent, through the present analysis of power within relationships, and the aim to make 'visible' taken-for-granted assumptions such as the so-called public-private spheres and the exclusion of relationship in the objective problem-solving frameworks of bioethics.

Continuity of midwifery carer is defined as getting to know the midwife. The general agree-

ment in the present narratives about the importance of carer continuity and of mother and midwife 'knowing' each other endorses the centrality of relationship in ethical midwifery practice. Women who birthed in mainstream hospital wards do not like a change of midwife, explaining that as labour progresses and pain increases it is difficult to communicate with someone new. It also takes time to develop a rapport with someone and often the change of shift means that the second midwife is with them for a relatively short period of time. Megan and Maree do wonder, however, if it might be a disadvantage to have the same midwife throughout if the mother does not like the midwife for some reason. Nevertheless, continuity of carer is overwhelmingly preferred to not knowing who the next carer is and not knowing that person prior to being in pain and vulnerable. As discussed above, procedure-dominated practices and practitioners are rejected as ethically inadequate or inappropriate for well, able women during a 'natural' but unique and intimate life experience. Individual choice is central to ethical childbirth practices. These findings concur with other research (Flint, Poulengeris & Grant 1989; Edwards 1998; Fraser 1999) but unlike recent literature, the current data are analysed for insight into the ethical nature of the mother-midwife relationship – the ethics of midwifery.

Most of these present women tend to view the midwives they respected and trusted as professionals with expertise rather than as 'experts' in the traditional, distant and elitist way. Similarly, many of the midwives see themselves as having a certain expertise and being a resource not an 'expert'. Kerry-Anne in particular believes that women who birth in mainstream hospital labour wards, in her experience, do not know what the midwife's role is, and she attributes this to midwives not making women aware of it. Mothers who perceive the midwife as 'expert' do so usually when collectively referring to birth attendants in a medicalised practice setting. This can also be related to the changing role of the hospital midwife when, as birth is imminent, the doctor and technology often assume control of the 'delivery'. For example, Judy tells of how with the actual birth, her second midwife's approach alters and she describes the more detached 'expert'. Caroline, too, birthed in a mainstream hospital ward and she speaks of the nurses as experts and the birth as the business end of things. Collington (1998) found that a small group of parents attending antenatal classes in England view the midwife as the expert, albeit s/he is a pregnancy adviser and supporter too. A larger scale study in England claims that approximately half of the women interviewed define the midwife's role as 'checks your blood pressure or checks that the baby is growing', 'delivers babies', 'gives information and advice about pregnancy and childbirth' and 'provides emotional and psychological support' (Leach et al 1998). Many women in the latter study were not clear about the role of the midwife, though, and the authors of the report postulate it may be because women were not able to identify the member of staff who carried out a task as a 'midwife'.

SUMMARY

Many of the themes in the present narratives are also found in contemporary literature on the experience of birth in an Anglo-Celtic culture and the approaches of midwives.

The birth – women's experiences

Mothers define 'safety' not in terms of mortality/morbidity but from a more holistic perspective. Their construct of safety encompasses the woman's feelings of comfort and personal 'security' during the vulnerable experience of childbearing. A lack of self-determination for the woman, and the misuse of science to mystify mothers and the public, are criticised by both these women and current literature. There is a lack of information and choice for women. When health professionals act as the experts on childbirth and consider that their decisions are more important than those of the woman, women feel disempowered and resent hospital policy and practices. Current literature also

concurs with what some of the women say, that the setting for labour changes to one of crisis at birth, using the powerful metaphor of the safety of science to sway even the most determined anti-interventionist.

Fear for baby with emergency caesarean sections is common to these narratives and the literature. Questions raised by evidence like these personal narratives however, are firstly, whether medicalised control of birth in the Western world leads to so-called emergency caesarean operations, and secondly, what are the ethical implications of practices that induce fear in women? Whilst current midwifery literature identifies dominance and submission, it does not analyse the implications of existing ethical frameworks for midwifery practice. When the woman and midwife are disempowered, the mother-midwife relationship is one of separateness, of disparate relationships. There is disengagement rather than engagement.

This present group of women is concerned about damage to their perineum. They fear tearing and do not wish to have an episiotomy. According to them, there is a marked difference between the hospital midwives and birth centre or independent practice midwives, in their orientation towards the perineum. Some of the women accept episiotomy almost as a given for mainstream hospital practice, but an intact perineum is highly valued and sought after by mothers and midwives in the birth centre or community-based midwifery services. An intact perineum was also a valued tradition of midwives in pre-medicalisation eras. Literature on women's experiences of perineal trauma in the immediate post-delivery period found that major influences were the doctor-'patient' relationship, particularly in relation to gender, not feeling heard, and a lack of information and advice.

Invasion of the birth canal is another vital part of these women's concept of self-determination and privacy. This fierce protection of the birth canal and ethical disapproval of its invasion could be related to the mother's protection of her baby, her prime relationship with the baby, as well as the integrity of her own body. If so, it requires further exploration in future research, as do 'prime relationships' generally, and the implication of cultural diversity.

Contrary to much of the current midwifery literature, the present narratives rarely use the term 'control'. Rather they speak of 'doing what is right for me', of the midwife as 'encouraging and supportive', she 'didn't get in the way', and of power and empowerment. These are terms of human engagement and are more positive expressions than that of 'control'. Furthermore, such positive terms suggest human engagement 'with' another, and therefore, may more accurately depict the nature of ethically adequate childbirth practices and mother-midwife relationships.

The woman will birth 'well' when and where she feels comfortable and secure, and that may mean different things and places for each woman. As midwives, we should be working with and supporting women to achieve this without judgement. Current literature, too, reports on the importance of women's mobility and 'control' over birthing positions, and of couples spending time alone with their baby undisturbed by their carers – something that Brenda is critical of with her mainstream hospital birth. Literature also discusses how medicalised childbirth practices and mainstream hospital settings create tension, render the birthing woman invisible and disempower both the midwife and the mother's support person. These concepts in the present analysis are incorporated into the themes of self-determination, freedom of space, and the woman's feeling of 'security', not mere physical safety.

Literature tends to discuss the concept of privacy, but these mothers speak of the midwife's 'presence' and 'being with' not 'doing to', concepts interpreted as sub-themes of 'knowing' and 'supporting' the woman. It is important that the woman and midwife know each other and that the midwife shares similar beliefs to the woman so there is mutual support and a continuity of philosophy of care. These themes reflect not only what women value about their birth experience but also what they value about the midwife's approach and engagement with them.

Midwife's approach – women's experiences

Earlier research (Flint, Poulengeris & Grant 1989; Edwards 1998; Fraser 1999) shows that individual choice is central to ethical childbirth practices. An aim of the present analysis is to examine the ethical nature of childbirth practices, in particular the mother-midwife relationship, and this means going beyond simply administering more choice for childbearing women. This analysis of mothers' and midwives' actual life experience, and examination of taken-for-granted assumptions in existing theoretical frameworks, has made explicit the implicit ethics of midwifery practice.

Current literature illustrates how procedure-dominated practices and practitioners are inappropriate for well, able, birthing women during what is mostly a 'natural' but unique and intimate life experience. Women in the present narratives discuss why those practices and approaches are inappropriate – they are rejected as ethically inadequate. Mothers' narrated experiences indicate that the midwifery ethics implicit in practice are the ethics of intimates and derive from a commitment to the particular person. It is an ethic of engagement. The individual midwife's practice, it seems, is embedded in the setting, context and orientation or 'way of seeing' that surrounds childbirth. What is identified in the present narratives, and which goes largely unidentified and unexplained in the current midwifery literature, is the ethical implication of settings and the exercise of power in relationships.

Professional-friendship often describes the mother-midwife relationship. When these women discuss the midwife's approach positively, they refer to it as being supportive and 'with' the woman – 'knowing' the woman as a professional friend. They tend to view the midwives they respected and trusted as professionals with expertise rather than 'experts' in the traditional, distant and elitist way. Current literature reports similar findings. Unlike the current literature, however, these narratives are analysed for insight into the ethical nature of the mother-midwife relationship, and findings illustrate that power in relationships and 'prime relationships' are major ethical features. The midwife who is 'being with' and supportive of the woman, has her prime relationship with the woman, facilitates the mother's prime relationship with her baby, and mostly exercises her power 'with' the woman through human engagement and the ethics of intimates. The mother and baby are not treated as adversaries, and there is congruence rather than a conflict of values in the mother-midwife relationship.

These narratives and current literature both identify that acknowledging the woman's achievement of birth, and sharing in the parents' emotions over their newborn, are important aspects of the midwife's role. Another crucial component to this role is the importance of the midwife's joining with parents in welcoming the baby and introducing the 'new' family to their existing family and social networks. Embodiment of the birthing woman, and embeddedness of birth for the family and midwife, are illustrated in the family-social-cultural role of the midwife.

It is also important that the midwife shares similar beliefs to the woman because of the continuity of philosophy of care. Both these women and current literature discuss the value and richness that friendship affords as opposed to the problem-solving principles and dilemma-oriented bioethics of medicalised childbirth. Examining the ethical implication highlights that gendered morality does not acknowledge care, personal relationships, and attentiveness to contextual detail. Friendship, on the other hand, is a close relationship in which trust, intimacy, and disclosure open us up to another's way of seeing. Our language and behaviour reflect our ways of seeing. Depersonalised terms such as she/he/they are used in statements about hospital caregivers during negative experiences, and illustrate the difference mothers experience between hospital births and birth centre or community-based midwifery births. The ethical nature of the mother-midwife relationship has to do with the human condition and the nature of human engagement.

REFERENCES

Berg M, Lundgren I, Hermansson E, Wahlberg V 1996 Women's experience of the encounter with the midwife during childbirth. Midwifery 12 (1) 11-15

Bondas-Salonen T 1998 How women experience the presence of their partners at the births of their babies. Qualitative Health Research 8 (6): 784-800

Clarke R A 1995 Ethics and midwifery practice: the links between moral responsibilities, midwives and homebirth. Midwives 108 (1292): 270-271

Collington V 1998 Do women share midwives' views of their educational role? British Journal of Midwifery 6 (9): 556-563

Edwards N 1998 Getting to know midwives. MIDIRS Midwifery Digest 8 (2): 160-163

Fleming V E M 1998 Women-with-midwives-with-women: a model of interdependence. Midwifery 14: 137-143

Flint C, Poulengeris P, Grant A 1989 The 'know your midwife' scheme: a randomised trial of continuity of care by a team of midwives. Midwifery 5 (1): 11-16

Fraser D M 1999 Women's perceptions of midwifery care: a longitudinal study to shape curriculum development. Birth 26 (2): 99-107

Friedman M 1993 What are friends for? Feminist perspectives on personal relationships and moral theory. Cornell University Press, Ithaca NY

Gilligan C 1982 In a different Voice: psychological theory and women's development. Harvard University Press, Cambridge

Hall S M, Holloway I M 1998 Staying in control: women's experiences of labour in water. Midwifery 14: 30-36

Halldorsdottir S, Karlsdottir S I 1996 Empowerment or discouragement: women's experience of caring and uncaring encounters during childbirth. Healthcare for Women International 17 (4): 361-379

Handler A, Raube K, Kelly M, Giachello A 1996 Women's satisfaction with prenatal care settings: a focus group study. Birth 23 (1): 31-39

Leach J, Dowswell T, Hewison J et al 1998 Women's perceptions of maternity carers. Midwifery 14: 48-53

Machin D, Scamell M 1997 The experience of labour: using ethnography to explore the irresistable nature of the biomedical metaphor during labour. Midwifery 13: 78-84

Morison S, Percival P, Huack Y, McMurray A 1999 Birthing at home: the resolution of expectations. Midwifery 15: 32-39

Noddings N 1984 Caring: a feminine approach to ethics and moral education. University of California Press, Berkeley

Norberg A, Uden G 1995 Gender differences in moral reasoning among physicians, registered nurses and enrolled nurses engaged in geriatric and surgical care. Nursing Ethics: An International Journal for Healthcare Professionals 2 (3): 233-242

Ogden J, Shaw A, Zander L 1998 Women's experience of having a hospital birth. British Journal of Midwifery 6 (5): 339-345

Rice P L 1999 What women say about their childbirth experiences: the case of Hmong women in Australia. Journal of Reproductive & Infant Psychology 17 (3): 237

Ryding E L, Wijma K, Wijma B 1998 Experiences of emergency cesarean section: a phenomenological study of 53 women. MIDIRS Midwifery Digest 9 (1): 67-72

Salmon D 1999 A feminist analysis of women's experiences of perineal trauma in the immediate post-delivery period. Midwifery 15: 247-256

Shields N, Turnbull D, Reid M et al 1998 Satisfaction with midwife-managed care in different time periods: a randomised controlled trial of 1299 women. Midwifery 14: 85-93

Spiby H, Henderson B, Slade P et al 2000 Strategies for coping with labour: does antenatal education translate into practice? Journal of Advanced Nursing 29 (2): 388-394

Tew M 1990 Safer childbirth? A critical history of maternity care. Chapman and Hall, London

Thompson F E 2001 The ethical nature of the mother-midwife relationship: a feminist perspective [unpublished PhD dissertation] University of Southern Queensland

Tong R 1993 Feminine and feminist ethics. Wadsworth Publishing Co, Belmont CA

Toulmin S 1986 How medicine saved the life of ethics. In: DeMarco J P, Fox R M (eds) New directions in ethics. Routledge and Kegan Paul, New York

van der Hulst L A M 1999 Dutch midwives: relational care and birth location. Health & Social Care in the Community 7 (4): 242-247

Walsh D 1999 An ethnographic study of women's experience of partnership caseload midwifery practice: the professional as a friend. Midwifery 15: 165-176

12

Mapping a new ethic for midwives – from 'Practice Estate' to the pool and back, now a return journey travelled in tandem

The journey began when I set off to find the pool of 'practice' or 'applied' ethics as opposed to the abstract theories of philosophy and the decontextualised problem-solving approach of dilemmic and 'bio' ethics. The traditions of medicine, nursing and midwifery were examined, and a critique presented on the medicalisation of childbirth. Bioethics typifies the ethics of strangers and is confirmed as a false trail for midwifery. Venturing further afield brought the pool into view. Feminism and postmodernism offer the advantage of inclusion and particularity, and their course or 'meaning' stands in parallel proximity to virtue ethics, for which engagement and the character of moral agents are imperative.

Through narratives of personal experience, mothers and midwives have provided insight into the ethical nature of the mother-midwife relationship and, therefore, a distinctive ethical response for midwifery practice. This next part of the discussion proposes a mapping strategy for constructing such a new ethic for midwives, based on the insight gained from those stories – the ethic of engagement. The discussion looks firstly at the nature of engagement in ethical responses and relationships, and, secondly, at the centrality of concepts that emerged from interviews and literature in the present analysis. Implications for practice are identified, and recommendations are formulated for refocusing our ethical 'gaze' on midwifery so that the implicit ethics evident in the mother-midwife relationship are made explicit in midwifery practice and theory.

THE ETHIC OF ENGAGEMENT – A MIDWIFERY ETHIC

The overall implication of the present analysis is that midwifery practice requires a different ethic to that of bioethics, to adequately respond to the needs of mothers and midwives. Mothers and midwives need an ethic which is responsive to women's moral theorising, and to the aspirations, values and lived reality of mothers who birth their babies and midwives who assist them.

The nature of engagement in ethical responses and relationships

Human engagement and the exercise of power in relationships are central to the ethical nature of the mother-midwife relationship. An ethical response which is adequately responsive to mothers and midwives, and distinctive to midwifery practice ought, therefore, to be based on human engagement and relationships, not on the 'rightness' or 'wrongness' of actions. What might such an ethic of midwifery look like? It may focus around the aspects of ethical responses and the types of ethical relationships.

Aspects of ethical responses

Context is an important aspect of ethical response because that is where the person stands, and s/he may or may not be an ethically committed individual. The human condition is a social construct and one's social relations include professional or role-based relationships, social practices, community or institutional settings and cultural structures. A person has

a history, a role, a culture, and an interlocking web of loyalties, commitments and obligations ... [and] most ethical situations involve encounters with or for others (Isaacs & Massey 1993 p.58).

The importance of context is demonstrated throughout the present narratives of mothers and midwives. The impact of practice setting and multiple contexts for the individual on the ethical response is evident. Context forms an essential part of deliberation for an adequate ethical response in midwifery.

Appreciating who the person is, is another crucial aspect of the mother-midwife relationship.

To appreciate the identity of another human being involves engaging with them – being with them – in a way that recognises and acknowledges their humanity (Isaacs & Massey 1994 p.4).

These mothers are united in their expectation of being valued as individuals. For them, an adequate ethical response is inclusive of difference and the midwife focuses on the woman – 'what is right for her'. There is open communication with time for the woman to talk and the midwife to listen. Whilst there is commitment to the abstract moral standard of 'respect', there is also a commitment to the particular person in the form of affection, a commitment that does not necessarily involve assumptions about the inherent moral worth of the person but rather attends to their unique particularity. A trusting relationship develops in which the mother and midwife 'know' each other's abilities and limitations. The mother's identity in particular, is constructed and acknowledged as an 'able' woman, through their narrative and dialogical engagement, their talk-in-interaction. The midwife's orientation or perspective is 'being with' the woman. It is not an instrumental orientation of objectifying, classifying and manipulating others.

It is important to appraise our relationships, practices, institutions and communities, not merely respond to ethical 'issues', problems and dilemmas. Ethical criteria such as the inclusion of women and difference, and the exercise of mutual power in relationships, are more helpful than pragmatic, technocratic or economic criteria – as the narratives, current literature and governmental inquiries discussed in this analysis show. Ethical frameworks that currently prevail in midwifery practice need to be critically examined to broaden the discourse about ethical matters and promote the ethical nature of virtues and relationship. Mothers and midwives relaying the present narratives overwhelmingly reject institutional dominance, paternalism and a lack of self-determination for the childbearing woman in what, for the vast majority, is a human experience and 'natural' life process. The language used and the approaches of birth attendants in medicalised birth settings reflect the objective, problem-solving orientation of bioethics and hospital protocols and procedures.

Transforming the dehumanising and wickedness of institutional dominance with criticism and resistance is the deconstructive change required:

dismantling of relationships, practices, institutions and cultures that are dominating, totalising, exploitative, manipulative, demeaning and dehumanising (Isaacs & Massey 1993 p.66).

Constructive change entails recognising and responding to conditions that limit what is possible. Ethically acceptable midwifery practice, according to these mothers and midwives, resembles the ethics of intimates, not strangers; the ethics of engagement. The task for midwives, therefore, is to develop understandings, competencies and dispositions that will enable us to transform ourselves, our relationships, practices, institutions, cultures and worlds in ways that are ethically acceptable to mothers and midwives. Some of the present mothers and midwives describe their personal transformation in terms of altered ways of seeing and changed practice or approach. These experiences give insight into the wider transformation needed.

Types of ethical relationships

The purpose of the relationship determines whether there is engaging 'over', 'for', 'with', 'alongside', or 'of the self' (Isaacs 1998a; 1998b;

1999). In some professional relationships, the practitioner engages 'for' others, or in certain circumstances unfortunately, 'over' others. An ethical relationship between midwifery and other colleagues involved in childbirth services is one wherein they engage 'alongside' each other. Similarly, as confirmed in these current narratives, an ethically adequate mother-midwife relationship exists when mothers and midwives engage 'with' each other.

Existing bioethical frameworks for nursing and midwifery seem to recommend 'restoring' the client/patient's autonomy. However, if the childbearing woman's self-determination were 'retained' and 'maintained' instead of 'restored', the adequate ethical response would be that the mother and midwife reposition themselves from the disparate relationships of the status quo, to that of exercising power 'with' the woman: engaging 'with' each other. The mother is the central and 'active' agent in birthing; the midwife is the 'inactive' agent, not exerting greater power than, or over, the mother. When the midwife does act as an advocate 'for' the woman, it is according to the woman's instruction rather than hospital procedures and disparate loyalties to colleagues and employer. The midwife's prime relationship is with the mother, as a partner rather than an institutional 'expert' or 'system worker'. The mother-midwife relationship should be woman-centred and the birthing woman should be empowered – not only through the relationship but most importantly, self-empowered through 'her' birthing of her baby. This engagement of 'self' plays a major role in birthing, as these mothers indicate with concepts such as 'going within myself', knowing 'what my body needs to do', and the enormous achievement felt by the woman after she has birthed her baby. The midwife enables the woman through their relationship but the woman empowers herself through her internal process and experience of birthing. The latter is unique to the birthing woman. No one else can take that part of the journey with or for her, but inequity in the distribution of power within practice relationships can deny her the experience.

The centrality of concepts which emerged from real life experience and literature, in an ethic of midwifery

The following discussion attempts to explain the interaction occurring between and amongst themes in mothers' and midwives' real life experiences. As detailed in earlier chapters, many of the concepts which emerged from these narratives are also discussed in current literature. The present analysis, however, examines the information for its ethical perspective and focuses on the mother-midwife relationship in particular.

Power

Power exists in all relationships. It is how one exercises the power that is ethically important. The practitioner's role is determined by the practice setting, and the setting impacts on the type of ethical response and relationship s/he has with others.

Institutional dominance

Institutional dominance of childbirth practices is the status quo in mainstream hospital services. Practice settings determine one's duty but our 'way of seeing' or orientation determines our concept of duty, and this can change. When institutional dominance through paternalism and lack of self-determination creates a conflict of values for the mother or midwife, this leads to a heightened awareness of their personal 'way of seeing' or orientation towards the practice. Once the individual's way of seeing has been altered or affirmed, the mother or midwife strives for transformation of practice to eliminate conflict and provide congruence.

Being 'with' woman

The implicit ethics of midwifery as demonstrated in ethically adequate mother-midwife relationships are based on the imperatives of feminist virtue ethics. Firstly, the personal is political and is seen in the way power in relationships is exercised to that end. Secondly, fully authentic caring only occurs in the absence of domination and subordination. Lastly, morality consists of more than conscientiousness and duty; it consists of caring and human engagement. The professional-friend description of the mother-midwife relationship indicates the centrality of a combination of trust, respect and affection for an appropriate and adequate ethical response in midwifery practice.

Relationships wherein mothers and midwives engage 'with' each other lead to a personal transformation of altered orientation towards the practice and a change in practice. Values-congruence occurs with affirmation of (i) embodied individuals, (ii) their embeddedness, and (iii) personal/ professional values, by the workplace/ service provider. Context, the particularity of the person, and character of moral agents are integral to ethical childbirth practice and deliberation. Woman-centred midwifery practice needs continuity of care and carer to provide the context and relationship characteristics necessary for optimum mutual outcomes.

Table 12.1 illustrates a mapping strategy for constructing a midwifery ethic based on the mother-midwife relationship – the ethic of engagement. It distinguishes between the gaze of a traditional hospital approach – that of medicalised birth – and the woman-centred, community approach of birth centres and independently practising midwives. Major themes are highlighted.

Concepts within the proposed approach derive from this analysis ('Practice Estate') and current literature on ethical theories (the pool or 'billabong' of ethics, not just the bioethics gaze).

IMPLICATIONS FOR PRACTICE AND RECOMMENDATIONS

One of the beginning premises of the present analysis is that the nature of midwifery is different from moral philosophy, medicine and nursing, and that the ethical frameworks from those other practices are not adequately responsive to midwifery practice. Except for Frith

(1996) who also questions the appropriateness of the ethics of other practices for midwifery, this concern is not publicly debated in the discourse on ethics and midwifery. Whilst bioethics and normative theories are critiqued generally, and technological dominance of women's reproductive health is condemned by feminists and midwives, there is a paucity of discussion on the ethics of everyday midwifery practice. More discourse on a distinctive ethical response for midwifery is needed. Another premise of the present analysis is that a distinctive midwifery ethic is implicitly available in the lived realities and shared engagement of mothers and midwives. Berg and colleagues (1996) express the belief that understanding the relationship between the birthing woman and midwife is tacit knowledge embedded in practice. Until the present analysis, there has been no attempt to explore whether or not such tacit and embedded knowledge reveals a distinctive ethical response for midwifery practice – the ethics that are implicit in mothers' and midwives' lived reality.

The concept of 'prime relationships' is identified in the present narratives as a central feature of the mother-midwife relationship. Probably the most significant implication of this analysis for practice is the required change of focus for midwives. Their focus needs to shift from loyalty and duty spread across disparate relationships to that of a professional-friend commitment and engagement with particular others: practice based on the ethics of intimates not strangers, and on human engagement in relationship. 'Strengthening' strategies which empower the woman during childbirth are (i) the provision and maintenance of privacy and self-determination to regress into herself if she wishes, (ii) an environment that is not 'time bound' or rules regulated, and (iii) a midwife who is present 'with' not 'doing to'; one who encourages self-confidence and courage in the woman. Disparate relationships on the other hand, render the woman invisible as a person and reinforce 'weakening' strategies such as self-denigration when the woman is grateful and/or apologetic.

Table 12.1 The ethic of engagement for midwifery, based on the mother-midwife relationship

Features	Medicalised Birth	Midwifery Birth
The embedded nature of the relationship in setting and context	**Power 'over'** Mother and midwife have disparate and adversarial relationships, i.e. loyalty to colleagues, doctors, hospital employer, and baby's versus mother's rights Mother and midwife are subordinate to medical authority	**Power 'with' and sometimes 'for'** Midwife's prime relationship is with mother, mother's prime relationship is with her baby Mother and midwife engage in a supportive partnership 'with' each other
The focus of the relationship – purpose or aim of the practice	**Institutional dominance** Institution-centred procedures Characterised by direction, paternalism, control and compliance for women, by experts, technology and biomedical assessment	**Being 'with' woman** Woman-centred engagement Characterised by supporting and 'knowing' the person and her needs/wishes, through a professional friendship between mother and midwife
Orientation and philosophy – the practice and practitioner's 'ways of seeing', also reflected in language	Abstract normative theory and principles – ethics of strangers Based on objective, scientific decision-making (problem-solving) and right/wrong actions, exclusive of experiential knowledge Language surrounding birth is 'normal', risk, fear and life-threatening Mother is in a patient/sick role, dependent and reliant on medicine/science to save her and her baby's lives	Feminist-virtue ethics and commitment to the particular person – ethics of intimates Interpretive and inclusive of multiple types of knowledge. Ethical practice occurs prior to and separately from 'problems': is based on relationship and human engagement – woman is embodied, and embedded in her social context Mother is 'able'. She determines assistance needed during the human and 'natural' life experience of birth
'Ways of seeing' – expressed as engagement in practice	Practice approach is impersonal and anonymous ('they') and unsupportive of the woman Emphasis is on fear and physical safety (mortality) The professional is in a privileged position; family are grateful for expert's services *Weakening strategies* – 'silencing' of subordinate, self-denegration (grateful, apologetic), woman rendered invisible as person and midwife as professional colleague, support person coaches woman according to hospital rules and becomes institution's ally	The person and identity are acknowledged (names) and practice is supportive of the woman Emphasis is on woman's ability, integrity and security not just physical safety Mother and midwife are proud of self and the 'other'. Family is interactive. *Strengthening strategies* – mother has privacy to regress into herself, midwife is 'present' does not 'do to', process of birth is not 'time bound' or rules-regulated, mother develops confidence and with trust can find strength
Emotions in practice – altered 'ways of seeing', personal transformation	**Conflict of values** Dissonance and disharmony of personal/professional values for woman-centred mothers and midwives	**Congruence of values** Consonance and harmony of personal/professional values for woman-centred mothers and midwives

REFERENCES

Berg M, Lundgren I, Hermansson E, Wahlberg V 1996 Women's experience of the encounter with the midwife during childbirth. Midwifery 12 (1): 11-15

Frith L (ed) 1996 Ethics and midwifery: issues in contemporary practice. Butterworth-Heinemann, Oxford

Isaacs P, Massey D 1993 Applied ethics: the nature of the engagement. Philosophy and Applied Ethics Re-Examined conference, University of Newcastle and the Australian Association for Professional and Applied Ethics, Department of Philosophy, Newcastle, NSW

Isaacs P, Massey D 1994 Mapping the applied ethics agenda. Third Annual Meeting, Australian Association for Practical and Professional Ethics

Isaacs P 1998a Social practices, medicine and the nature of medical ethics. Society for Health and Human Values Spring Regional Meeting, Youngston State University, Youngston, Ohio

Isaacs P 1998b Notes from advanced seminar in applied ethics research methods [unpublished]. Queensland University of Technology, Queensland

Isaacs P 1999 Lecture notes for nurses [unpublished]. Queensland University of Technology, Queensland

Conclusion

This analysis set out to investigate the ethical nature of the mother-midwife relationship and, therefore, the nature of a distinctive ethical response for midwifery practice. Personal narratives reveal that an ethically adequate mother-midwife relationship is one that is open and honest; trusting and respectful of persons, and of the woman's ability to birth.

Mothers and midwives both reject institutional dominance over childbirth practices, and describe a range of feelings that are manifest as the result of conflicting values between the workplace or service provider ethics and their personal and professional midwifery ethics. This emotional response to ethical conflict supports the claim that emotions and feelings are integral to ethical deliberation, and should not be excluded in the way that normative theory and reductionist problem-solving does. To exclude context is to oversimplify the situation. Birth is a social construction, and language, personal experience and emotions all indicate identity and embedded context. Our lived reality is of human beings acting and interacting in social, cultural and historical context. The ethics of intimates such as casuistry, contextualism, virtue ethics, and feminist ethics that also focus on context, character of moral agent, the nature of relationships, and our responsibility to particular others, offer valid alternatives to contemporary applied ethics and problem-solving bioethics.

Imperatives for ethical midwifery practice are that the childbearing woman should be valued as an individual, afforded the dignity of informed choice and self-determination, and should feel 'secure' not merely have her and her baby's lives 'saved'. The implicit ethics in midwifery practice derive from human engagement, not simply the rightness or wrongness of 'actions'. The most adequate ethical responses occur within consultative, woman-centred relationships or partnerships, when the mother and midwife have developed a knowledge and understanding of each other through continuity of carer and philosophy of care. In such relationships, the midwife's power is mostly exercised 'with' the woman. When the midwife acts 'for' the woman, the balance of power reverts back to the woman quite quickly as soon as the woman's vulnerability is reduced.

Midwifery does need an ethic that is different from the existing bioethical and problem-solving principlist frameworks, and such an ethic should be based on the ethics that have previously been implicit in practice but which these mothers' and midwives' narratives have made explicit.

The proposed new ethic – the Ethic of Engagement for Midwifery – is situated within the practice of midwifery and resembles those promoted by feminist-virtue ethics. The latter not only redress the politics of the existing hegemonic maternity services system, but they also place women's concerns central to practice and deliberation. The aspirations, values and lived reality of mothers and midwives, and the commitment of the professional-friend midwife to the particularity of the birthing woman, are the focus of this reconstructed ethic for midwifery practice, an ethic which reunites morality and personal interest. The impact on practice of human engagement, and the centrality of concepts identified in mothers' and midwives' narratives, are integral to such a strategy.

Midwifery needs to refocus its ethical 'gaze' from the abstract to the particular, and from right or wrong 'action' to the nature of relationships. Midwives need to reposition themselves to engage 'with' childbearing women and to change their focus from loyalty and duty across disparate relationships to that of a professional-friend commitment with particular others – the 'able' women they attend. Such an approach will result in the implicit ethics evident in this analysis being explicit in midwifery practice, education and theory.

GLOSSARY OF TERMS

Casuistry

The study of cases and precedents - can be helpful in ethics as it is in law, but does not decide things for us ... [it] is an attempt to help us bridge the gulf between the universal and the particular, between moral absolutes and the relativities of everyday life, general moral rules and specific problems in concrete cases. Historically, casuistry in ethics evolved with attempts of confessors to deal with the problems presented to them by penitents in the confessional ... The debate about the need for casuistry has revived in the past decade (Jonsen & Toulmin 1988 cited in Thompson, Melia & Boyd 1994 p.85).

Constructivism

The aim of inquiry is understanding and reconstruction of the constructions that people (including the inquirer) initially hold, aiming toward consensus but still open to new interpretations as information and sophistication improve ... Knowledge consists of those constructions about which there is relative consensus (or at least some movement toward consensus) among those competent (and in the case of more arcane material, trusted) to interpret the substance of the construction. Multiple 'knowledges' can coexist when equally competent (or trusted) interpreters disagree, and/or depending on social, political, cultural, economic, ethnic, and gender factors that differentiate the interpreters. These constructions are subject to continuous revision, with changes most likely to occur when relatively different

constructions are brought into juxtaposition in a dialectical context (Denzin & Lincoln 1994 p.113).

Deontological ethics

The equal and uncompromising application of fixed principles, regardless of changing circumstances. Immanuel Kant (1724-1804) proposed that an act is good if everyone ought, for rational reasons and in similar circumstances, to act in the same way without exception (universalisability principle) (Bandman & Bandman 1995). Deontology claims 'duty' is the basis of morality and that some acts are obligatory regardless of their consequences.

Dualism

The belief in two antagonistic principles governing human life. The dualisms of Enlightenment/modernist/positivist thought include rational/irrational, subject/object, and culture/nature (Heckman 1990).

Embedded

Refers to being within one's personal and social context.

Embodiment

Refers to how human beings perceive or constitute their world. It represents the subject's own view of her/his body as it has to be lived with subjectively, and represents the exact opposite of one's body as perceived by others in the objective outer world.

Epistemology

[H]ow we conceptualise our reality and our images of the world (Denzin & Lincoln 1994 p.6).

Ethics

Each participant defined for herself what constituted 'ethics' in midwifery practice. For the author, the terms ethics and morals are being used interchangeably throughout this analysis, in accord with the original Greek and Latin meanings (Bandman & Bandman 1995; Jones 1994; Johnstone 1994; Thompson, Melia & Boyd 1994; Veatch 1989).

Contrary to popular nursing opinion, there is no philosophically significant difference between the terms 'ethics' and 'morality' (Ladd 1978, p.400) ... 'ethics' coming from the ancient Greek ethikos (originally meaning 'pertaining to custom or habit'), and 'morality' coming from the Latin moralitas (also originally meaning 'custom' or 'habit'). Bioethics, in essence, is a subclass of ethics, which, in turn, is a branch of philosophy. Medical ethics and nursing ethics, on the other hand, are distinctive specialized fields of inquiry naturally born of the practices of medicine and nursing respectively (p.37-8) ... Western moral philosophy ... illuminate[s] what we ought to do by asking us to consider and reconsider our ordinary actions, judgments and justifications (Beauchamp & Childress 1983 p.xii).

['Ethics' and 'morals'] originally meant much the same thing, 'ethics' coming from Greek and 'morals' coming from its Latin equivalent. Both words referred to the general area of the rights and wrongs, in theory and practice, of human behaviour. In everyday usage moral and ethical can still be used more or less interchangeably, but a distinction has grown up between the two terms in more formal usage. Morals (and also morality) now tends to refer to the standards of behaviour actually held or followed by individuals and groups, while ethics refers to the science or study of morals - an activity, in the academic context, also often called moral philosophy (Thompson, Melia & Boyd 1994 p.3).

In this analysis however, 'ethics' does not refer only to moral philosophy but in a broader and applied sense includes the ethics of the professional practice and practitioners. Neither is the research limited to 'morals' meaning the values and beliefs of the individual childbearing woman or midwife. Rather, in seeking stories about the 'ethical' aspects surrounding childbirth the aim is to hear the voices of mothers and midwives in the context of their interaction, to extrapolate ethical nuances and, from these, to attempt to construct the ethical nature of their relationship. A knowledge of the ethical nature of the mother-midwife relationship may help to identify some of the characteristics which are important for a distinctive ethical response for midwifery practice.

Hegemony

The permeation throughout civil society ... of an entire system of values, attitudes, beliefs, morality, etc. that is in one way or another supportive of the established order and the class interests that dominate it ... to the extent that this prevailing consciousness is internalized by the broad masses, it becomes part of 'common sense' ... For hegemony to assert itself successfully in any society, therefore, it must operate in a dualistic manner: as a 'general conception of life' for the masses and as a 'scholastic programme' (Boggs quoted in Greer 1982:305; also in Martin 1987:23).

Heterogeneous

Different in kind; unlike; incongruous (The Macquarie Dictionary 1981).

Homogenous

Of the same kind or nature; not heterogeneous (The Macquarie Dictionary 1981).

Midwife

Midwifery practice has been broadly defined according to linguistic derivations of the term midwife: that is, midwife in Anglo-Saxon meaning 'with woman' and 'comare' in the old Italian meaning 'with mother' (Donnison 1988 p.11).

The international definition of a midwife is:

A midwife is a person who, having been regularly admitted to a midwifery educational programme, duly recognised in the country in which it is located, has successfully completed the prescribed course of studies in midwifery and has acquired the requisite qualifications to be registered and/or legally licensed to practice midwifery.

Sphere of practice of a midwife is:

She must be able to give the necessary supervision, care and advice to women during pregnancy, labour and the postpartum period, to conduct deliveries on her own responsibility and to care for the newborn and the infant. This care includes preventative measures, the detection of abnormal conditions in mother and child, and the procurement of medical assistance and the execution of emergency measures in the absence of medical help.

She has an important task in health counselling and education, not only for patients but also within the family and the community. The work should involve antenatal education and preparation for parenthood and extends to certain areas of gynaecology, family planning and child care.

She may practice in hospitals, clinics, health units, domiciliary conditions or in any other service.

Definition adopted by the International Confederation of Midwives (ICM), Federation of International Gynaecologists & Obstetricians (FIGO), World Health Organisation (WHO) and Australian College of Midwives Incorporated (ACMI). Adopted at the 2nd Biennial General Meeting, National Midwives' Association (now ACMI), 2/81. Reviewed 6/89 (ACMI philosophy and position statements).

In accord with the international definition, this analysis uses the term 'midwife' to describe a practitioner whose role enables her/him to exercise professional midwifery judgement and a degree of independent practice in caring for childbearing women. The term 'obstetric nurse' refers to the healthcare professional whose scope of practice is limited to assisting medical personnel in the practice of obstetrics and whose role constrains her/him from exercising professional midwifery judgement.

Modernism

Modernism is deeply committed to the view that the facts of the world are essentially there for study. They exist independently of us as observers, and if we are rational we will come to know the facts as they are. Constructivists are deeply committed to the contrary view that what we take to be objective knowledge and truth is the result of perspective. Knowledge and truth are created, not discovered by mind (Denzin & Lincoln 1994 p.125).

Mother-midwife relationship

This analysis is primarily interested in the mother-midwife dyad relationship but acknowledges that there is a triad of 'others' such as family and support persons, medical and allied health practitioners, and employers who influence the dyad.

From the organisational viewpoint, the midwife-mother relationship is the medium through which the service is provided ... For the service user, the relationship is about feeling safe and able (Kirkham 2000 p.227).

The mother-baby relationship is also a major focus. The present analysis interprets that the midwife-baby relationship generally exists through the mother-midwife relationship unless the baby's physical condition requires a decision in which the mother is unable to participate because of her physical or mental status. The midwife-baby relationship in the latter circumstance would operate via the baby's father or next of kin, in consultation with medical and allied health professionals.

Moral relativism

Moral beliefs are relative, relative either to the individual or his culture (Thompson, Melia & Boyd 1994).

Ontology

The science of being, as such (The Macquarie Dictionary 1981.

Epistemology asks, how do we know the world? What is the relationship between the inquirer and the known? Ontology raises basic questions about the nature of reality (Denzin & Lincoln 1994 p.99).

Personal values: justice: supremacy

Justice has many interpretations, but for the purposes of this analysis it is not merely the balancing of economic cost-benefit. It refers more to a relational concept and social construct.

Personal values are not merely cognitive beliefs but include an emotional or affective component and are enacted in everyday life in multiple arenas. In this way, they also come to constitute one's identity [and] help to build a moral vocabulary by which we evaluate ourselves and others as praiseworthy or blameworthy. They shape how we participate in the world at multiple levels from intimate to associate to citizen ... [and are] informed by emotions [which] provide the link between personal values and justice because they assume a critical role in the evaluative structures of the self as well as social organizations ... Personal values are understood not as arbitrary preferences, but, rather, as reflective of our commitments ... Justice is a relational concept binding together people from different social positions within a certain social order ... supremacy does imply the negation of the perspectives of others. To be supreme is to stand outside the relational configuration of justice and to demonstrate an unwillingness or inability to get the big picture, to negotiate a new moral space (Liaschenko 1999 p.35).

Power, trust, inclusion, role flexibility and inquiry

For employees to engage in ethical reflection, the conditions of power, trust, inclusion, role flexibility and inquiry must be present. Workers should have the right to receive relevant information, to be free to say what is needed to be said about an issue (power), and to be free to disagree with one another in order to increase their understanding of issues (trust) (Olson 1998).

This reflects the author's interpretation of power and trust, during childbirth in particular.

Pragmatism

The theory that something is right because it works - confines attention to means - to rational planning based on the calculation of available means and resources - to achieve aims [e.g. Sartre] (Thompson, Melia & Boyd 1994).

Principlism

Normative ethical theories include deontology and utilitarianism, and claim that moral principles (such as proposed by Beauchamp & Childress in their principlism framework) apply in any and all circumstances. Tong (1993) draws the distinction between universal moral principles and concrete moral rules; the latter apply only to recurring specific situations.

Reductionism

The tendency to make supposedly comprehensive explanations of complex phenomena simply by analysing and describing their parts (The Macquarie Dictionary 1981).

Relationship

Relationship in the present analysis refers to the connection between one person and another or others; for example, between mother and child, or mother and midwife. A connection or association; an emotional association between two people (The Australian Oxford Dictionary 1999).

Social construct

The terms by which the world is understood are social artifacts, products of historically situated interchanges among people (Gergen 1985 cited in Denzin & Lincoln 1994 p.127). A social construct aids analysis and understanding of social phenomena. It is a deliberate abstraction from reality which focuses on particular aspects and ignores others in order to open up new lines of thought and new areas of investigation. Examples are the concepts of status and role.

Temporality

Refers to changes over time.

Totalitarian

Pertaining to a centralised government in which those in control grant neither recognition nor tolerance to parties of differing opinion (The Macquarie Dictionary 1981).

Tradition and shared tradition

The term 'tradition' refers

more generally, to any settled manner of doing things ... What a tradition gives [to the practitioner] is a way of seeing the world ... ways of seeing must be acquired from and are therefore shared with others [shared tradition] (Langford 1985, p.8).

Utility ethics

The consequences of one's action in balancing the greatest amount of pleasure (good) against the greatest amount of pain (evil) is the basis of the utility argument.

Virtue ethics

They focus on the goodness or badness of the individual's moral character. Aristotle's virtue ethics originate from the fifth century BC.

CONTEXT OF THE ANALYSIS

The nature of narrative inquiry means that no generalisations can or should be made from the findings. The narratives detail personal experiences of a small number of mothers and midwives and are intended to provide insight only, into the ethical nature of the mother-midwife relationship. However, concepts and values identified by these informants are echoed in other recent midwifery research as noted herein, and therefore may be acknowledged as commonly shared traditions of childbearing practices. The present analysis is also confined to an Anglo-Celtic framework of theory and practice.

REFERENCES

Bandman E L, Bandman B 1995 Nursing ethics: through the life span, 3rd edn. Appleton & Lange, Norwalk, Connecticut

Beauchamp T L, Childress J F 1983 Principles of biomedical ethics, 2nd edn. Oxford University Press, New York

Denzin N K, Lincoln Y S (eds) 1994 Handbook of qualitative research. Sage, Thousand Oaks, California

Donnison J 1988 Midwives and medical men: a history of the struggle for the control of childbirth, 2nd edn. Historical Publications, London

Greer E 1982 Antonio Gramsci and legal hegemony. In: Kairys D (ed) The politics of law: a progressive critique. Pantheon, New York

Heckman S J 1990 Gender and knowledge: elements of a postmodern feminism. Polity Press, Cambridge

Johnstone M J 1994 Bioethics: a nursing perspective, 2nd edn. Saunders, Sydney

Jones S R 1994 Ethics in midwifery. Mosby-Year Book Europe Ltd, London

Kirkham M 2000 The midwife-mother relationship. Macmillan, Basingstoke

Langford G 1985 Education, persons and society: a philosophical inquiry. Macmillan, London

Liaschenko J 1999 Can justice coexist with the supremacy of personal values in nursing practice? Western Journal of Nursing Research 21 (1): 35-50

Martin E 1987 The woman in the body: a cultural analysis of reproduction. Open University Press, Milton Keynes

More B (ed) 1999 The Australian Oxford dictionary. Oxford University Press, Melbourne

The Macquarie Dictionary 1981. Macquarie Library Pty Ltd, McMahons Point, New South Wales

Thompson I K, Melia K M, Boyd K M 1994 Nursing ethics. Churchill Livingstone, Melbourne

Tong R 1993 Feminine and feminist ethics. Wadsworth Publishing Co, Belmont, California

Veatch R M 1989 Medical ethics. Jones and Bartlett Publishers, Boston, Massachusetts

Index